Chronic Non-communicable Diseases in Low- and Middle-income Countries

FSC
www.fsc.org
MIX
Paper from
responsible sources
FSC® C013604

Chronic Non-communicable Diseases in Low- and Middle-income Countries

Edited by

Ama de-Graft Aikins

and

Charles Agyemang

www.cabi.org

CABI is a trading name of CAB International

CABI
Nosworthy Way
Wallingford
Oxfordshire OX10 8DE
UK

Tel: +44 (0)1491 832111
Fax: +44 (0)1491 833508
E-mail: info@cabi.org
Website: www.cabi.org

CABI
745 Atlantic Avenue
8th Floor
Boston, MA 02111
USA

T: +1 617 682 9015
E-mail: cabi-nao@cabi.org

A catalogue record for this book is available from the British Library, London, UK.

Library of Congress Cataloging-in-Publication Data

Chronic non-communicable diseases in low and middle-income countries / [edited by] Ama de-Graft Aikins and Charles Agyemang.
p. ; cm.
Includes bibliographical references and index.
ISBN 978-1-78064-332-8 (alk. paper)
I. Aikins, Ama de-Graft, editor. II. Agyemang, Charles, editor.
[DNLM: 1. Chronic Disease. 2. Developing Countries. WT 500]

RM108
616'.044091724--dc23

2015029400

ISBN-13: 978 1 78064 332 8

Commissioning editors: Caroline Makepeace
Editorial assistant: Emma McCann
Production editor: Tracy Head

Typeset by AMA DataSet, Preston, UK.
Printed and bound in the UK by CPI Group (UK) Ltd, Croydon, CR0 4YY, UK.

Contents

Contributors

About the Editors

Ama de-Graft Aikins, PhD

Ama de-Graft Aikins is an Associate Professor of Social Psychology at the Regional Institute for Population Studies, University of Ghana and Visiting Senior Fellow at the Department of Social Policy, London School of Economics and Political Science (LSE). She received her PhD in Social Psychology from the LSE and completed post-doctoral training at the University of Cambridge. Her research focuses on representations and experiences of chronic physical and mental illnesses among Ghanaians in Ghana, Europe and the USA, and on Africa's chronic non-communicable disease (NCD) burden. She is engaged in NCD advocacy and has served on NCD committees convened by the Ghana Health Service and the World Health Organization. Since 2006, she has co-directed the Academic Partnership on Chronic Conditions in Africa (APCCA), a British Academy-supported partnership of multi-disciplinary NCD researchers based in Africa, Europe and North America (http://www.apccafrica.org). The partnership has produced a series of flagship publications on the global burden of NCDs including special journal issues on the burden of NCDs in Ghana (*Ghana Medical Journal*, 2012, 46(2)), Africa (*Globalization and Health*, 2009/2010, 5/6) and low- and middle-income countries (*Ethnicity and Health*, 2012, 17(6)).

Charles Agyemang, MPH, PhD

Charles Agyemang is a Principal Investigator and Associate Professor at Amsterdam Medical Centre, University of Amsterdam. He received his PhD from Erasmus Medical Centre, University of Rotterdam. Prior to this, he studied and did his Master's degree in Public Health at Edinburgh Medical School, University of Edinburgh. He has vast research experience in cardiovascular diseases (CVDs) among ethnic minority groups in Europe and has conducted numerous studies on CVDs in low-resource settings. He is a project leader and scientific coordinator of the

RODAM project – a European Commission (EC)-funded project on gene–environmental interactions on obesity and diabetes among African migrants (http://www.rod-am.eu) – and co-investigator of the EC-funded InterConnect project (http://www.interconnect-diabetes.eu). He was a member and a rapporteur of the Planning Committee for the World Health Organization Global Consultation on Migrant Health. He is currently a Vice President of the Migrant Health section of the European Public health Association.

About the Authors

Juliet Addo, MD, PhD

Juliet Addo is a Clinical Lecturer in Epidemiology in the Department of Non-communicable Disease Epidemiology at the London School of Hygiene and Tropical Medicine. She is the module organizer for the Distance Learning MSc in Global Epidemiology of Non-communicable Disease. Juliet's research has focused on cardiovascular diseases and their risk factors including stroke, hypertension and diabetes. She is particularly interested in the ethnic and socio-economic differences and inequalities in their risks, management and outcome. She is currently leading the UK recruitment of participants for a multi-centre study researching diabetes and obesity in black Africans in Europe compared with in sub-Saharan Africa (RODAM).

Davies Adeloye, MBBS, PhD

Davies Adeloye is a medical doctor and epidemiologist with extensive clinical and research experience in Nigeria and the UK. He received his PhD from the University of Edinburgh under the prestigious Charles Darwin International Fellowship. Davies has been involved with the Global Health Epidemiology Reference Group based at the Usher Institute, University of Edinburgh, for about 5 years. He led research on the burden of non-communicable diseases in Africa, and has co-authored a number of publications on this in respected international journals. He is a member of the European Respiratory Society, Medical and Dental Council of Nigeria, and Editorial Board of the *Journal of Global Health*. Davies currently lectures at Covenant University, Ota, Nigeria. He is also an Adjunct Research Fellow and external consultant at the Centre for Global Health Research, University of Edinburgh. His research interests include evidence-based medicine, global health metrics, non-communicable diseases, cancers and non-infectious causes of child mortality.

Ernest Afrifa-Anane, MPhil

Ernest Afrifa-Anane is a doctoral student at the Regional Institute for Population Studies, University of Ghana. His research interests include examining the social, cultural and environmental determinants of physical (in)activity and their inter-relationships with major chronic diseases such as diabetes and hypertension across all age groups in Ghana and sub-Saharan Africa. His MPhil thesis focused on the inter-relationship between physical inactivity, body mass index and blood pressure among poor urban youth in Accra, Ghana.

Dickens H. Akena, MBChB, MMed Psych, PhD

Dickens H. Akena is a Lecturer and Psychiatrist in the Department of Psychiatry, School of Medicine, College of Health Sciences, Makerere University-Kampala, Uganda. Dickens earned his Medical Doctorate (MBChB) and Master of Medicine in Psychiatry (MMed Psych) from Makerere University, and his PhD in Psychiatry from the University of Cape Town, South Africa. He has expertise in epidemiological research and integrated mental health intervention and service research. He also has expertise in depression instrument development and validation for diverse African populations. His research has focused on depression in human immunodeficiency virus-positive persons and in patients with non-communicable diseases in Uganda.

Pascale Allotey, PhD, FRSPH, FRSH, MMedSci, PGDip, BA(Hons), RN, SCM, PHN

Pascale Allotey is Professor of Public Health, the lead of Global Public Health and Associate Director of the South East Asia Community Observatory (SEACO) at Monash University's campus in Malaysia. She is a medical anthropologist and epidemiologist with research expertise in gender and other marginalizing factors on diseases of poverty including tropical diseases and non-communicable diseases. Other areas of research expertise are sexual and reproductive health and rights, health policy, health systems, implementation research and public health research capacity building. Pascale has established research and training programmes in Australia, Africa, the UK and Malaysia, and was appointed a Professorial Fellow and Member of the Academy of Experts of the Royal Society for Public Health in the UK. Pascale publishes across a range of public health disciplines with over 130 peer-reviewed papers, book chapters and reports to her name. She has served as a technical expert on several committees for various United Nations organizations and is on the board of trustees for several international non-governmental organizations.

Kofi A. Anie, PhD, AFBPsS

Kofi A. Anie is a Consultant Psychologist responsible for Haemoglobinopathy Psychological Services at London North West Healthcare NHS Trust, and Honorary Senior Clinical Lecturer at Imperial College London. He is an international expert in sickle cell disease with a track record in research and collaboration in low- and middle-income countries including Ghana and Nigeria. His special areas of current interest are behavioural medicine and telehealth, and the application of mobile technology to chronic non-communicable diseases and psychosocial interventions. Kofi is a Fellow of the Royal Society of Medicine and Associate Fellow of the British Psychological Society. He is also a Haemoglobinopathies Editor for the Cochrane Cystic Fibrosis and Genetics Disorders Review Group of the Cochrane Collaboration.

Lilian Lem Atanga, PhD

Lilian Lem Atanga is an Associate Professor of Gender and Discourse Studies in the Department of Linguistics of the University of Bamenda. She is the Coordinator of the Applied Linguistics Programme of the University of Bamenda. Her research has focused on the discursive representation of chronic diseases in

Cameroon and also in the area of gender and language and politics. Lem gained a PhD in Gender and Language from Lancaster University, examining discursive gender and power relations within the Cameroonian parliament, and has since collaborated on research projects spanning gender to discourse and representation of non-communicable diseases. She is currently examining the discursive representation of non-communicable diseases focusing on epilepsy in the Northwest region of Cameroon.

Raphael Baffour Awuah, MPhil
Raphael is a PhD student at the Regional Institute for Population Studies, University of Ghana. His research interest focuses on the prevalence, awareness, treatment, control, perceptions and determinants of hypertension and diabetes at the community level in Ghana and African countries. He also has an interest in chronic disease intervention programmes.

Besa H. Bauta, MSW, LSW, MPH
Besa H. Bauta is the Senior Director of Research and Evaluation at the Center for Evidence Based Implementation and Research (CEBIR) at the Catholic Guardian Services and Adjunct Assistant Professor at the New York University (NYU) Silver School of Social Work. Under her direction, CEBIR facilitates the implementation of evidence-based practices in social-service settings through system alignment, fidelity assessments, analysis of programme outcomes and training in evidence-based models. Besa has extensive expertise in refugee mental health, trauma and child maltreatment. Her current research interests focus on health systems, global mental health, and integrated maternal and child health services. She holds a BA in Anthropology from Rutgers University in New Brunswick, New Jersey, an MSW in Clinical Social Work from the Silver School of Social Work and an MPH in Global Public Health from the Global Institute of Public Health at NYU. She is currently completing her Doctorate in Clinical Social Work at NYU, and is expecting to graduate in 2016.

Sabrina Cheng, MPH
Sabrina Cheng is an Associate Research Scientist with the Department of Population Health at NYU Langone Medical Center. She holds an MPH in Epidemiology from Mailman School of Public Health at Columbia University. She has strong interests in health disparities and population health research. Her work has focused on psychiatric epidemiology, programme evaluation, and health service and quality improvement research in international contexts.

Oleg Chestnov, MD, PhD
Oleg Chestnov is Assistant Director-General for Non-communicable Diseases and Mental Health at the World Health Organization (WHO), Geneva. Prior to that, Oleg was the Deputy-Director for International Relations at the Ministry of Health and Social Development of the Russian Federation, a post he occupied from 2005. He earned a degree in Medicine in 1979 from the Saratov State Medical Institute and a Doctorate of Philosophy in Medical Sciences from the Russian Federation in 2008. He joined the Red Cross and Red Crescent Movement in 1987, and worked in several countries affected by conflict as well as by natural and technical disasters where he was engaged in managing the delivery of humanitarian aid assistance.

Ernestina Coast, PhD

Ernestina Coast is an Associate Professor in Population Studies in the Department of Social Policy at the London School of Economics, where she is the Programme Director for the MSc in Population and Development. She has led interdisciplinary social science research projects on sexual and reproductive health, households and poverty, all focused on low-income countries. Ernestina is currently leading: a research programme on women's health in the occupied Palestinian Territories; a research project on abortion in Zambia; and commissioned research for the WHO on the role of culture in maternity care. She currently serves as a member of the WHO Guideline Development Group for Maternal and Newborn Health. As a social scientist with training in demography and anthropology, Ernestina's research focuses on using mixed methods (quantitative and qualitative) to research the inter-relationships between social context and demographic behaviour, with a focus on sexual and reproductive health. Recent research has been funded externally by the Economic and Social Research Council (ESRC), Department for International Development (DFID), Wellcome Trust and the Nuffield Foundation. She has acted as adviser to a number of organizations, including DFID, the joint United Nations Programme on HIV and Aids (UNAIDS), Marie Stopes International and Danish International Development Agency (DANIDA), and has been a Visiting Scholar at the African Population and Health Research Centre, Nairobi, Kenya.

Justin Basile Echouffo-Tcheugui, MD, PhD

Justin Basile Echouffo-Tcheugui specializes in general internal medicine and is Assistant Professor of Public Health at Emory University, Atlanta. Justin's research focuses on diabetes, obesity and cardiovascular diseases. He has a particular interest in cardiovascular complications of metabolic disorders across populations in various continents including Europe, Africa, Asia and America.

Rajni Gathibandhe, MD

Rajni Gathibandhe is a trained psychiatrist from India with more than 10 years of international experience in public health and clinical and research psychiatry. She is currently pursuing an MPH in Public Health–Global Health Leadership at NYU. Rajni's primary research interest is global mental health, especially in improving access to mental health care and developing programmes to promote the human rights of people with mental disorders. She has experience in serving as a psychiatric consultant and being a member of the Mental Health Advisory Council for the Ministry of Health in the Republic of Maldives. In these positions, she advised the ministry in preparing the draft bill on the 'Mental Health Act', focusing on the delivery of mental healthcare, accountability and patient rights. Through an interdisciplinary collaboration, she also initiated and delivered a mental health training framework for paramedic, community health and mental health workers, in collaboration with the WHO, aiding in strengthening the mental health system. In association with the Ministry of Education and Health in the Republic of Maldives, she pioneered task shifting and task sharing for mental health to school teachers and counsellors through a focused mental health training platform to aid early identification of mental illness in school children.

Liz Grant, PhD

Liz Grant is Assistant Principal Global Health and Director of the Global Health Academy at the University of Edinburgh. She co-directs the MSc in Global Health Non Communicable Diseases, the MSc in Global eHealth and the online Master's in Family Medicine, which focuses on strengthening the primary care medical workforce in low- and middle-income countries. Liz's main research is in palliative care and health system strengthening. She leads a DFID programme integrating palliative care within the health systems of Kenya, Rwanda, Uganda and Zambia, and works with partners in Malawi, South India and Chile on cancer care and Information and Communications Technology (ICT) for health. Liz is interested in the intersection of faith and health, and local community resilience building.

Ricardo Queiroz Gurgel, MD, PhD

Ricardo Queiroz Gurgel is an Associate Professor of Paediatrics at the Federal University of Sergipe. Trained as a paediatrician, Ricardo completed his medical degree at the Federal University of Sergipe in 1981 and did his Residency, Master's and PhD at the Medical School of Ribeirão Preto – São Paulo University, Brazil. He completed 1 year of a Post-Doc Fellowship at the Liverpool School of Tropical Medicine in 2007. Ricardo works with infectious diseases in children (mostly diarrhoea and respiratory infections) and environmental and social risk factors during perinatal and childhood periods. Nutritional aspects of child health are one of his topics of interest, within the context of Brazil's epidemiological transition. He has coordinated the country-wide ERICA Study (Adolescents Cardiovascular Risk Study) in his state.

Keng-Yen Huang, PhD, MPH, CPH

Keng-Yen Huang is an Associate Professor of Population Health at the NYU School of Medicine. She is also a Faculty Affiliate at the NYU Global Institute of Public Health. Ken-Yen has expertise across several disciplines, including psychiatric epidemiology, mental health systems and policy, prevention and implementation science, quantitative modelling, and immigrant and global public health. Her research focuses on investigating mechanisms of mental health disparities; testing cost-effective family, community and systems approaches of preventive strategies to address health disparities; and broadening evidence-based programme implementation and dissemination in underserved populations and low-income countries (e.g. Uganda, Kenya and Ghana). Ken-Yen is a principal investigator and co-investigator on numerous prevention and longitudinal research projects that focus on vulnerable populations both in the USA and in low-income countries.

Eleanor Hukin, PhD

Eleanor Hukin is an anthropological demographer and researcher whose work has focused on reproductive and maternal health in low-income countries in South-east Asia and sub-Saharan Africa. Her expertise lies in reproductive, maternal and newborn health; contraception and abortion across cultures; mixed methods research; the fertility transition; and medical anthropology. Eleanor gained her PhD in Demography from the London School of Economics, conducting an ethnography of Cambodian women's fertility intentions and unmet needs for contraception. She is now a Technical Advisor at Options Consultancy on the MamaYe Evidence for Action programme, which uses a strategic combination of evidence, advocacy and accountability to improve maternal and newborn survival in six African countries.

Rohina Joshi, MBBS, MPH, PhD
Rohina Joshi is a Senior Research Fellow at The George Institute for Global Health, Australia, and Senior Lecturer at the University of Sydney. She is a cardiovascular epidemiologist who works in the area of effective models of care for chronic disease management and disease surveillance in resource-poor settings. Rohina teaches public health at the School of Public Health, University of Sydney. She is a member of the Technical Advisory Group for the Civil Registration and Vital Statistics programme of the Bloomberg Data for Health Initiative. Her research interests are in global health, task sharing for chronic disease management and verbal autopsy-based surveillance in low- and middle-income countries.

Nahid Kamal, PhD
Nahid Kamal has been a Research Associate with MEASURE Evaluation, University of North Carolina at Chapel Hill, since 2011. She is on secondment to the International Centre for Diarrhoeal Disease Research, Bangladesh (icddr,b), collaborating on nationally representative surveys on urban health and maternal mortality. Her work for the past 4 years has focused largely on impact evaluation of health programmes. Her recent publications include studies on early marriage and equity in healthcare. Nahid has a Doctoral degree in Demography from the London School of Economics. Her 15-year career in public health includes work with the Global Fund in Geneva, Marie Stopes International in London and the Population Council in Dhaka. Her research interests include the demography of South Asia, and reproductive health policy and health systems strengthening.

Andre Pascal Kengne, MD, PhD
Andre Pascal Kengne is the Director of the Non-Communicable Diseases Research Unit at the South African Medical Research Council and Associate Professor at the Department of Medicine of the University of Cape Town in South Africa. He is a physician with specialization in internal medicine. His research interest is on chronic non-communicable diseases, with a major focus on developing countries, and those in Africa in particular.

Kwadwo Ansah Koram, MB, ChB, MPH&TM, PhD
Kwadwo Koram is a Professor of Epidemiology and the current Director of the Noguchi Memorial Institute for Medical Research, University of Ghana. He is a public health physician with an interest in the epidemiology and control of malaria including intervention studies and the nature of the health transition in the country. He teaches at the School of Public Health, University of Ghana, and collaborates with colleagues working on cancers and other non-communicable diseases.

Shanthi Mendis, MBBS, MD, FRCP, FACC
Shanthi Mendis is Senior Adviser, Prevention and Management of Non-communicable Diseases in WHO, Geneva, Switzerland. She is a physician with

specialization in cardiology. She is a Fellow of the Royal College of Physicians of London and Edinburgh and of the American College of Cardiology. Prior to joining the WHO 17 years ago, she engaged in clinical practice and medical education in the UK, the USA and Sri Lanka. She also held the post of Professor of Medicine at the University of Sri Lanka for more than a decade, engaging in undergraduate and postgraduate medical education. Shanthi's areas of expertise include global public health, internal medicine, cardiology, health research, and health policy development and implementation in developing countries.

Pietro Amedeo Modesti, MD, PhD
Pietro Modesti gained his degree in Medicine and Surgery at the University of Florence in 1981. He specialized in internal medicine cardiology in 1986. He gained his PhD in Clinical Pathophysiology in 1992 and specialized in cardiology in 1995 at the University of Florence. In 1996 and 1998, he was a Visiting Scholar at the New York Medical College. Pietro is a member of numerous national and international scientific societies. He is the founder and chairman of the European Society of Hypertension Working Group on Cardiovascular Risk in Low Resource Settings. He is also a Chairman of the Interregional Section (Tuscany and Umbria) of the Italian Society of Internal Medicine, and Vice Chairman of the Interregional Section (Tuscany and Umbria) of the Italian Society of Cardiology. He has coordinated various national and international research projects on clinical cardiology, cardiovascular prevention, arterial hypertension and diabetes, with research and educational projects in Yemen, Libya and Eritrea. He is currently coordinating the CHIP project (Chinese in Prato, on behalf of the Regione Toscana).

Belinda Afriyie Nimako, MB, ChB, MPH
Belinda Nimako qualified as a physician at the University of Ghana Medical School in 2006. She has a strong interest in population health. She has experience spanning clinical work, leadership, project management, teaching and research, especially in the changing patterns of diseases in Ghana. She also holds an MPH from the University of Ghana and is currently serving as a District Director of Health in Ghana, responsible for the health of a district population of over 50,000 individuals.

Gbenga Ogedegbe, MD, MPH, FACP
Gbenga Ogedegbe is Vice Dean and Chief Medical Officer for New York University Global Institute of Public Health. He is a Professor of Medicine and Population Health, Chief Division of Health and Behavior, and Director of the Center for Healthful Behavior in the Department of Population Health, New York University School of Medicine. He is a clinical epidemiologist, hypertension specialist and behavioural scientist with expertise in development, implementation and translation of evidence-based behavioural interventions (targeted at cardiovascular risk reduction) into primary care practices and community-based settings. A leading expert in health disparities research, Gbenga has expanded his work globally, to reduce the burden of cardiovascular disease in sub-Saharan Africa, where he is funded by the National Institutes of Health to build research capacity in non-communicable diseases, and implement task-shifting strategies to improve cardiovascular diseases in primary care practices in Ghana and Nigeria.

Tolu Oni, MBBS, MRCP, MPH, DFPH, MD(Res)
Tolu Oni is a Public Health Physician and Clinical Epidemiologist. After postgraduate clinical training in internal and HIV medicine in the UK and Australia, she completed her doctorate in the clinical epidemiology of HIV-associated tuberculosis. Her research area of expertise is in population health transition and the epidemiology of the interaction between HIV, tuberculosis and non-communicable diseases in urban unplanned settings. She is a Senior Lecturer in the School of Public Health and Family Medicine, University of Cape Town, is responsible for the undergraduate public health curriculum and co-convenes the Epidemiology of Non-communicable Disease module of the Master's in Public Health programme. She is a member of the South African Young Academy of Science, and aims to promote translation of science for society and the generation of evidence to inform healthy public policy.

Olutobi A. Sanuade, MPhil
Olutobi Sanuade is a PhD student at the Regional Institute for Population Studies (RIPS), University of Ghana. He has participated in research projects on 'urban health and poverty' in poor urban communities in Ghana as field supervisor and editor. He is currently participating in a project on hypertension intervention in urban poor communities in Accra, Ghana. His research interests include: population and health, with a specific focus on lived experience, management and rehabilitation of stroke as well as stroke caregiving in Africa; community-based cardiovascular disease interventions; and the health and well-being of the elderly.

Nigel Unwin, BA, BM, BCh, MSc, DM, FRCP, FFPH
Nigel Unwin is a Professor of Public Health and a public health physician, with a track record in studying the burden, prevention and control of diabetes and cardiovascular diseases, including the interaction between diabetes and tuberculosis. Much of this work has been in low- and middle-income country settings. His academic career began at Newcastle University in 1993. He has worked with the International Diabetes Federation and the WHO, including 2 years as Medical Officer with the diabetes group in Geneva. In August 2010, he moved to the University of West Indies (UWI), at the Cave Hill Campus, in Barbados, where he currently holds the Chair of Population Health Sciences at the Chronic Disease Research Centre. At UWI, he has helped to develop graduate public health training and new research addressing the prevention and control of diabetes and cardiovascular diseases.

Steven van de Vijver, MD, MIH
Steven van de Vijver combines his position as Director of Urban Health at the Amsterdam Institute for Global Health and Development (AIGHD) with clinical work at the Onze Lieve Vrouwe Gasthuis (OLVG) in Amsterdam. Steven specializes in tropical medicine and family medicine, and is associated with the African Population and Health Research Center (APHRC) with his research on prevention of cardiovascular diseases in the slums of Nairobi, Kenya.

Sanni Yaya, MSc, PhD
Sanni Yaya is Associate Professor of Economics and Global Health at the University of Ottawa. He is the Editor of the *Innovation Journal* and is currently leading a

series on Society and Health at the University of Ottawa Press. Sanni was post-doctoral research fellow at Yale University and Senior Visiting Scholar at New York University. He has experience in the design and implementation of randomized controlled trials and observational epidemiological studies of maternal and child health, infectious diseases and chronic diseases. He and his research team focus their work on the following topics: improving access and use of health services in low-and middle-income countries; health systems reform; global health financing; effects of globalization; health and economic evaluation of interventions; and interaction between economic development and healthcare.

Abbreviations

AD	Alzheimer's disease
AORTIC	African Organization for Research and Training in Cancer
APCA	African Palliative Care Association
ART	antiretroviral therapy
CARRS	Centre for Cardiometabolic Risk Reduction in South Asia
CCDRFS	China Chronic Disease and Risk Factor Surveillance
CDC	US Centers for Disease Control and Prevention
CHD	coronary heart disease
CHNS	China Health and Nutrition Survey
CHPS	Community-Based Health Planning and Services Programme
CIG	Common Interest Group
CKD	chronic kidney disease
COPD	chronic obstructive pulmonary disease
CORIS	Coronary Risk Factor Study
CPHA	Canadian Public Health Association
CPS	Contraceptive Prevalence Survey
CRA	Comparative Risk Factor Assessment
CVD	cardiovascular disease
DALYs	disability adjusted life years
DHS	Demographic Health Survey
FCTC	Framework Convention on Tobacco Control
GATS	Global Adult Tobacco Survey
GAVI	Global Alliance for Vaccines and Immunization
GBD	Global Burden of Disease
GFATM	Global Fund to fight AIDS, Tuberculosis and Malaria
GHPSS	Global Health Professions Student Survey
GICR	Global Initiative for Cancer Registries Development
GSPS	Global School Personnel Survey

GTF.CCC	Global Task Force on Expanded Access to Cancer Care and Control in Developing Countries
GTSS	Global Tobacco Surveillance System
GYTS	Global Youth Tobacco Survey
HBA1c	glycated haemoglobin
HBV	hepatitis B virus
HDSS	health and demographic surveillance system
HIV	human immunodeficiency virus
HPV	human papilloma virus
IARC	International Agency for Research on Cancer
ICD	International Classification of Diseases
ICMR-INDIAB	Indian Council of Medical Research – India Diabetes
ID	infectious disease
INDEPTH	International Network for the Demographic Evaluation of Populations and Their Health
IUHPE	International Union for Health Promotion and Education
KTL	Finnish National Public Health Institute
LMIC	low- and middle-income country
LSMS	Living Standards Measurement Study
MHaPP	Mental Health and Poverty Project
MHHP	Minnesota Heart Health Program
mhLAP	Mental Health Leadership and Advocacy Program
MNS	Mental Neurological and Substance (disorders)
NCD	non-communicable disease
NGO	non-governmental organization
NHNES	National Health and Nutrition Examination Survey
NPHP	non-physician healthcare provider
NRTI	nucleoside reverse transcriptose inhibitor
OECD	Organisation for Economic Co-operation and Development
PD	Parkinson's disease
PI	protease inhibitor
PWD	people with dementia
SAGE	WHO Study on global AGEing and adult health
SDH	social determinants of health
STEPS	WHO's STEPwise approach to Surveillance
T2DM	type 2 diabetes mellitus
TB	tuberculosis
UMHCP	Uganda Minimum Health Care Package
UN	United Nations
USAID	United States Agency for International Development
VaD	vascular dementia
WARFS	World Alliance for Risk Factor Surveillance
WFS	World Fertility Survey
WHA	World Health Assembly
WHO	World Health Organization
WHO-AIMS	WHO-Assessment Instrument for Mental Health Systems

Introduction: Addressing the Chronic Non-communicable Disease Burden in Low- and Middle-income Countries

AMA DE-GRAFT AIKINS* AND CHARLES AGYEMANG

Chronic non-communicable diseases (NCDs) are non-infectious diseases that progress over the lifetime of affected individuals and require long-term treatment and care [1, 2].[1] Left undiagnosed, untreated or poorly managed, they often progress into serious disabling and life-threatening conditions. The four major types of chronic NCDs are cardiovascular diseases (CVDs), cancers, chronic respiratory diseases and diabetes. Other types include musculoskeletal conditions like arthritis, neurodegenerative conditions like dementia, mental health disorders and injuries.

Low- and middle-income countries (LMICs) in Africa, Asia and Latin America and the Caribbean bear a significant proportion of the global burden of NCDs. We define burden as the cumulative medical, economic and psychosocial costs of the conditions. For example, 90% of people dying under the age of 70 from NCDs live in LMICs and 80% of deaths attributable to CVDs occur in LMICs [3]. The majority of new cases of some conditions like cancer and dementia are found in LMICs. The cost of NCD care in LMICs is higher compared with the cost in high-income countries (HICs) for individuals, health systems and governments [1, 2, 4, 5]. Globally, long-term illnesses cause complex disruptions to the lives of affected individuals and their families. However, in LMICs, NCDs create a vicious cycle of ill-health and poverty that undermines psychological health, social support and other psychosocial outcomes for affected communities [1, 6, 7].

There have been a number of important reviews on the NCD burden in Africa, Asia and Latin America in international journals such as the *Lancet*, *Bulletin of the World Health Organization*, *Globalization and Health*, *Ethnicity and Health* and *Global Health Action*. However, there is no authoritative text that synthesizes the research evidence on the NCD burden across countries and regions that share similar public health, socio-economic and developmental patterns. This edited

*E-mail: adaikins@ug.edu.gh

volume aims to present the first comprehensive synthesis of the context and impact of NCDs in LMICs and to offer insights on successful and sustainable interventions and policies that work for at-risk populations.

NCD Burden in Low- and Middle-income Countries: Context and Responses

Over the last decade, a series of high-level global health discussions on the global burden of NCDs have been convened by the World Health Organization (WHO), the United Nations (UN), the World Health Assembly and other global health institutions. These discussions have shaped the development of a global agenda for NCD control that underscores the need for a 'multi-faceted and multi-institutional' framework and 'a whole of government, whole of society' approach for developing sustainable interventions [1, 8, 9]. There is a consensus that NCDs are a developmental issue and are fast becoming diseases of poverty. As a result, there is a strong recommendation for addressing the social determinants of NCDs, as well as the biological determinants [7]. Social determinants are defined as 'economic, environmental, political and social conditions in which people are born, live, work, and age' [10]. One important aspect of a social determinants approach to health intervention and policy is the relationship between the 'social gradient' and the structure, level and impact of health inequality [11]. As poverty increases at the level of country or community, the social determinants of NCD risk, experiences and care become more crucial in the development of solutions. Another aspect is the role played by 'structural drivers' of everyday life conditions. These drivers include 'poor social policies, inequitable economic arrangements and bad politics that fashion the way societies are organized under the authorities of governments, as well as between countries under the effects of globalization' [12]. Within the context of NCDs, the 'policy regime' of the global health and the global NCD agenda also counts as a structural driver. The shared or contested ideological framework of global and local policy actors, as well as the structural arrangements within which ideas are embedded and operationalized, play a central role in the formulation, uptake and implementation of NCD policies across countries.

Most experts recommend interventions that tackle the medical, social, economic and political aspects of the NCD burden. For example, the Lancet Commission on Investing in Health recommends 'a combination of inexpensive population-based and clinical interventions, strengthening of health systems and fiscal policies such as taxation, regulation, subsidies and other legislation to curtail the health and economic effects of NCDs' [7].

The key factors underpinning the burden of NCDs in LMICs are known. They include urbanization, ageing, globalization, unhealthy lifestyle practices and poverty [8]. These factors arise from the intersection of demographic, epidemiological and nutrition transitions unique to LMICs. Demographically, LMICs have the fastest rate of urbanization and ageing. Countries are experiencing a 'protracted and polarised' epidemiological transition characterized by the co-existence of infectious and chronic diseases and by the poor facing a double jeopardy of both conditions [13]. A combination of food market globalization and weak governance has created a double burden of undernutrition and overnutrition within countries, households and individuals [14]. The solutions proposed by the global agenda on NCDs are also known by LMIC governments and policy makers. The challenge has been to translate these well-known and politically endorsed recommendations into concrete context-specific solutions.

Introduction to the Chapters

The volume is presented in three parts. Part I focuses on the state of the problem and state of knowledge on the epidemiology and burden of the major NCDs. Three chapters review the epidemiology and burden of cardiovascular diseases and diabetes (Awuah *et al.*, Chapter 1), cancers (Adeloye and Grant, Chapter 2) and neurodegenerative diseases (de-Graft Aikins *et al.*, Chapter 4). Two chapters focus on the co-morbid and multi-morbid interactions between the major NCDs and infectious diseases (Oni and Unwin, Chapter 3) and mental health disorders (Huang *et al.*, Chapter 5). For each chapter, authors review the roots and impact of the burden of their focal condition(s) and discuss available evidence on: (i) prevalence, morbidity and mortality; (ii) social determinants; and (iii) the major questions for future research, intervention and policy. The cross-cutting themes that emerge from Part I are presented in Box I.1.

Part II focuses on best practices and innovation in research and intervention. Four chapters discuss key issues on this theme including health systems strengthening (Coast *et al.*, Chapter 6), population surveillance (Kengne *et al.*, Chapter 7), community-based interventions (Addo and van de Vijver, Chapter 8) and self-help approaches to NCD care (de-Graft Aikins *et al.*, Chapter 9). Cross-cutting themes from evidence on interventions are presented in Box I.2.

Policy development, implementation and evaluation are crucial but neglected aspects of health systems responses to the NCD burden in LMICs. Part III focuses on policy development and implementation. Three chapters offer a comprehensive analysis of existing policies relevant to NCD prevention and control. They focus on policies that work, as well as discussing the lessons that can be learned from infectious disease control (Koram and Nimako, Chapter 10), NCD control in HICs (Agyemang *et al.*, Chapter 11) and the current policy issues and activities arising from the 2011 UN High Level Meeting on NCDs and leading to a post-2015 global health agenda (Mendis and Chestnov, Chapter 12). Cross-cutting themes emerging from Part III are presented in Box I.3.

The majority of chapters apply the WHO health systems model to examine the challenges and opportunities in NCD research, prevention, control and policy. With this model, strong health systems have six building blocks – service delivery, health workforce, medicines and technology, information systems, financing, and leadership and governance – that work synergistically to provide accessible, equitable, responsive and quality health services to the general population [15]. Strong health systems are also driven by people and their participatory power as both recipients and producers of healthcare. Most LMIC health systems do not meet the criteria set by the WHO model. The chapters provide insights into particular health systems failures within the context of NCD. They also offer evidence

Box I.1. Cross-cutting themes on the state of the problem and state of knowledge on the NCD burden in LMICs.

- The burden of conditions like CVD and cancers is higher in LMICs compared with HICs.
- Some conditions, like cancers and neurodegenerative diseases, constitute a complex of discrete diseases with their unique epidemiological and medical profiles and implications for primary, secondary and tertiary care.
- The major NCDs share the following risk factors: physical inactivity, unhealthy diets, alcohol overconsumption and smoking. For some conditions like asthma and cancers, environmental risk factors (such as pollution) are important.
- Regional differences exist in the epidemiology of NCDs. For example, hypertension prevalence rates are highest in sub-Saharan Africa and lowest in Latin America; and physical activity levels are higher in South-east Asia compared with sub-Saharan Africa.
- NCDs and their risk factors are gendered for some conditions like diabetes and hypertension and some risk factors like physical inactivity and obesity.
- NCDs interact in complex bidirectional ways with infectious diseases (such as human immunodeficiency virus, malaria and tuberculosis) and mental health conditions (such as depression and anxiety).
- Cultural and community resources are central to the development of successful interventions – in terms of knowledge, beliefs and attitudes, health-seeking behaviours, community responses to people living with NCDs, competing systems of health and healing systems, and empowering communities and patients to advocate for better formal care and improved self-care.
- Effective solutions require a life course approach, taking into account age, gender and environmental mediators/modifiers.
- Health systems are weak across the six building blocks of service delivery, medicines and technology, health workforce, information, financing and leadership/governance.
- Innovative strategies are emerging to address health systems deficiencies including integrated and collaborative care models, partnership approaches, task-shifting, advocacy for cheaper treatment and disease surveillance. These trends are particularly strong for cancer, mental health and neurodegenerative disease care.

of interventions or initiatives that seek to strengthen or reorient health systems to provide more competent NCD care. In Fig. I.1, we present a synthesis of chapter insights on concepts and models for developing NCD-competent health systems in LMICs.

Summary and Conclusions

This edited volume captures at least five unique challenges that LMICs face with respect to the burden of NCDs. First, the double burden of infectious and chronic diseases in many countries compounds the complexity of NCDs in terms of their co-morbid and multi-morbid interactions with other chronic and infectious conditions (Oni and Unwin, Chapter 3; Huang *et al.*, Chapter 5). As more individuals live with two or more conditions, the medical, psychosocial and health systems impact of NCDs increases. Secondly the structure and speed of the demographic

Box I.2. Cross-cutting themes on best practices and innovation in research and intervention.

- For the majority of LMICs, health systems are fragmented and weak.
- Best-practice models and promising pilot studies exist in some LMICs that suggest health systems can be strengthened or reoriented to address the NCD burden. Models and studies exist across the six building blocks and include *task-shifting* (health workforce), *collaborative care models* (service delivery), *NCD surveillance systems* (information), *advocacy for access to medicines by research groups and civil society organizations* (medicines and technology), *social insurance and social franchising approaches to NCD care financing* (financing) and *political investments in population-based interventions* (leadership and governance).
- Prioritizing prevention is critical for minimizing the financial, medical and psychosocial costs of NCDs.
- A 'multi-faceted and multi-institutional' approach to NCD prevention and control requires equitable partnerships between patients, communities, health workers, mass media, civil society, policy makers, politicians and development partners.
- Empowering people as both recipients and producers of healthcare is central to health systems strengthening. Civil society organizations and patient and self-help groups are an emerging phenomenon at present but are expected to be drivers of change in the future.
- Leadership and governance are critical to driving/sustaining initiatives and in scaling up effective/cost-effective interventions. Good and replicable models of NCD leadership and governance are reported in Bangladesh, Ethiopia and Thailand.

Box I.3. Cross-cutting themes on NCD policy development and implementation.

- NCDs are a developmental challenge.
- Social determinants of NCDs are central to understanding burden and developing solutions.
- Cost-effective and sustainable NCD policies and interventions require finding a balance between prevention and management and drawing intelligently on existing resources.
- Partnerships are central to NCD policy development and implementation. These partnerships must be multi-disciplinary, multi-sectoral and equitable.
- Service delivery has to be modelled on the ideal of universal health coverage and a diagonal and integrated approach to care will be essential.
- Understanding the synergies between the health systems building blocks and broader structural factors will inform more context-specific and sustainable interventions.
- Patients and communities have to play a greater role in advocating for health systems change and addressing the structural drivers relating to NCDs.
- A major challenge to leadership and governance in LMICs is the persistent gap between NCD policy development and implementation.
- Global frameworks for NCDs are important, but local ownership is crucial in implementing cost-effective and sustainable solutions across countries.

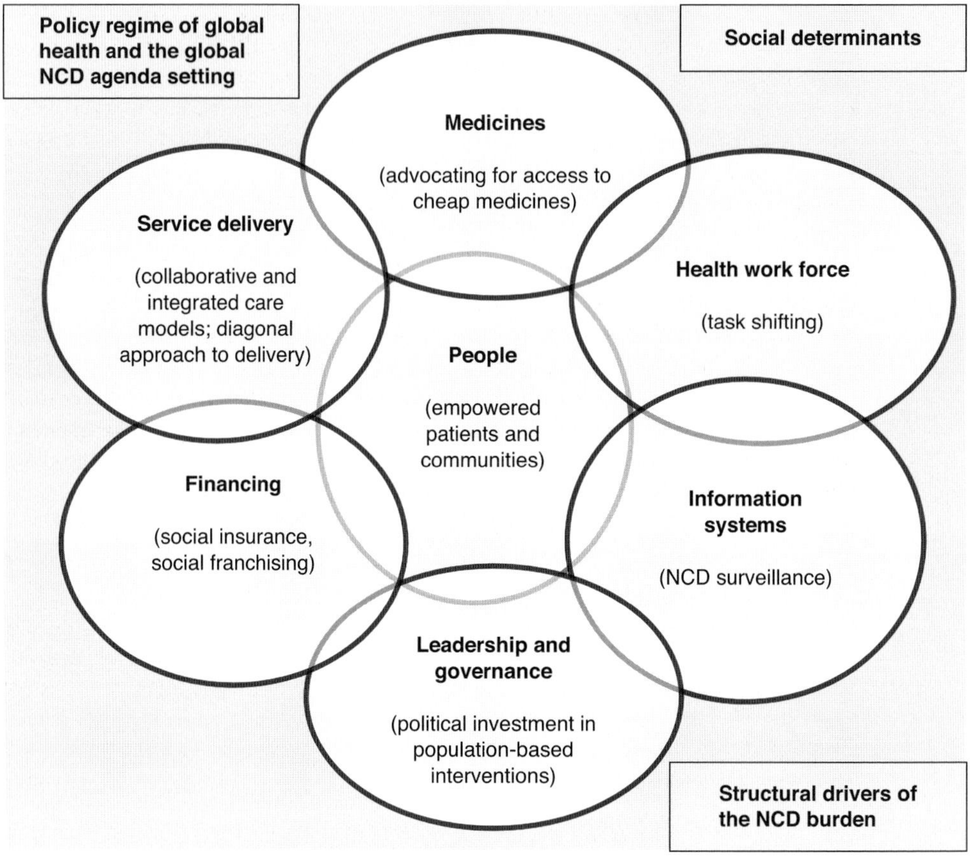

Fig. I.1. Concepts and models for developing NCD-competent health systems in LMICs.

transition in LMICs have led to rapid urbanization and ageing. Urbanization and urban poverty create conditions of high risk, such as unhealthy diets, physical inactivity, alcohol use, smoking, environmental pollution, psychosocial stress and infections. As populations age, there is a corresponding increase in the prevalence of diseases of ageing and of experiences of co-morbid and multi-morbid conditions. Thirdly, poverty – at national, community and household levels – engenders an interaction of social, economic and political barriers to good health, general well-being and optimal healthcare. Fourthly, LMIC health systems are weak and struggle to cope with complex public health problems due to inadequate financial, material and human resources. Health systems are also weakened by their ideological and practical orientation to treating acute infectious diseases, and this is partly responsible for the limited attention to the social determinants of NCDs in health systems responses. Finally, the policy regime of global health and the global NCD agenda engenders hierarchical relationships and inequitable sharing of resources between global and local actors. This undermines local commitment to and ownership of potential solutions and excludes the participation of individuals and communities affected by NCDs.

Most chapters have presented 'best-practice' responses and solutions to these challenges. Some chapters have presented evidence of health systems strengthening or reorienting initiatives that have yielded productive outcomes for NCD prevention and control in countries like India, Haiti, Malawi, Mauritius, Rwanda, South Africa and Thailand (Coast *et al.*, Chapter 6; Addo and van de Vijver, Chapter 8). Community-based interventions have been implemented with some success in Brazil, China, India, Mauritius and Peru, demonstrating that sustainable interventions can be developed in conditions of poverty and that empowered communities can contribute to these efforts (Addo and van de Vijver, Chapter 8; Koram and Nimako, Chapter 10). Some chapters have provided examples of how leadership and governance reshapes national responses to NCDs in countries like Bangladesh, Ethiopia, Mauritius and Thailand (Coast *et al.*, Chapter 6; Addo and van de Vijver, Chapter 8). Lessons from infectious disease control (Koram and Nimako, Chapter 10) and NCD interventions in high income countries (Agyemang *et al.*, Chapter 11) are informing NCD control activities in some LMICs. Countries like Burma, Cambodia, Ethiopia, Malawi, Thailand and Vietnam have used human immunodeficiency virus/AIDS control as a platform for improving NCD care (Coast *et al.*, Chapter 6). The review of the global agenda on NCDs by Mendis and Chestnov (Chapter 12) suggests that most LMIC governments are signatories to the current global recommendations on NCD prevention and control. The challenge for the future is replicating and scaling up existing best-practice models for specific conditions and affected communities in different countries. This will require a commitment to bridging the gap between policy development and implementation. Existing leadership and governance efforts in NCD control in LMICs provide important lessons for policy development and implementation.

Note

[1]There are debates over terminology. Some experts prefer to use chronic diseases instead of non-communicable diseases because chronic disease 'suggests important shared features: chronic disease epidemics take decades to become fully established; given their long duration, there are many opportunities for prevention; they require a long-term and systematic approach to treatment; and health services must integrate the response to these diseases with the response to acute, infectious diseases' [1]. The use of 'chronic disease' can be problematic in the sense that 'some diseases referred to as "chronic" . . . may actually be acute (such as some forms of heart disease), just as some communicable diseases (such as HIV/AIDS) may assume "chronic" characteristics' [2].

References

1. WHO (2005) *Preventing Chronic Disease. A Vital Investment.* World Health Organization, Geneva, Switzerland <http://www.who.int/chp/chronic_disease_report/contents/en>.
2. Suhrcke, M., Nugent, R.A., Stuckler, D. and Rocco, L. (2006) *Chronic Disease: An Economic Perspective.* Oxford Health Alliance, London, UK.

3. WHO (2011) *Global Status Report on Noncommunicable Diseases 2010*. World Health Organization, Geneva, Switzerland.
4. Samb, B.N., Desai, N., Nishtar, S., Mendis, S., Bekedam, H., Wright, A., Hsu, J., Martiniuk, A., Celletti, F., Patel, K., Adshead, F., McKee, M., Evans, T., Alwan, A. and Etienne, C. (2010) Prevention and management of chronic disease: a litmus test for health-systems strengthening in low-income and middle-income countries. *Lancet* 376, 1785–1797.
5. Allotey, P., Reidpath, D.D., Yasin, S., Chan, C. and de-Graft Aikins, A. (2010) Rethinking health systems: a focus on chronicity. *Lancet* 377, 450–451.
6. de-Graft Aikins, A., Pitchforth, E., Allotey, P., Ogedegbe G. and Agyemang, C. (2012) Culture, ethnicity and chronic conditions: reframing concepts and methods for research, intervention and policy in low and middle income countries. *Ethnicity & Health*, 17, 551–561.
7. Clarke, J. (2014) Medicalization of global health 3: the medicalization of the non-communicable diseases agenda. *Global Health Action* 7, 24002.
8. WHO (2014) *Global Status Report on NCDs*. World Health Organization, Geneva, Switzerland <http://www.who.int/chp/ncd_global_status_report/en>.
9. UN (2011) *Draft Political Declaration of the High-level Meeting on the Prevention and Control of Non-Communicable Diseases*. United Nations, New York <http://www.un.org/en/ga/ncdmeeting2011/pdf/NCD_draft_political_declaration.pdf>.
10. Cheng, J.K. (2012) Confronting the social determinants of health – obesity, neglect, and inequity. *New England Journal of Medicine* 367, 1976–1977.
11. Marmot, M. (2005) Social determinants of health inequalities. *Lancet* 365, 1099–1104.
12. Commission for Social Determinants of Health (2008) *Closing the Gap in a Generation: Health Equity through Action on the Social Determinants of Health*. World Health Organization, Geneva, Switzerland.
13. Frenk, J., Bobadilla, J.L., Sepulveda, J. and Cervantes, M.L. (1989) Health transition in middle-income countries: new challenges for health care. *Health Policy and Planning* 4, 29–39.
14. Popkin, B.M., Adair, L.S. and Ng, S.W. (2011) Global nutrition transition and the pandemic of obesity in developing countries. *Nutritional Reviews* 70, 3–21.
15. Gonzàlez Block, M.A., Akosa, A.B. and Chowdhury, M. (2012) Health systems research and infectious diseases of poverty: from the margins to the mainstream. In: *Global Report for Research on Infectious Diseases of Poverty*. 2012, WHO/WHO Special Programme for Research and Training in Tropical Diseases, Geneva, Switzerland.

1 Cardiovascular Diseases and Established Risk Factors in Low- and Middle-income Countries

Raphael Baffour Awuah[1], Ernest Afrifa-Anane[1] and Charles Agyemang[2*]

[1]*Regional Institute for Population Studies, University of Ghana, Accra, Ghana;* [2]*Department of Public Health, Academic Medical Center, University of Amsterdam, Amsterdam, The Netherlands*

1.1 Introduction

Cardiovascular diseases (CVDs) are the leading cause of mortality worldwide, with more deaths from CVDs than from any other cause annually [1]. In 2008, it was estimated that CVDs accounted for over 17 million deaths worldwide from a total of 57 million [1]. The CVD burden varies across different world regions. In high-income countries, CVD-related deaths have declined progressively since the mid-20th century because of successful preventive strategies and improved treatment for acute CVD events [2]. By contrast, in many low- and middle-income countries (LMICs), CVD rates are increasing rapidly, and CVD is already the leading cause of death in many countries [3]. It is estimated that over 80% of deaths attributable to CVDs occur in LMICs, with the occurrence being equally distributed among men and women [1]. Estimates show that LMICs experience 300–600 CVD deaths per 100,000 of the population, which is higher than in most high-income countries [1]. This is an unfortunate paradox because many years of progress in the fight against CVD in most high-income countries is being superseded by the rapidly increasing CVD burden in many LMICs [4].

*E-mail: c.o.agyemang@amc.uva.nl

The total number of CVD deaths (mainly stroke and coronary heart disease (CHD)) increased globally from 14.4 million in 1990 to 17.5 million in 2005. Of these deaths, 7.6 million were attributed to CHD and 5.7 million were attributed to stroke [5]. About 51% of deaths due to stroke and 45% of deaths due to CHD are also attributable to hypertension [6, 7].

The burden of CVD in LMICs is expected to increase further. It is estimated that over 23 million people will die from CVD by 2030 [1, 8] and it will remain the single leading cause of mortality and morbidity [8], more than infectious diseases (including human immunodeficiency virus/AIDS, tuberculosis and malaria), maternal and perinatal conditions, and nutritional disorders combined [9]. The largest increase in terms of percentage will occur in the Eastern Mediterranean region and the largest increase in number of deaths in the South-east Asia region.

The main drivers of the increasing burden of CVD in LMICs are the increasing trends in the prevalence of risk factors such as hypertension, obesity and diabetes. Time trend analyses, for example, indicate that the prevalence of obesity in urban West Africa has more than doubled over the last 15 years [10]. The most important behavioural risk factors of CVD are unhealthy diet, physical inactivity and tobacco use. The effects of unhealthy diet and physical inactivity may lead to hypertension, diabetes, dyslipidaemia, overweight and obesity, and subsequent CVDs. This clearly reflects the changing lifestyles in most LMICs, such as consumption of energy-dense foods and refined sugars complemented by less-energy-demanding jobs, particularly in the urban settings. The changing lifestyle is driven mainly by rapid economic growth coupled with the rapid pace of urbanization in LMICs. It has been suggested that it is the rapid development and resulting changes in the social fabric and physical environment that are accelerating the CVD and other chronic diseases epidemic in LMICs [4]. The potentially devastating effects of this trend are magnified by a detrimental economic impact on households and nations, where poverty can be both a contributing cause and a consequence of CVDs and other chronic diseases [2].

The increasing burden of CVD is occurring at a time when communicable diseases are still highly prevalent, particularly in Africa and South-east Asia, placing a great demand on the overburdened and impoverished healthcare systems in many of these countries.

Below we describe the current burden of the main CVDs (i.e. stroke and CHD) and their main risk factors (i.e. hypertension, diabetes, obesity, smoking, physical inactivity, excessive alcohol consumption) in the last 15 years using data from individual studies and systematic review articles known to the authors. Literature searches were performed using electronic databases (PubMed, PsycINFO and Google Scholar) that reported data on the epidemiology of stroke, CHD, hypertension and diabetes, overweight and obesity, smoking, physical inactivity and alcohol consumption in Africa, Asia, the Middle East, Latin America and the Caribbean. The articles used in this review consist of scholarly papers published between 2000 and 2014.

1.2 The Burden of CVD

Stroke

The prevalence of stroke in LMICs in the period between 2000 and 2014 ranged from 114 per 100,000 people in an urban community in Nigeria [11] to 9300 per 100,000 people in an urban area in China [12]. In rural areas of LMICs, the prevalence of stroke ranged from 243 per 100,000 in South Africa [13] to 6500 per 100,000 in Mexico [12]. The prevalence of stroke varied between different studies for some countries. For example, in Egypt, the prevalence of stroke ranged from 508 per 100,000 [14] to 963 per 100,000 [15]. The incidence of stroke ranged from 25 per 100,000 in Nigeria [16] to 250 per 100,000 in Egypt [17]. The prevalence and incidence of stroke was higher in men than in women.

The estimates indicated that stroke prevalence and mortality rates were 25% greater in LMICs relative to high-income countries [18]. Furthermore, a study of 56 population-based registries worldwide showed that there was a 42% decrease in stroke incidence in high-income countries, whereas LMICs experienced a 100% increase in stroke incidence from 1970 to 2008 [19]. In the absence of any meaningful clinical or public health interventions, it is expected that the incidence of stroke will increase further in LMICs.

Coronary heart disease

CHD, the principal component of CVD, is the leading cause of death in all World Health Organization (WHO) regions of the world except for the African region [20]. CHD is not only a disease of the elderly in high-income countries but also has a major global impact on the economically active population, and is a growing concern for LMICs [21]. Even in sub-Saharan Africa, where CHD was not considered as a major public health concern, it now ranks eighth among the leading causes of death in men and women in the region [22]. More importantly, among people aged >60 years, CHD is already the leading cause of death in men and the second leading cause of death in women in the African region. Mensah's study showed the age-adjusted mortality rate for CHD ranged from 111 per 100,000 in Algeria to 277 per 100,000 in Mauritius in men, and 49 per 100,000 in the Seychelles to 161 per 100,000 in Mauritius among women [22]. Additionally, in China, the age-adjusted death rate from CHD in the period under review was 80–128 per 100,000 for men and 57–98 per 100,000 for women [23]. Furthermore, among men aged 35–64, CHD mortality rates were 64–106 per 100,000 in China [24]. High mortality levels have also been reported in many LMICs. Age-standardized mortality due to CHD was 110 per 100,000 in the Federated States of Micronesia, 125 per 100,000 in Samoa and 181 per 100,000 in Nauru [7]. In Mexico, the age-adjusted mortality due to CHD in the year 2000 was 82 per 100,000 in men and 53 per 100,000 in women [25]. In India, it was estimated that 31.8 million people were living with CHD in 2001 [26].

The age-adjusted prevalence of CHD in Iran was 12.7% [27], 5.5% in Saudi Arabia [28] and 5.9% in Jordan [29]. The rising prevalence of risk factors such as hypertension and diabetes, as well as the weak and overstretched health systems in most LMICs, will most likely exacerbate the burden of CHD in these regions.

1.3 Risk Factors of CVD

1.3.1 Metabolic risk factors

Hypertension

We considered articles that defined hypertension as a measured blood pressure of >140 mmHg systolic and/or >90 mmHg diastolic or as those receiving antihypertensive therapy. The prevalence of hypertension ranged from 6.8% in a rural community in Mexico [30] to 69.9% in an urban study among individuals aged 70 and above in Tanzania [31]. The prevalence in rural areas ranged between 6.8% in Mexico [30] and 42.9% in Brazil [32]. The prevalence of hypertension in urban areas, on the other hand, ranged from 12.3% in Kenya [33] to 69.9% in Tanzania [31]. There was a higher hypertension prevalence among males than among females. There were considerable differences in the prevalence of hypertension in studies conducted in the same country. For example, the prevalence of hypertension ranged from 21.9% [34] to 42.1% [35] in China, from 9.3% [36] to 30.3% [37] in Ethiopia and from 15% [38] to 30.3% [39] in India. The evidence from the studies included in this review suggests that the prevalence of hypertension is comparable to that found in high-income countries. The African region has the highest prevalence rate, 46% of adults aged 25 and above, whereas the Americas have the lowest prevalence, at 35%.

Despite the increasing burden of hypertension in LMICs, a large number of people with hypertension are undiagnosed, untreated and uncontrolled [40]. As of 2008, almost 1 billion people had uncontrolled hypertension worldwide [41]. This means that a large number of people in LMICs will be affected by hypertension-related complications unless major efforts are made to halt or reduce the current rising prevalence of hypertension and its poor control.

Diabetes

With regard to diabetes (type 2), articles were included if they reported the prevalence of the condition, impaired fasting glucose and/or impaired glucose tolerance. The prevalence of diabetes in LMICs was as low as 0.4% in a rural community in Uganda [42] and as high as 26.3% in a study conducted in an urban community in South Africa [43]. Most of the studies reported a higher diabetes prevalence among men compared with women. The prevalence in rural settings ranged between 0.4% in Uganda [42] and 17.5% in Sri Lanka [44]. In the studies that focused on urban communities, the prevalence was from 4.4% in Peru [45] to 26.3% in South Africa [43]. The prevalence of impaired glucose tolerance was from 2.2% in an urban community in Nigeria [46] to 21.6% in Ethiopia [47], while the prevalence of impaired fasting glucose ranged from 1.2% in an urban town in South Africa [48] to 12.1% in a study conducted in a rural community in

Angola [49]. Studies conducted in the same country showed some variation in the prevalence of diabetes. For example, the prevalence of diabetes ranged from 4.3% in rural India [50] to 24.6% in urban India [51].

The review of studies on diabetes in LMICs indicated that the rates are as high as rates observed in high-income countries [52]. The number of individuals with diabetes in LMICs is likely to be even higher than current estimates because of a substantial proportion of people living with diabetes who are undetected [53]. This leads to an increase in diabetes complications (principally nephropathy, retinopathy, neuropathy and small-vessel vasculopathy causing lower extremity amputation). These complications account for much of the social and financial burden of diabetes in LMICs [52]. According to the latest estimates from the International Diabetes Federation, the African region has the highest proportion of undiagnosed type 2 diabetes (63%), and over half a million people in the region died from diabetes-related causes in 2013 [53]. This represents 8.6% of deaths from all causes in adults in the region. Moreover, despite the predominantly urban impact of the epidemic, diabetes is fast becoming a major health problem in rural communities in LMICs [54].

The rising prevalence of diabetes in LMICs is, to a large extent, attributed to rapid globalization and urbanization, with subsequent changes in diet, a reduction in physical activity levels and the adoption of sedentary lifestyles. The diabetes epidemic has increased in line with the worldwide rise in overweight and obesity.

Obesity

The prevalence of overweight and obesity is increasing at an alarming rate in both high-income countries and LMICs throughout the globe. WHO estimates indicate that the undernourished population in the world has declined, whereas the overnourished population has increased significantly [55]. Data from WHO show that, globally, there are more than 1 billion adults who are overweight and 300 million obese people. LMICs have been particularly affected, with obesity rates having increased more than threefold since 1980 in the Pacific Islands, Australasia and China [55]. Overweight and obesity are important risk factors for diabetes, CVD, cancer and premature death. In a review of CHD among LMICs, Gaziano *et al.* found a high population attribution factor of 10 and 5%, respectively, for Eastern Asia and Pacific and South Asia and 8% for sub-Saharan Africa [25]. In addition, Kelly *et al.* reported an average prevalence of overweight of 20.4% among women and 16.8% among men for Asian countries compared with those of sub-Saharan Africa, which were 17.5 and 12.1% for women and men, respectively [56]. Although explanations for the high prevalence are complex, it can be attributed to factors such as changes in dietary patterns, low physical activity levels and sedentary behaviours due to increased used of motorized vehicles as urbanization increases [57]. The gender-based prevalence from the studies indicates that women have been more affected by overweight and obesity than men. In India, 30% of females aged 25 and above were considered to be obese compared with 18% of their male counterparts [58]. Urban residents have also been more affected by overweight and obesity compared with rural residents.

For example, in Cameroon, 17.1% versus 5.4% of urban women and men and 3% versus 0.5% of rural women and men, respectively, were found to be obese [59].

As the overweight and obesity epidemic positively correlates with the rising burden of CVD in LMICs, their reduction will have a major impact in reducing the current CVD burden worldwide.

Dyslipidaemia

High cholesterol levels increase the risks of heart disease and stroke [60]. About one-third of CHD is attributable to high cholesterol globally. High cholesterol is estimated to cause 2.6 million deaths and 29.7 million disability-adjusted life years [61]. High cholesterol is a major cause of disease burden in both high-income countries and LMICs as a risk factor for CHD and stroke [62]. In 2008, the global prevalence of high total cholesterol among adults was 39%. The prevalence was higher in women (40%) than in men (37%). In general, raised cholesterol is higher in high-income countries than in LMICs. However, evidence suggests that the levels are increasing in LMICs. The prevalence of high total cholesterol was highest in the WHO European Region (54% for both men and women), followed by the WHO Region of the Americas (48% for both men and women). The WHO African Region and the WHO South-east Asia Region showed the lowest prevalence of high cholesterol (23 and 30%, respectively). Reduction of high cholesterol levels will have a major impact in reducing CHD and stroke in LMICs. It has been found that a 10% reduction in serum cholesterol in men aged 40 and above resulted in a 50% reduction in heart disease within 5 years [63].

1.3.2 Behaviour risk factors

Alcohol consumption

Harmful use of alcohol is an important contributor to the global burden of disease and is the third leading risk factor for premature deaths and disabilities in the world [61]. It is estimated that about 2.5 million people worldwide die of alcohol-related causes every year. Harmful use of alcohol is a major avoidable risk factor for neuropsychiatric disorders and other non-communicable diseases such as CVD, cirrhosis of the liver and various cancers. The prevalence of alcohol consumption is generally higher in males than in females, and in urban residents than in rural residents in LMICs. The proportion of males who regularly consume alcohol is more than twice the number of females (35% versus 13%, respectively) [64, 65].

A considerable scientific knowledge base is available for policy makers on the effectiveness and cost-effectiveness of strategies and interventions to prevent and reduce alcohol-related harm. However, much of the evidence comes from high-income countries and suggests the need for more work on this topic in LMICs. Nevertheless, the current evidence gives sufficient knowledge to inform policy in terms of comparative effectiveness and cost-effectiveness of selected policy measures [66].

Tobacco

Tobacco use is an important risk factor for CVD, cancer and respiratory mortality. Worldwide, 12% of all deaths among adults aged 30 years and over are attributed to tobacco. It kills nearly 6 million people each year [61]. Over 5 million of these deaths are due to direct tobacco use, while more than 600,000 are due to non-smokers being exposed to second-hand smoke. About 80% of the world's 1 billion smokers reside in LMICs. The prevalence of tobacco use ranges from 8.9 to 41.8% [65]. Generally, men in LMICs constitute higher proportions of individuals who use tobacco compared with their female counterparts. This high proportion is among Asian countries such as Nepal and the Federated States of Micronesia compared with sub-Saharan Africa. In the Federated States of Micronesia, one study reported that 37.7% of males compared with 16.7% of females had used tobacco [67]. Knowledge about the health consequences of tobacco use was found to be high among some sub-Saharan African countries like Ghana. In a faith-based study in Ghana, 97% of 167 congregants of some selected churches in Accra had the knowledge that cigarette smoking could cause heart disease and stroke [68].

Considerable progress has been made in global tobacco control since the adoption of the WHO Framework Convention on Tobacco Control. The *WHO Report on the Global Tobacco Epidemic* in 2013 demonstrated that any country can introduce an effective tobacco control programme to reduce tobacco use, irrespective of its political structure or income level [69]. This means that efforts to incorporate all provisions of the WHO Framework Convention into national tobacco control programmes will save more lives in LMICs.

Physical inactivity

Evidence strongly indicates that physical inactivity increases the risk of many adverse health conditions such as CHD, type 2 diabetes and cancers, and also shortens life expectancy. It has been estimated that a 10 or 25% reduction in physical inactivity, for example, could avert 533,000 and more than 1.3 million deaths every year [70]. However, physical inactivity remains a major problem across the world. Globally, 31% of adults aged 15 years and above were insufficiently active in 2008 [1]. In a review by Hallal *et al.*, individuals living in LMICs had lower levels of physical inactivity compared with those living in high-income countries (20% for LMICs compared with more than 40% for high-income countries) [71]. They also found that, in LMICs, there were more individuals who were physically inactive in sub-Saharan Africa compared with those from South-east Asia [71]. Generally, there is an important gender difference in the prevalence of physical inactivity in LMICs. The prevalence of physical inactivity was high among females compared with their male counterparts. For instance, about 88.6% of females compared with 72.6% of males from the Federated States of Micronesia were physically inactive [67]. Similarly, Nepalese females were more physically inactive than their male counterparts (21.9 versus 17.9%). In contrast, Yusuf *et al.* found among four LMICs that higher proportions of males (22.5%) compared with females (17.1%) were physically inactive [65]. Physical inactivity rates are also relatively high in urban areas compared with rural areas [72]. In Nigeria, physical activity was found to be lower among individuals with a higher income [73]. In addition, neighbourhood safety from traffic and crime at night and during the day were found to be promoters of physical activity [74].

1.4 Implications for the Increasing Burden of CVDs in LMICs

CVDs come with a huge economic burden. Besides the disruption of life functions/activities and loss of life associated with CVD, LMICs face immense economic challenges associated with the epidemic. The costs are twofold: the indirect cost to the national economy (which includes time and productivity loss), and that to individuals and households (which includes income loss of individuals living with CVD and family members, usually the caregivers) [75]. For example, in India, it has been estimated that loss of income of individuals living with CVD and caregivers was 60.5 and 39.5%, respectively [76].

There is also a direct cost to the healthcare system. For example, in China, annual direct costs of CVD are estimated at over US$40 billion, which is about 4% of its gross national income [77]. In addition, estimated losses to gross domestic product as a result of CVD ranged from US$20 million dollars in Ethiopia to nearly US$1 billion in China and India in 2005 [18]. The economic impact is further compounded by the fact that a high proportion of the CVD burden in LMICs occurs earlier among adults in the economically active population [78]. An evaluation of the potential loss due to early onset of CVD in Brazil, India, China, South Africa and Mexico indicated that about 21 million years of future productive life are lost because of CVD each year [79].

Although the economic impact of CVD in LMICs is high, the resources devoted toward healthcare are inadequate. Most LMICs devote about 6% of their gross national income to healthcare compared with 10% in high-income countries [78]. Considering the limited resources available in LMICs, only the interventions that can lead to substantial reductions in the mortality and morbidity of CVD at relatively low cost are likely to be sustainable.

It has been suggested that the prevention of CVD risk factors is a more cost-effective and sustainable approach in dealing with the CVD epidemic in LMICs [80]. Furthermore, paying attention to the prevention and management of CVD risk factors will lower costs of care, foster effective treatment and reduce the burden of CVD, particularly morbidity and mortality [81]. Prevention and management strategies will be more effective if they are structured and integrated [81] (see Koram and Nimako, Chapter 10, this volume). In most LMICs, it is difficult to implement such structured and integrated programmes because of overstretched and poorly resourced health systems and the lack of political commitment or will [82]. To overcome some of these challenges, stakeholders in the health sector in LMICs should draw on the most effective programmes from high-income countries and other LMICs who have managed and reduced the CVD burden in the planning and implementation of CVD intervention programmes [82] (see Koram and Nimako, Chapter 10, and Agyemang *et al.*, Chapter 11, this volume).

1.5 Conclusion

CVDs have increased to approximately 50% of the total disease burden in LMICs undergoing the epidemiological transition. This burden has financial implications for individuals and governments in LMICs. A focus on prevention of CVD may be a more efficient strategy given the limited resources in LMICs. The challenges that LMICs face in the prevention and control of CVD are enormous, including the under-appreciation of the magnitude of the disease burden, poorly resourced healthcare systems for provision of comprehensive preventive and primary healthcare, and increasing urbanization accompanied by the adoption of less healthy lifestyles. Although daunting, these challenges are not insurmountable. Effective intervention programmes or policies will require a multi-disciplinary approach of key national and international players with a strong political commitment.

References

1. WHO (2011) *Global Status Report on Noncommunicable Diseases 2010*. World Health Organization, Geneva, Switzerland.
2. Institute of Medicine (2010) *Promoting Cardiovascular Health in the Developing World: a Critical Challenge to Achieve Global Health*. The National Academies Press, Washington, DC.
3. Bovet, P. and Paccaud, F. (2012) Cardiovascular disease and the changing face of global public health: a focus on low and middle income countries. *Public Health Reviews* 33, 397–415.
4. Paradis, G. and Chiolero, A. (2011) The cardiovascular and chronic diseases epidemic in low- and middle-income countries: a global health challenge. *Journal of the American College of Cardiology* 57, 1775–1777.
5. WHO (2009) *World Health Statistics 2009*. World Health Organization, Geneva, Switzerland.
6. Lim, S.S., Vos, T., Flaxman, A.D., Danaei, G., Shibuya, K., Adair-Rohani, H., AlMazroa, M.A., Amann, M., Anderson, H.R., Andrews, K.G. *et al.* (2012) A comparative risk assessment of burden of disease and injury attributable to 67 risk factors and risk factor clusters in 21 regions, 1990–2010: a systematic analysis for the Global Burden of Disease Study 2010. *Lancet* 380, 2224–2260.
7. WHO (2008) *The Global Burden of Disease: 2004 Update*. World Health Organization, Geneva, Switzerland.
8. Mathers, C.D. and Loncar, D. (2006) Projections of global mortality and burden of disease from 2002 to 2030. *PLoS Medicine* 3, e442.
9. Beaglehole, R. and Bonita, R. (2008) Global public health: a scorecard. *Lancet* 372, 1988–1996.
10. Abubakari, A.R., Lauder, W., Agyemang, C., Jones, M., Kirk, A. and Bhopal, R.S. (2008) Prevalence and time trends in obesity among adult West African populations: a meta-analysis. *Obesity Reviews* 9, 297–311.
11. Danesi, M., Okubadejo, N. and Ojini, F. (2007) Prevalence of stroke in an urban, mixed-income community in Lagos, Nigeria. *Neuroepidemiology* 28, 216–223.
12. Ferri, C.P., Schoenborn, C., Kalra, L., Acosta, D., Guerra, M., Huang, Y., Jacob, K.S., Llibre Rodriguez, J.J., Salas, A., Luisa Sosa, A., Williams, J.D., Liu, Z., Moriyama, T., Valhuerdi, A. and Prince, M.J. (2011) Prevalence of stroke and related burden among older people living in Latin America, India and China. *Journal of Neurology, Neurosurgery and Psychiatry* 82, 1074–1082.

13. Connor, M. (2004) Prevalence of stroke survivors in rural South Africa: results from the Southern Africa Stroke Prevention Initiative (SASPI) Agincourt Field Site. *Stroke* 35, 627–632.
14. Kandil, M.R., El-Tallawy, H.N., Farawez, H.M., Khalifa, G., Ahmed, M.A., Hamed, A. and Ali, A.M. (2006) Epidemiology of cerebrovascular stroke and TIA in Upper Egypt (Sohag) – relative frequency of stroke in Assiut University Hospital. *Egyptian Journal of Neurology and Neurosurgery* 43, 593–602.
15. Khedr, E.M., Elfetoh, N.A., Al Attar, G., Ahmed, M.A., Ali, A.M., Hamdy, A., Kandil, M.R. and Farweez, H. (2013) Epidemiological study and risk factors of stroke in Assiut Governorate, Egypt: community-based study. *Neuroepidemiology* 40, 288–294.
16. Danesi, M.A., Okubadejo, N.U., Ojini, F.I. and Ojo, O.O. (2013) Incidence and 30-day case fatality rate of first-ever stroke in urban Nigeria: the prospective community based Epidemiology of Stroke in Lagos (EPISIL) phase II results. *Journal of the Neurological Sciences* 331, 43–47.
17. Farghaly, W.M.A., El-Tallawy, H.N., Shehata, G.A., Rageh, T.A., Abdel-Hakeem, N.M., Elhamed, M.A., Al-Fawal, B.M. and Badry, R. (2013) Epidemiology of nonfatal stroke and transient ischemic attack in AlKharga District, New Valley, Egypt. *Neuropsychiatric Disease and Treatment* 9, 1785–1790.
18. Mukherjee, D. and Patil, C.G. (2011) Epidemiology and the global burden of stroke. *World Neurosurgery* 76 (Suppl.), S85–S90.
19. Feigin, V.L., Lawes, C.M., Bennett, D.A., Barker-Collo, S.L. and Parag, V. (2009) Worldwide stroke incidence and early case fatality reported in 56 population-based studies: a systematic review. *Lancet Neurology* 8, 355–369.
20. WHO (2002) *The World Health Report 2001: Reducing Risks, Promoting Healthy Life*. World Health Organization, Geneva, Switzerland.
21. Abegunde, D.O., Mathers, C.D., Adam, T., Ortegon, M. and Strong, K. (2007) The burden and costs of chronic diseases in low-income and middle-income countries. *Lancet* 370, 1929–1938.
22. Mensah, G.A. (2008) Ischaemic heart disease in Africa. *Heart* 94, 836–843.
23. Zhang, X.H., Lu, Z.L. and Liu, L. (2008) Coronary heart disease in China. *Heart* 94, 1126–1131.
24. Liu, L. (2007) Cardiovascular diseases in China. *Biochemistry and Cell Biology* 85, 157–163.
25. Gaziano, T.A., Bitton, A., Anand, S., Abrahams-Gessel, S. and Murphy, A. (2010) Growing epidemic of coronary heart disease in low- and middle-income countries. *Current Problems in Cardiology* 35, 72–115.
26. Gupta, R. (2005) Burden of coronary heart disease in India. *Indian Heart Journal* 57, 632–638.
27. Nabipour, I., Amiri, M., Imami, S.R., Jahfari, S.M., Shafeiae, E., Nosrati, A., Iranpour, D. and Soltanian, A.R. (2007) The metabolic syndrome and nonfatal ischemic heart disease; a population-based study. *International Journal of Cardiology* 118, 48–53.
28. Al-Nozha, M.M., Arafah, M.R., Al-Mazrou, Y.Y., Al-Maatouq, M.A., Khan, N.B., Khalil, M.Z., Al-Khadra, A.H., Al-Marzouki, K., Abdullah, M.A., Al-Harthi, S.S., Al-Shahid, M.S., Nouh, M.S. and Al-Mobeireek, A. (2004) Coronary artery disease in Saudi Arabia. *Saudi Medical Journal* 25, 1165–1171.
29. Nsour, M., Mahfoud, Z., Kanaan, M.N. and Balbeissi, A. (2008) Prevalence and predictors of nonfatal myocardial infarction in Jordan. *Eastern Mediterranean Health Journal* 14, 818–830.
30. Guerrero-Romero, F., Rodríguez-Morán, M., Sandoval-Herrrera, F. and Alvarado-Ruiz, R. (2000) Prevalence of hypertension in indigenous inhabitants of traditional communities from the north of Mexico. *Journal of Human Hypertension* 14, 555–559.
31. Dewhurst, M.J., Dewhurst, F., Gray, W.K., Chaote, P., Orega, G.P. and Walker, R.W. (2013) The high prevalence of hypertension in rural-dwelling Tanzanian older adults and the disparity between detection, treatment and control: a rule of sixths? *Journal of Human Hypertension* 27, 374–380.

32. Matozinhos, F.P., Mendes, L.L., Oliveira, A.G., Velásquez-Meléndez, G. (2011) Factors associated with arterial hypertension in rural populations. *Revista Mineira de Enfermagem* 15, 333–340.
33. van de Vijver, S.J., Oti, S.O., Agyemang, C., Gomez, G.B. and Kyobutungi, C. (2013) Prevalence, awareness, treatment and control of hypertension among slum dwellers in Nairobi, Kenya. *Journal of Hypertension* 31, 1018–1024.
34. Ruixing, Y., Weixiong, L., Hanjun, Y., Dezhai, Y., Shuquan, L., Shangling, P., Qiming, F., Jinzhen, W., Jianting, G. and Yaju, D. (2008) Diet, lifestyle, and blood pressure of the middle-aged and elderly in the Guangxi Bai Ku Yao and Han populations. *American Journal of Hypertension* 21, 382–387.
35. Zhang, J., Huang, Q., Yu, M., Cha, X., Li, J., Yuan, Y., Wei, T. and Zhong, H. (2013) Prevalence, awareness, medication, control, and risk factors associated with hypertension in Bai ethnic group in rural China: the Yunnan Minority Eye Study. *PLoS One* 8, e70886.
36. Muluneh, A.T., Haileamlak, A., Tessema, F., Alemseged, F., Woldemichael, K., Asefa, M. *et al.* (2012) Population based survey of chronic non-communicable diseases at Gilgel Gibe Field Research Center, southwest Ethiopia. *Ethiopian Journal of Health Sciences* 22 (Suppl.), 7–18.
37. Tesfaye, F., Byass, P. and Wall, S. (2009) Population based prevalence of high blood pressure among adults in Addis Ababa: uncovering a silent epidemic. *BMC Cardiovascular Disorders* 9, 1471–2261.
38. Madhu, B., Srinath, K.M. and Ashok, N.C. (2012) Hypertension: prevalence and its associated factors in a rural South Indian population. *Indian Journal of Public Health Research & Development* 3, 105–109.
39. Asgary, R., Galson, S., Shankar, H., O'Brien, C. and Arole, S. (2012) Hypertension, pre-hypertension, and associated risk factors in a subsistent farmer community in remote rural central India. *Journal of Public Health* 21, 251–258.
40. Ataklte, F., Erqou, S., Kaptoge, S., Taye, B., Echouffo-Tcheugui, J.B. and Kengne, A.P. (2015) Burden of undiagnosed hypertension in sub-saharan Africa: a systematic review and meta-analysis. *Hypertension* 65, 291–298.
41. WHO (2013) *A Global Brief on Hypertension. Silent Killer, Global Public Health Crisis.* World Health Organization, Geneva, Switzerland.
42. Maher, D., Waswa, L., Baisley, K., Karabarinde, A., Unwin, N. and Grosskurth, H. (2011) Distribution of hyperglycaemia and related cardiovascular disease risk factors in low-income countries: a cross-sectional population-based survey in rural Uganda. *International Journal of Epidemiology* 40, 160–171.
43. Erasmus, R.T., Soita, D.J., Hassan, M.S., Blanco-Blanco, E., Vergotine, Z., Kegne, A.P. and Matsha, T.E. (2012) High prevalence of diabetes mellitus and metabolic syndrome in a South African coloured population: baseline data of a study in Bellville, Cape Town. *South African Medical Journal* 102, 841–844.
44. Wijewardene, K., Mohideen, M.R., Mendis, S., Fernando, D.S., Kulathilaka, T., Weerasekara, D. and Uluwitta, P. (2005) Prevalence of hypertension, diabetes and obesity: baseline findings of a population based survey in four provinces in Sri Lanka. *Ceylon Medical Journal* 50, 62–70.
45. Escobedo, J., Buitrón, L.V., Velasco, M.F., Ramírez, J.C., Hernández, R., Macchia, A. *et al.* (2009) High prevalence of diabetes and impaired fasting glucose in urban Latin America: the CARMELA Study. *Diabetic Medicine* 26, 864–871.
46. Nyenwe, E.A., Odia, O.J., Ihekwaba, A.E., Ojule, A. and Babatunde, S. (2003) Type 2 diabetes in adult Nigerians: a study of its prevalence and risk factors in Port Harcourt, Nigeria. *Diabetes Research and Clinical Practice* 62, 177–185.
47. Nshisso, L.D., Reese, A., Gelaye, B., Lemma, S., Berhane, Y. and Williams, M.A. (2012) Prevalence of hypertension and diabetes among Ethiopian adults. *Diabetes and Metabolic Syndrome* 6, 36–41.
48. Peer, N., Steyn, K., Lombard, C., Lambert, E.V., Vythilingum, B. and Levitt, N.S. (2012) Rising diabetes prevalence among urban-dwelling black South Africans. *PLoS One* 7, e43336.

49. Evaristo-Neto, A.D., Foss-Freitas, M.C. and Foss, M.C. (2010) Prevalence of diabetes mellitus and impaired glucose tolerance in a rural community of Angola. *Diabetology & Metabolic Syndrome* 2, 63.
50. Pandey, R.M., Gupta, R., Misra, A., Misra, P., Singh, V., Agrawal, A., Dey, S., Rao, S., Menon, V.U., Kamalamma, N., Devi, K.P., Revathi, K. and Sharma, V. (2013) Determinants of urban-rural differences in cardiovascular risk factors in middle-aged women in India: a cross-sectional study. *International Journal of Cardiology* 163, 157–162.
51. Boddula, R., Yadav, S., Bhatia, V., Genitta, G., Pandey, D., Kumar, A., Singh, H.K., Ramesh, V., Julka, S., Bansal, B., Srikant, K. and Bhatia, E. (2008) High prevalence of type 2 diabetes mellitus in affluent urban Indians. *Diabetes Research and Clinical Practice* 81, e4–e7.
52. van Dieren, S., Beulens, J.W., van der Schouw, Y.T., Grobbee, D.E. and Neal, B. (2010) The global burden of diabetes and its complications: an emerging pandemic. *European Journal of Cardiovascular prevention and Rehabilitation* 17 (Suppl. 1), S3–S8.
53. IDF (2013) *Diabetes Atlas*, 6th edn. International Diabetes Federation, Brussels, Belgium.
54. Mbanya, J.C., Motala, A.A., Sobngwi, E., Assah, F.K. and Enoru, S.T. (2010) Diabetes in sub-Saharan Africa. *Lancet* 375, 2254–2266.
55. WHO (2008) *Controlling the Global Obesity Epidemic*. World Health Organization, Geneva, Switzerland.
56. Kelly, T., Yang, W., Chen C.-S., Reynolds, K. and He, J. (2008) Global burden of obesity in 2005 and projections to 2030. *International Journal of Obesity* 32, 1431–1437.
57. Popkin, B.M. and Gordon-Larsen, P. (2004) The nutrition transition: worldwide obesity dynamic and their determinants. *International Journal of Obesity and Related Metabolic Disorders* 28, S2–S9.
58. Gallieni, M., Aiello, A., Tucci, B., Sala, V., Mandal, S.K.B., Doneda, A. and Genovesi, S. (2014) The burden of hypertension and kidney disease in Northeast India: the Institute for Indian Mother and Child Noncommunicable Diseases Project. *Scientific World Journal* 2014, 320869.
59. Sobngwi, E., Mbanya, J.-C.N., Unwin, N.C., Kengne, A.P., Fezeu, L., Minkoulou, E.M., Aspray, T.J. and Alberti, K.G. (2002) Physical activity and its relationship with obesity hypertension and diabetes in urban and rural Cameroon. *International Journal of Obesity* 26, 1009–1016.
60. Ezzati, M., Lopez, A.D., Rodgers, A., Vander Hoorn, S., Murray, C.J. and the Comparative Risk Assessment Collaborating Group (2002) Selected major risk factors and global and regional burden of disease. *Lancet* 360, 1347–1360.
61. WHO (2009) *Global Health Risks: Mortality and Burden of Disease Attributable to Selected Major Risks*. World Health Organization, Geneva, Switzerland.
62. Meyer, K.A., Lawrence, H.K., Jacobs, D.R. and Folsom, A.R. (2001) Dietary fat and incidence of type 2 diabetes in older Iowa women. *Diabetes Care* 24, 1528–1535.
63. Law, M.R., Wald, N.J. and Thompson, S.G. (1994) By how much and how quickly does reduction in serum cholesterol concentration lower risk of ischaemic heart disease? *British Medical Journal* 308, 367–372.
64. Vaidya, A. and Krettek, A. (2014) Physical activity level and its sociodemographic correlates in a peri-urban Nepalese population: a cross-sectional study from the Jhaukhel-Duwakot health demographic surveillance site. *International Journal of Behavioral Nutrition and Physical Activity* 11, 39.
65. Yusuf, S., Rangarajan, S., Teo, K., Islam, S., Li, W., Liu, L., Bo, J., Lou, Q., Lu, F., Liu, T. *et al.* (2014) Cardiovascular risk and events in 17 low-, middle-, and high-income countries. *New England Journal of Medicine* 371, 818–827.
66. WHO (2009) *Evidence for the Effectiveness and Cost-effectiveness of Interventions to Reduce Alcohol-related Harm*. World Health Organization, Regional Office for Europe, Copenhagen, Denmark.
67. Hosey, G.M., Samo, M., Gregg, E.W., Padden, D. and Bibb, S.G. (2014) Socioeconomic and demographic predictors of selected cardiovascular risk factors among adults living in Pohnpei, Federated States of Micronesia. *BMC Public Health* 14, 895.

68. Abanilla, P.K.A., Huang, K.-Y., Shinners, D., Levy, A., Ayernor, K., de-Graft Aikins, A. and Ogedegbe, O. (2011) Cardiovascular diseases prevention in Ghana: feasibility of a faith-based organizational approach. *Bulletin of the World Health Organization* 89, 648–656.
69. WHO (2013) *WHO Report on the Global Tobacco Epidemic, 2013: Enforcing Bans on Tobacco Advertising, Promotion and Sponsorship*. World Health Organization, Geneva, Switzerland.
70. Lee, I.M., Shiroma, E.J., Lobelo, F., Puska, P., Blair, S.N., Katzmarzyk, P.T. and the Lancet Physical Activity Series Working Group (2012) Effect of physical inactivity on major non-communicable diseases worldwide: an analysis of burden of disease and life expectancy. *Lancet* 380, 219–229.
71. Hallal, P.C., Andersen, L.B., Bull, F.C., Guthold, R., Haskell, W., Ekelund, U. and the Lancet Physical Activity Series Working Group (2012) Global physical activity levels: surveillance progress, pitfalls and prospects. *Lancet* 380, 247–257.
72. Abubakari, A.R., Lauder, W., Jones, M.C., Kirk, A., Agyemang, C. and Bhopal, R.S. (2009) Prevalence and time trends in diabetes and physical inactivity among adult West African populations: the epidemic has arrived. *Public Health* 123, 602–614.
73. Oyeyemi, A.L., Oyeyemi, A.Y., Jidda, Z.A. and Babagana, F. (2013) Prevalence of physical activity among adults in a metropolitan Nigerian city: a cross-sectional study. *Journal of Epidemiology* 23, 169–177.
74. Oyeyemi, A.L., Adegoke, B.O., Sallis, J.F., Oyeyemi, A.Y. and Bourdeaudhuij, I.D. (2012) Perceived crime and traffic safety is related to physical activity among adults in Nigeria. *BMC Public Health* 12, 294.
75. Kankeu, H.T., Saksena, P., Xu, K. and Evans, D.B. (2013) The financial burden from non-communicable diseases in low- and middle-income countries: a literature review. *Health Research Policy and Systems* 11, 31.
76. Grover, S., Avasthi, A., Bhansali, A., Chakrabarti, S. and Kulhara, P. (2005) Cost of ambulatory care of diabetes mellitus: a study from north India. *Postgraduate Medical Journal* 81, 391–395.
77. Gaziano, T.A. (2007) Reducing the growing burden of cardiovascular disease in the developing world. *Health Affairs (Millwood)* 26, 13–24.
78. Gaziano, T.A. (2005) Cardiovascular disease in the developing world and its cost-effective management. *Circulation* 112, 3547–3553.
79. Leeder, S., Raymond, S., Greenberg, H., Liu, H. and Esson, K. (2004) *A Race Against Time: the Challenge of Cardiovascular Disease in Developing Countries*. Trustees of Columbia University, New York.
80. WHO (2007) *Prevention of Cardiovascular Disease: Guidelines for Assessment and Management of Total Cardiovascular Risk*. World Health Organization, Geneva, Switzerland.
81. Fuster V and Kelly, B.B. (2010) *Promoting Cardiovascular Health in the Developing World*. National Academies Press, Washington, DC.
82. van de Vijver, S., Oti, S., Addo, J., de-Graft Aikins, A. and Agyemang, C. (2012) Review of community-based interventions for prevention of cardiovascular diseases in low- and middle-income countries. *Ethnicity & Health* 17, 651–676.

2 A Review of Cancers in Africa

DAVIES ADELOYE AND LIZ GRANT*

University of Edinburgh, Edinburgh, UK

2.1 Introduction

The burden of cancers is increasing worldwide and is a major contributor to global morbidities and mortalities [1]. Cancer was previously thought to be a disease of the industrialized nations [1, 2]; however, evidence now shows that most new cases of cancers are found in low- and middle-income countries (LMICs), increasing from 15% in 1970 to 56% in 2008, and projected to reach about 70% by 2030 [3]. One major challenge is in the overall response to this growing burden in many LMICs, with late presentations, a poor health system response and consequently low survival rates reported in many LMICs compared with improved responses and survival rates in developed countries [4, 5]. Rapid population growth, increasing life expectancy and progressively westernized lifestyles in many developing countries are driving the burden of cancers, which will continue to rise [6], with about 27 million incident cases, 17 million deaths and over 75 million prevalent cases of cancers expected by 2030 [7]. According to the 2011 United Nations High-Level Meeting on Non-Communicable Diseases, the focus of many stakeholders has turned towards addressing this growing burden of cancers and other non-communicable diseases (NCDs) [8], especially in Africa and other LMICs, where the existing high burden from infectious diseases is exacerbating the cancer profile and contributing to double and triple burdens of disease [9].

Cancer is not a single disease but a group of chronic diseases characterized by the uncontrolled growth of abnormal cells within the body. These abnormal cells often spread to other parts of the body (e.g. liver, lymph nodes, lungs and brain) – a process called metastasis. Most cancers arise from damage to genes or genetic mutations, which themselves are influenced by both internal and environmental factors. There is no one cause of cancer; rather, there are many causes and many

*E-mail: liz.grant@ed.ac.uk

contributing factors, with each cancer type having its own specific set of drivers and risk factors. However, there are also shared factors that together influence the cancer burden inordinately. These include environmental factors such as tobacco, radiation, chemicals, dietary factors and infectious diseases. Alongside these external factors, there are a set of internal factors linked to cancer including hormones, immune conditions, metabolic disorders and inherited genetic abnormalities.

2.2 Global Summary of Cancers

2.2.1 LMICs

Table 2.1 presents a set of different cancers ranked over the past 20 years [10, 11]. Parkin *et al.* noted that there were 10.1 million new cancer cases and 6.2 million deaths in 2000. Lung cancer was the main cancer globally, with over 1.2 million new cases and 1.1 million deaths, and breast cancer was the second most common with about 1.05 million new cases and about 373,000 deaths [10]. Other cancers dominating the landscape include colorectal cancer with 876,000 new cases and 492,000 deaths, stomach cancer with 876,000 new cases and 647,000 deaths, and liver cancer with 564,000 new cases and 549,000 deaths [10]. Oncologists have noted that the relatively favourable prognosis of breast cancer has been shaped by better responses from many health sectors, and this has resulted in a relatively lower death rate compared with other cancers with higher incidence rates [4]. However, Jemal *et al.* argued that, despite a relatively lower cancer incidence in the developed world compared with less developed countries, the overall mortality rates are virtually the same [14]. The 2002 GLOBOCAN study reported estimates underpin this increasing burden of cancers globally [13]. By 2008, GLOBOCAN estimates rose to a total of 12.7 million new cancer cases and 7.6 million deaths, with Africa accounting for 5.6 and 7.1% of global new cancer cases and deaths, respectively [7]. For specific cancers, the pattern remained the same as the estimates reported in 2000 and 2002. Lung cancer presented with the highest burden with 1.61 million new cases and 1.38

Table 2.1. Reported new cases and deaths for the top five cancers globally (1990–2008).

	Year (estimate in millions)							
	1990 [12]		2001 [10]		2002 [14]		2008 [7]	
Site	New cases	Deaths	New cases	Deaths	New cases	Deaths	New cases	Deaths
All	–	–	10.1	6.2	10.9	6.7	12.7	7.6
Lung	1.04	–	1.2	1.1	1.35	1.18	1.61	1.38
Breast	0.796	–	1.05	0.373	1.15	0.411	1.38	0.458
Colorectal	0.782	–	0.945	0.492	1.02	0.529	1.23	0.608
Stomach	0.798	–	0.876	0.647	0.934	0.7	0.989	0.738
Liver	0.437	–	0.564	0.549	0.626	0.598	0.748	0.696

million deaths, followed by breast cancer with 1.38 million new cases and 458,000 deaths, colorectal cancer with 1.23 million new cases and 608,000 deaths, stomach cancer with 989,000 cases and 738,000 deaths, and liver cancer with 748,000 cases and 696,000 deaths [7].

According to Soerjomataram *et al.*, about 169.3 million years were lost due to cancers in 2008, with colorectal, lung, breast and prostate cancers, respectively, being the main contributors to global disability-adjusted life years [15]. As noted above, the 2008 CONCORD study of cancers in five continents showed the 5-year survival rate was highest for breast cancer, followed by colorectal and prostate cancers, respectively [4]. Meanwhile, the incidence of paediatric solid tumours also varies across world regions, with leukaemia, brain tumours and nephroblastoma prevalent in industrialized countries, while Burkitt's lymphoma was more prevalent in Africa [16].

2.2.2 Agenda setting for cancer and key global players

Since 2000, key global stakeholders have been advocating for detailed agenda settings on cancer-related health issues aiming towards ensuring an improved response to the rising burden of cancers globally [8]. The following are among the key global players involved in agenda setting for the control, treatment and overall management of cancers globally [3, 8, 17]:

- 2005 World Health Assembly resolution on cancer prevention and control;
- 2007 Institute of Medicine of the National Academies report on cancer in LMICs;
- 2008 International Agency for Research on Cancer (IARC) and World Health Organization (WHO) World Cancer Report;
- 2011 United Nations High-level Committee on NCDs;
- Global Task Force on Expanded Access to Cancer Care and Control in Developing Countries (GTF.CCC), convened by the Dana-Farber Cancer Institute, Harvard Global Initiative, Harvard Medical School and Harvard School of Public Health in 2009, focusing on designing and implementing global and regional initiatives for the financing and the procurement of affordable cancer drugs, vaccines and good health services; and
- others include various non-governmental organizations (NGOs), research institutions, and health facilities.

Largely, most global players and stakeholders in cancer management have been involved in the following [7, 8, 17]:

- capacity building for the health systems at country and international levels;
- training and quality assurance in the delivery of cancer care;
- raising awareness on cancers (with active community engagement);
- redesigning health architecture (with infrastructural development);
- improving cancer research (and registration) through detailed data capture, monitoring and evaluation; and
- building healthy public policies for sustainable cancer care.

2.3 Prevalence, Morbidity and Mortality in Africa

2.3.1 An overview of cancer epidemiology and mapping of prevalence

Cancer is increasingly becoming a major public health burden in Africa due to the prevalence of human immunodeficiency virus (HIV)/AIDS, rapid urbanization and associated lifestyle changes, as well as increasing life expectancies [18]. The prevalence of cancers in Africa varies across countries, and it is still difficult to say, with certainty, what the true prevalence of cancers is in many parts of Africa due to the lack of data [11]. Experts still report that, with the few data available, the evidence indicates an increasing burden [11]. In 2008, the WHO reported that the annual diagnosis of cancer in Africa was estimated at 650,000 cases out of a total population of 965 million [19]. Variations have been observed in the patterns of cancers in Africa, especially between northern Africa and sub-Saharan Africa [20], as reports have shown that the burden of cancers is rising at a faster rate in sub-Saharan Africa compared with the northern parts of Africa due to relatively higher prevalence of infectious disease, unhealthy diets and poverty in sub-Saharan Africa [2]. The WHO estimated there were about 551,000 new cases of cancers in sub-Saharan Africa in 2008 with about 421,000 deaths [2]. However, the GLOBOCAN 2008 study reported a total of 715,600 new cases of cancers and 541,800 deaths, with eastern Africa accounting for the highest burden at 221,000 new cancer cases and 173,700 deaths, followed by western Africa at 184,100 new cancer cases and 139,300 deaths [7] (see Table 2.2 for details).

Africa accounts for 6.3 and 6.4% of the global new cancer cases and deaths, respectively [21]. The incidence of cancers in Africa has changed with the burden of HIV [22]. Instances of cervical cancer, Kaposi's sarcoma and non-Hodgkin's lymphoma, all AIDS-defining illnesses, have increased in the last two decades [22]. According to Parkin *et al.*, the top five cancers among women in Africa in 2008 were cervical cancer (23.3%), breast cancer (19.2%), Kaposi's sarcoma (5.1%), liver cancer (5.0%) and non-Hodgkin's lymphoma (3.7%), while among men, it was Kaposi's sarcoma (12.9%), liver cancer (14.8%), prostate cancer (9.5%), bladder cancer (6.1%) and non-Hodgkin's lymphoma (5.7%) [19]. Morhason-Bello *et al.* reported that the incidence of breast cancer showed regional variation between northern Africa and sub-Saharan Africa; breast cancer was the leading cancer among women in northern Africa but was second to cervical

Table 2.2. Distribution of cancer new cases and deaths in Africa [7].

	New cases (×1000)			Deaths (×1000)		
African region	Men	Women	Total	Men	Women	Total
All Africa	324.9	390.7	715.6	267.0	274.8	541.8
Eastern Africa	100.8	120.2	221.0	85.4	88.3	173.7
Central Africa	29.5	37.4	66.9	25.6	27.6	53.2
Northern Africa	81.5	82.9	164.4	65.4	55.4	120.8
Southern Africa	40.6	38.6	79.2	29.3	25.5	54.8
Western Africa	72.5	111.6	184.1	61.3	78.0	139.3

cancer in sub-Saharan Africa [20]. In addition, prostate cancer was reported as the leading cancer among African men, especially in the northern parts, while Kaposi's sarcoma was the leading cancer in sub-Saharan Africa [20, 23].

The multiple challenges faced in Africa include late presentation of patients to health facilities (usually at advanced stages of malignancy), poor and inappropriate treatment, the high cost of medications, lack of adequate follow-up, and the innate social norms and beliefs, poverty and poor standards of living [24]. First-care options are often traditional healers or herbalists, followed by local for-profit clinics where there is little quality control or governance of practitioner practice, before people attend a government or faith-based health service.

2.3.2 Causes of cancers in Africa

While the causes of cancers in Africa vary and have been linked to several factors, epidemiologists report that infections are the main causes of cancer in Africa, responsible for 25.0–32.7% of new cancer cases in 2008 [7, 25].

Infections

As noted, HIV is a main cause of cancer in Africa, responsible for Kaposi's sarcoma, cervical cancer and other AIDS-defining cancers [26]. In 2007, 22.5 million people were living with HIV/AIDS in Africa, with the prevalence ranging from 5% in Nigeria to 38% in Botswana [22]. HIV ranks among the leading causes of death in Africa, accounting for about 1.6 million deaths in 2007, with AIDS-defining cancers contributing hugely to this [24]. However, other infectious agents include hepatitis B and C viruses (liver cancers), human papilloma virus (cervical cancer), Epstein–Barr virus (Burkitt's lymphoma), *Helicobacter pylori* (stomach cancer), Kaposi's sarcoma-associated herpesvirus (human herpesvirus type 8; Kaposi's sarcoma and primary effusion lymphoma), human T-lymphotropic virus (adult T-cell leukaemia) and human polyomaviruses (brain tumours and mesotheliomas) [27].

Smoking and harmful use of alcohol

Tobacco is regarded as the most preventable cause of cancer globally [30]. In Africa, the prevalence of smoking has been increasing, especially in the younger population age groups, owing to the new targeting of the African population by tobacco countries squeezed from western markets, and the lack of effective government policies on tobacco sales and consumption [28, 29]. According to Pampel, the prevalence of smoking in Africa ranges from 8.0% to about 27.3% [28]. Moreover, the consumption of alcohol in many African countries is increasing [30], with about 20–30% of liver cancers related to this [25].

Unhealthy diets, physical inactivity and obesity

Due to rapid urbanization in many African countries, there has been a corresponding increase in related western lifestyles, which are main risk factors for many NCDs, including cancers [31]. The changing nature of industrialization in Africa also means that many people are increasingly becoming physically inactive due to sitting for many hours (mostly in offices). Cars are a key status symbol of wealth and success, and the use of cars corresponds with reduced walking and exercise [31]. Consequently, there is an increased prevalence of overweight and obesity. Efforts to focus on weight reduction and the risks of obesity have been met with scorn and refusal in many quarters, as weight is seen not as a sign of poor health but as a sign of healthy and wealthy living in some African settings [32]. Fried foodstuffs, high-meat diets, and high sugar and salt content dominate the African diet. About 30–40% of cancers are related to unhealthy diets, physical inactivity and obesity [25].

Industrialization and environmental pollution

In many African countries, there are almost no policies on environmental pollution [33]. Carbon monoxide and many industrial toxic wastes are well-established carcinogens [24, 34]. Albrecht further reported that, in some African settings, up to 90% of cancers may be due to chemicals released into the atmosphere from various sources of environmental pollution [35]. Recent reports emerging from the northern Kenyan region of Marsabit of large numbers of throat and lung cancers appear to be directly related to contaminants buried in the ground by mining industries.

2.3.3 Data capture

Cancer registries

The WHO advocate that the main objective of a cancer registry is to provide timely, complete and comparable data on cancer with the aim of providing researchers, experts and policy makers with the required information on how to address the cancer burden effectively [2, 36]. A major problem in understanding and acting on the cancer burden in Africa is the lack of data and poor record keeping [36]. Reports show that few countries have population-based cancer registries, with the few available data sourced from the few hospital-based registries, which are not regularly updated [36, 37]. Largely, this has resulted in a poor response from the health system, and obviously is reflected in greater morbidity and mortality rates in Africa compared with other world regions [18]. Data capture is characterized by the lack of a regularly updated, comprehensive and reliable data collation system [20]. Jedy-Agba *et al.* reported that there is a need for improvement in data collation on cancers in Africa, as in recent times data sources have been based mostly on a few case series estimates, medical records, mortality records and hospital-based cancer registries [37].

Parkin notes that the incidence data on cancers are better sourced jointly from hospital-based and population-based cancer registries, as this will allow new cancer cases to be sourced from within and outside hospitals [36]. However, many African countries do not have functional cancer registration systems [2]. The few cancer registries in these regions cover only the urban cities and do not generally spread to the rural areas [38]. In fact, only five cancer registries from five African countries contributed to the first volume of *Cancer Incidence in Five Continents* [39, 40]. In 1990, only 5% of African countries were covered by functional cancer registries, with this increasing to about 20% in 2008 [7]. Resource allocation for cancer registration is low in many developing countries, as this is perceived to be a luxury amid other challenging health issues [40].

Vital registration systems

Vital registration systems are important sources of mortality data on cancers [21]. Indeed, they are regarded as the most reliable source of mortality data when deaths are certified by a medical practitioner, with reported causes of death conforming to the uniform coding of the International Classification of Diseases (ICD) [36]. Despite about 42% global vital registration coverage as at 1990, the current coverage in Africa has been reported to be incomplete and implausibly low [21].

Meanwhile, survival statistics and prevalence data are also important in the public health response to cancers [4] (see also Kengne *et al*, Chapter 7, this volume). The cancer registries are important in ensuring these data are regularly updated, as data collation may involve regular follow-up of registered cases, active matching of death certificates with cancer notifications and a general assumption that the unmatched cases are still living [36]. Reports show that active collation of survival data on cancers has been lacking in Africa, obviously due to an alarming expansion of cancer cases in urban African centres without a proper health system capacity response [40]. Follow-up systems for tracking patients are negligible and are a major course of failure on the cancer pathway.

2.4 Patients' Journeys

2.4.1 Diagnosis

The WHO has championed the screening and early detection of cancers globally, especially in developing countries where the burden of cancers is highest [2]. Research findings show that one-third of cancers are preventable and/or treatable in developing countries if detected early, thus making the presence of an effective screening and diagnosis system across countries a vital component in cancer management [41]. However, this is rarely the case in Africa, as resources are regarded as far too limited to be diverted to cancer diagnosis in the face of other health challenges [20]. For example, Albrecht reported a lack of cancer screening programmes in Africa, citing that 80% of South African women have never had a pap smear, which is a reflection of the lack of a national cytology plan in many African countries [35, 42]. Cronjé *et al.* reported that, in some African countries, minimal screening infrastructure does exist [42]; however, due to a lack of trained health staff, active cancer screening has been poor and even decreasing in some settings [43].

2.4.2 Cancer management and treatment options

Generally, cancer management involves any or a combination of chemotherapy, surgery and radiotherapy [44].

Chemotherapy

Chemotherapy has been proven to be effective in treating many cancers and is usually indicated for cancers that have spread to other body parts [41]. However, its use in Africa is subject to availability, accessibility and affordability, and few patients can afford to pay [44]. Reports show that only 5% of cancer patients undergo chemotherapy in Africa [43].

Surgery

Surgery is indicated for cancers at early stages, as the tumour is usually localized and easy to remove, with chemotherapy or radiotherapy mainly serving as adjuvant therapies [44]. The challenge in many African settings is that many medical practitioners lack the expertise to perform surgeries, and thus post-surgery prognosis is usually poor [43]. There is also a challenge from a lack of effective analgesics and follow-up after surgery [45, 46]. Failure to see early-stage presentations is the greatest barrier to effective surgery, usually because surgeons capable of operating are based in central or provincial hospitals, and patients journey through local health providers (formal and informal), traditional healers, clinics and district hospitals before being referred to national hospitals where surgery is possible.

Radiotherapy

In sub-Saharan Africa, radiotherapy has been shown to improve surgical outcomes for cancers including breast and colorectal cancer [47]. However, oncologists have reported that the use of radiotherapy is limited owing to a lack of adequate medical infrastructure, specialty centres, radiologists and technical expertise in many African regions [45]. In 2013, research findings showed that only 23 countries in Africa offered radiotherapy, with external beam radiotherapy being the most widely used [48]. Other types of radiotherapy that are rarely used in Africa include brachytherapy, which is highly indicated for cervical cancers [44].

2.4.3 Care pathways and palliative care

Palliative care has attracted substantial interest globally and has been indicated by the WHO as an important component of the cancer care pathway [49–51]. Research findings have shown that about 80% of cancer cases are detected late in Africa [52]; hence chemotherapy, radiotherapy and surgical treatments are no longer viable options for many patients. Thus, to ensure improved management of cancer, particularly in Africa, palliative care is imperative and is now believed to be a practical and humane solution to Africa's cancer burden [50, 52, 53]. The African Palliative Care Association (APCA) and Hospice Africa (Uganda) are working with many African healthcare providers to establish national palliative care initiatives in a large number of African countries, and to relieve the pains and improve overall well-being of people at advanced stages of cancers and with other terminal illnesses [46, 50]; however, reports have shown that these initiatives have been limited by the unavailability and unaffordability of effective pain-relieving medications [46]. A 2004 survey noted that only five African countries had cancer palliative care programmes and/or allowed the dispensing of oral morphine [50, 54]. This had increased to 28 out 57 African countries in 2010 [55]. It was further observed that with strong political will, increased funding, capacity building and establishment of improved treatment facilities, sustainable palliative care programmes may be established in Africa [55], as was the case in Uganda, which is one of the very few African countries where nurses are allowed to prescribe morphine [49].

2.5 Cancer and the African Health System

2.5.1 Architecture for cancer care

Governance and policies

As noted above, tobacco smoking is increasing in many African countries due to the lack of regulatory policies on its sales and use [56]. In fact, due to the support many tobacco companies give to African governments, they have been able to manoeuvre policy makers in favour of tobacco sales and use [29, 56]. Experts have clamoured for better public awareness of the need for increased taxation on tobacco products, with the money derived diverted into useful health promotion measures [57]. In addition, many African countries do not offer patient-friendly policies related to taxes on cancer medications and screening technology, and, as such, some chemotherapy drugs have been found to cost about 1000% more than the costs in UK and other parts of Europe [43]. Due to this high taxation and the associated high cost of cancer treatment, the African Organization for Research and Training in Cancer (AORTIC) is now fronting continent-wide lobbying to convince African governments to cut taxes on drugs, including those on medical equipment [58].

Programmes

Recent studies show that some African countries are beginning to step up efforts to address cancers by convening awareness campaigns programmes on cancers and their risk factors [25]. In addition, screening programmes for cervical cancer, breast cancer and Burkitt's lymphoma have been established in countries such as Kenya, Uganda and Zambia [35, 49]. However, the major challenge lies in the sustainability, as ongoing programmes have been aborted abruptly in many cases [43]. As noted, palliative care programmes do exist in some settings but are not well equipped to offer pain-relieving medications and help the overall well-being of cancer patients [18, 50, 55].

Training

Training programmes specific for cancer management are rare in Africa [24, 58]. This is one of the major challenges that has resulted in the high mortalitics from cancers in Africa, as many medical practitioners do not have the requisite expertise to manage cancers, especially in rural Africa [18].

Funding

The budget allocation for cancers by many African governments is low, as this is rarely considered a priority due to the high burden from HIV/AIDS, tuberculosis and malaria [45]. In the wake of cost-effective measures for cancer control, including vaccination against infectious causes, donor funding (from international organizations and NGOs) for cancer control has been greatly advocated [24].

2.5.2 Infrastructure for cancer care

Health system

Generally, the healthcare systems of many African countries are poorly equipped to deal with cancers, despite accounting for a greater proportion of the global cancer burden [43] (see Coast *et al.*, Chapter 6, this volume). From the 2009 Oxford Declaration, it was clearly evident that many African governments do not recognize the growing cancer epidemics within the continent and, as such, many health systems are not adequately equipped to address this [59].

Health workforce

Health workers are too few to meet the increasing demand from many diseases, and certainly far too few to respond to the pandemic of cancers [19]. Only 3% of the total world health workers currently live and work in sub-Saharan Africa [60]. In recent times, with the strong push–pull factors influencing retention and attrition, there has been an increase in the influx of medical practitioners to high-income countries due to poor welfare and conditions of services in their own countries [61]. Although ethical recruitment agreements have been established in countries such as the UK to prevent this brain drain, loopholes in the law mean that many are still leaving their countries to seek employment in nursing homes or in private medicine.

Health service delivery

Cancer treatment is gradually improving in Africa, but cancer screening and detection, especially in rural areas, remains an important public health issue [44]. The Oxford Declaration calls for African governments to work with international partners and NGOs to implement effective cancer screening programmes using appropriate medical technology [59].

2.5.3 Paradigm in which cancer care is understood and delivered

Health service delivery and healthcare-seeking behaviour among Africans are affected by a wide range of socio-cultural behaviours, including inherent beliefs and norms [62].

Healthcare-seeking behaviour

A survey in Lagos, Nigeria, showed that 81.7% of cervical cancer patients had never heard of the disease prior to diagnosis, 98% believed that the cancer was not serious and could be cured, and 50% thought the symptoms were due to irregular menses or a sexually transmitted infection, while only 9% knew that the disease was cervical cancer and could have a poor prognosis [63]. Moreover, many African women with cervical and breast cancers present late to healthcare facilities because their husbands have not allowed them to attend earlier, refusing travel or refusing travel money [63]. This further highlights the gender inequality plaguing many indigenous African communities [19].

It is also important to recognize that some inherent traditional practices are putting many African women at risk of cancer, as early marriage and high parity are dominant in a number of societies, with girls being bought for a bride price at the age of 13 or 14 years [25]. The use of traditional leaves in sexual intercourse, particularly common among commercial sex workers, has been linked by women themselves as a cause of cervical cancer.

Health service delivery

The behavioural challenge facing the delivery of health services may also be related to stigmatization and discrimination [43]. Many, in the course of receiving care and treatment, have been subjected to varying degrees of stigmatization, especially from health workers who have linked cancers to witchcraft and to immoral sexual practices [25], and this further reduces the patronage of standard health services. Indeed, as noted when care is eventually sought, many cancer patients prefer to be taken to traditional healers, where they believe their illnesses are kept secret and the services rendered are thought to be comparatively cheaper, and only present to standard health facilities when the cancer is too advanced for any curative treatment [25].

2.6 Opportunities to Change the Landscape

Lingwood *et al.* noted that, to establish a comprehensive cancer care programme in Africa, an integrated effort of clinicians, oncologists, epidemiologists and public health experts within an effective health system is paramount, as these are opportunities that can prompt effective control, detection and management of cancer in the region [43]. While this may be anticipated, there are still other opportunities for change, notably in research, technical training and the availability of new treatments for cancers.

2.6.1 Research and technical training

Experts have clamoured for more rigorous research that will inform better care of cancer patients in Africa [20]. A bottom-up approach is thought to be helpful, especially from detailed vital statistics and cancer registration at rural hospital levels, which can then be synergized with larger population-based cancer registries in urban centres [36]. With this, appropriate estimation of the burden can be expected, which can then help in policy planning and practices for cancer management in Africa. Importantly, studies can be more effective if they tackle problems that address native health needs, which can be transferable to other comparable health systems in Africa [24]. Improved technology should be advocated, especially for cancer detection and screening, standard radiotherapy machines and other related medical equipment. Finally, there is a huge opportunity in the advancement of health to begin to give patients a voice in their own early diagnosis and treatment, in building a linked professional network of cancer-skilled health workers including community health workers who can begin to refer and support patients, and in establishing patient referral and follow-up pathways for continuity of care. Technologies can also begin to improve the rapid training of health workers on the current management of cancer patients.

2.6.2 New treatments

Most advancements in cancer treatments in Africa have been based on new and effective vaccines [45]. Vaccinations are important in the management of cancers in Africa due to the high prevalence of cancers with infectious aetiologies [64]. Assessing current vaccination programmes, monitoring vaccine effectiveness, and ensuring sustainable and affordable vaccination with active community participation are believed to be vital for the successful treatment of cancers [44].

2.7 Conclusion

Cancer contributes hugely to the public health burden in Africa. Yet, due to data gaps, the exact burden is still far from known. With continued urbanization, population growth and increasing life expectancies in Africa, the burden of cancer is expected to increase. The response from the governments of many African nations remains a huge concern. There is a need for urgent reprioritization of health programmes in Africa towards improving research and training, screening, diagnosis and treatment, cancer registration and data handling, and the overall management of cancer in the region.

References

1. Arbyn, M., Castellsague, X., de Sanjosé, S., Bruni, L., Saraiya, M., Bray, F. and Ferlay, J. (2011) Worldwide burden of cervical cancer in 2008. *Annals of Oncology* 22, 2675–2686.
2. WHO (2013) *Cancer: Fact Sheets*. World Health Organization, Geneva, Switzerland.
3. Farmer, P., Frenk, J., Knaul, F.M., Shulman, L.N., Alleyne, G., Armstrong, L., Atun, R., Blayney, D., Chen, L., Feachem, R., Gospodarowicz, M., Gralow, J., Gupta, S., Langer, A., Lob-Levyt, J., Neal, C., Mbewu, A., Mired, D., Piot, P., Reddy, K.S., Sachs, J.D., Sarhan, M. and Seffrin, J.R. (2010) Expansion of cancer care and control in countries of low and middle income: a call to action. *Lancet* 376, 1186–1193.
4. Coleman, M.P., Quaresma, M., Berrino, F., Lutz, J.M., Angelis, R.D., Capocaccia, R., Baili, P., Rachet, B., Gatta, G., Hakulinen, T., Micheli, A., Sant, M., Weir, H.K., Elwood, J.M., Tsukuma, H., Koifman, S., Azevedo e Silva, G., Francisci, S., Santaquilani, M., Verdecchia, A., Storm, H.H., Young, J.L. and the CONCORD Working Group (2008) Cancer survival in five continents: a worldwide population-based study (CONCORD). *Lancet Oncology* 9, 730–756.
5. Murray, C.J.L., Vos, T., Lozano, R., Naghavi, M., Flaxman, A.D., Michaud, C., Ezzati, M., Shibuya, K., Salomon, J.A., Abdalla, S. *et al.* (2012) Disability-adjusted life years (DALYs) for 291 diseases and injuries in 21 regions, 1990–2010: a systematic analysis for the Global Burden of Disease Study 2010. *Lancet* 380, 2197–2223.
6. Chan, K.Y., Adeloye, D., Grant, L., Kolcic, I. and Marusic, A. (2012) How big is the 'next big thing'? Estimating the burden of non-communicable diseases in low- and middle-income countries. *Journal of Global Health* 2, 020101.
7. Ferlay, J., Shin, H.R., Bray, F., Forman, D., Mathers, C. and Parkin, D.M. (2010) Estimates of worldwide burden of cancer in 2008: GLOBOCAN 2008. *International Journal of Cancer* 127, 2893–2917.
8. Beaglehole, R., Bonita, R., Alleyne, G., Horton, R., Li, L., Lincoln, P., Mbanya, J.C., McKee, M., Moodie, R., Nishtar, S., Piot, P., Reddy, K.S., Stuckler, D. and the Lancet NCD Action Group (2011) UN high-level meeting on non-communicable diseases: addressing four questions. *Lancet* 378, 449–455.
9. de-Graft Aikins, A., Unwin, N., Agyemang, C., Allotey, P., Campbell, C. and Arhinful, D. (2010) Tackling Africa's chronic disease burden: from the local to the global. *Globalization and Health* 6, 5.
10. Parkin, D.M., Bray, F.I. and Devesa, S.S. (2001) Cancer burden in the year 2000. The global picture. *European Journal of Cancer* 37 (Suppl. 8), S4–S66.
11. Bray, F., Jemal, A., Grey, N., Ferlay, J. and Forman, D. (2012) Global cancer transitions according to the Human Development Index (2008–2030): a population-based study. *Lancet Oncology* 13, 790–801.
12. Parkin, D.M., Pisani, P. and Ferlay, J. (1999) Estimates of the worldwide incidence of 25 major cancers in 1990. *International Journal of Cancer* 80, 827–841.
13. Parkin, D.M., Bray, F., Ferlay, J. and Pisani, P. (2005) Global cancer statistics, 2002. *CA: A Cancer Journal for Clinicians* 55, 74–108.
14. Jemal, A., Bray, F., Centre, M.M., Ferlay, J., Ward, E. and Forman, D. (2011) Global cancer statistics. *CA: A Cancer Journal for Clinicians* 61, 69–90.
15. Soerjomataram, I., Lortet-Tieulent, J., Parkin, D.M., Ferlay, J., Mathers, C., Forman, D. and Bray, F. (2012) Global burden of cancer in 2008: a systematic analysis of disability-adjusted life-years in 12 world regions. *Lancet* 380, 1840–1850.
16. Hadley, L.G.P., Rouma, B.S. and Saad-Eldin, Y. (2012) Challenge of pediatric oncology in Africa. *Seminars in Pediatric Surgery* 21, 136–141.
17. Mensah, G.A. and Mayosi, B.M. (2013) The 2011 United Nations high-level meeting on non-communicable diseases: the Africa agenda calls for a 5-by-5 approach. *South African Medical Journal* 103, 77–79.

18. Jemal, A., Bray, F., Forman, D., O'Brien, M., Ferlay, J., Center, M. and Parkin, D.M. (2012) Cancer burden in Africa and opportunities for prevention. *Cancer* 118, 4372–4384.
19. Parkin, D.M., Sitas, F., Chirenje, M., Stein, L., Abratt, R. and Wabinga, H. (2008) Part I: Cancer in indigenous Africans – burden, distribution, and trends. *Lancet Oncology* 9, 683–692.
20. Morhason-Bello, I.O., Odedina, F., Rebbeck, T.R., Harford, J., Dangou, J.M., Denny, L. and Adewole, I.F. (2013) Challenges and opportunities in cancer control in Africa: a perspective from the African Organisation for Research and Training in Cancer. *Lancet Oncology* 14, 142–151.
21. Parkin, D.M. (2001) Global cancer statistics in the year 2000. *Lancet Oncology* 2, 533–543.
22. Hirschhorn, L.R., Kaaya, S.F., Garrity, P.S., Chopyak, E. and Fawzi, M.C.S. (2012) Cancer and the 'other' noncommunicable chronic diseases in older people living with HIV/AIDS in resource-limited settings: a challenge to success. *AIDS* 26 (Suppl. 1), S65–S75.
23. Center, M.M., Jemal, A., Lortet-Tieulent, J., Ward, E., Ferlay, J., Brawley, O. and Bray, F. (2012) International variation in prostate cancer incidence and mortality rates. *European Urology* 61, 1079–1092.
24. Adebamowo, C.A. and Akarolo-Anthony, S. (2009) Cancer in Africa: opportunities for collaborative research and training. *African Journal of Medicine & Medical Sciences* 38 (Suppl. 2), 5–13.
25. Sitas, F., Parkin, D.M., Chirenje, M., Stein, L., Abratt, R. and Wabinga, H. (2008) Part II: Cancer in indigenous Africans – causes and control. *Lancet Oncology* 9, 786–795.
26. Chokunonga, E., Levy, L.M., Bassett, M.T., Borok, M.Z., Mauchaza, B.G., Chirenje, M.Z. and Parkin, D.M. (1999) AIDS and cancer in Africa: the evolving epidemic in Zimbabwe. *AIDS* 13, 2583–2588.
27. Pagano, J.S., Blaser, M., Buendia, M.-A., Damaniad, B., Khalili, K., Raab-Traub, N. and Roizman, B. (2004) Infectious agents and cancer: criteria for a causal relation. *Seminars in Cancer Biology* 14, 453–471.
28. Pampel, F. (2008) Tobacco use in sub-Sahara Africa: estimates from the demographic health surveys. *Social Science & Medicine* 66, 1772–1783.
29. Saloojee, Y. and Dagli, E. (2000) Tobacco industry tactics for resisting public policy on health. *Bulletin of the World Health Organization* 78, 902–910.
30. Pisa, P.T., Kruger, A., Vorster, H.H., Margetts, B.M. and Du, T.L. (2010) Alcohol consumption and cardiovascular disease risk in an African population in transition: the Prospective Urban and Rural Epidemiology (PURE) study. (Special Issue: Alcohol consumption in South Africa: from molecules to society.) *South African Journal of Clinical Nutrition* 23(Suppl. 1), S29–S37.
31. Assah, F.K., Ekelund, U., Brage, S., Mbanya, J.C. and Wareham, N.J. (2011) Urbanization, physical activity, and metabolic health in sub-Saharan Africa. *Diabetes Care* 34, 491–496.
32. Cecchini, M., Sassi, F., Lauer, J.A., Lee, Y.Y., Guajardo-Barron, V. and Chisholm, D. (2010) Tackling of unhealthy diets, physical inactivity, and obesity: health effects and cost-effectiveness. *Lancet* 376, 1775–1784.
33. Wichmann, J. and Voyi, K. (2012) Ambient air pollution exposure and respiratory, cardiovascular and cerebrovascular mortality in Cape Town, South Africa: 2001–2006. *International Journal of Environmental Research & Public Health* 9, 3978–4016.
34. Mortimer, K., Gordon, S.B., Jindal, S.K., Accinelli, R.A., Balmes, J. and Martin, I.W.J. (2012) Household air pollution is a major avoidable risk factor for cardiorespiratory disease. *Chest* 142, 1308–1315.
35. Albrecht, C. (2011) *Ninety Percent of Cancers are Caused by Environmental Factors of Which Most are Chemicals.* Cancer Association of South Africa, Gauteng, South Africa <http://drcarlalbrecht.com/documents/2013/90percent-of-cancers.pdf>.
36. Parkin, D.M. (2006) The evolution of the population-based cancer registry. Nature Reviews Cancer 6, 603–612.
37. Jedy-Agba, E., Curado, M.P., Ogunbiyi, O., Oga, E., Fabowale, T., Igbinoba, F., Osubor, G., Otu, T., Kumai, H., Koechlin, A., Osinubi, P., Dakum, P., Blattner, W. and Adebamowo, C.A. (2012)

Cancer incidence in Nigeria: a report from population-based cancer registries. *Cancer Epidemiology* 3, 271–278.
38. Awadelkarim, K.D., Mariani-Costantini, R. and Elwali, N.E. (2010) Cancer in the Sudan: an overview of the current status of knowledge on tumor patterns and risk factors. *Science of the Total Environment* 423, 214–228.
39. Whelan, S.L. and Ferlay, J. (1992) Cancer incidence in five continents. Age-specific and standardized incidence rates. *IARC Scientific Publications* 1992, 178–861.
40. Valsecchi, M.G. and Steliarova-Foucher, E. (2008) Cancer registration in developing countries: luxury or necessity? *Lancet Oncology* 9, 156–167.
41. Cazap, E. (2012) Screening and cancer prevention in underdeveloped environments: a global view. In: *Cancer Research Conference: 103rd Annual Meeting of the American Association for Cancer Research*, Chicago, Illinois, 31 March–4 April, 2012. *Cancer Research* 72, Abstract SY26-01.
42. Cronjé, H.S. and Beyer, E. (2007) Screening for cervical cancer in an African setting. *International Journal of Gynecology and Obstetrics* 98, 168–171.
43. Lingwood, R.J., Boyle, P., Milburn, A., Ngoma, T., Arbuthnott, J., McCaffrey, R., Kerr, S.H. and Kerr, D.J. (2008) The challenge of cancer control in Africa. *Nature Reviews Cancer* 8, 398–403.
44. Kingham, T.P., Alatise, O.I., Vanderpuye, V., Casper, C., Abantanga, F.A., Kamara, T.B., Olopade, O.I., Habeebu, M., Abdulkareem, F.B. and Denny, L. (2013) Treatment of cancer in sub-Saharan Africa. *Lancet Oncology* 14, e158–e167.
45. Boyle, P., Anderson, B.O., Andersson, L.C., Ariyaratne, Y., Auleley, G.R., Barbacid, M., Bartelink, H., Baselga, J., Behbehani, K., Belardelli, F. *et al.* (2008) Need for global action for cancer control. *Annals of Oncology* 19, 1519–1521.
46. O'Brien, M., Mwangi-Powell, F., Adewole, I.F., Soyannwo, O., Amandua, J., Ogaja, E., Okpeseyi, M., Ali, Z., Kiwanuka, R. and Merriman, A. (2013) Improving access to analgesic drugs for patients with cancer in sub-Saharan Africa. *Lancet Oncology* 14, e176–e182.
47. Barton, M.B., Frommer, M. and Shafiq, J. (2006) Role of radiotherapy in cancer control in low-income and middle-income countries. *Lancet Oncology* 7, 584–595.
48. Abdel-Wahab, M., Bourque, J.-M., Pynda, Y., Iewska, J., Merwe, D., Zubizarreta, E. and Rosenblatt, E. (2013) Status of radiotherapy resources in Africa: an International Atomic Energy Agency Analysis. *Lancet Oncology* 14, e168–e175.
49. Morris, K. (2003) Cancer? In Africa? *Lancet Oncology* 4, 5.
50. Harding, R., Selman, L., Powell, R.A., Namisango, E., Downing, J., Merriman, A., Ali, Z., Gikaara, N., Gwyther, L. and Higginson, I. (2013) Research into palliative care in sub-Saharan Africa. *Lancet Oncology* 14, e183–e188.
51. World Health Assembly (2005) *Cancer Prevention and Control*. World Health Organization, Geneva, Switzerland.
52. Wakabi, W. (2007) Africa's increasing efforts to control cancer. *Lancet Oncology* 8, 1057.
53. Stjernswärd, J., Foley, K.M. and Ferris, F.D. (2007) The public health strategy for palliative care. *Journal of Pain and Symptom Management* 33, 486–493.
54. Wright, M., Wood, J., Lynch, T. and Clark, D. (2008) Mapping levels of palliative care development: a global view. *Journal of Pain and Symptom Management* 35, 469–485.
55. Grant, L., Downing, J., Namukwaya, E., Leng, M. and Murray, S.A. (2011) Palliative care in Africa since 2005: good progress, but much further to go. *BMJ Supportive & Palliative Care* 1, 118–122.
56. Otañez, M.G., Mamudu, H.M. and Glantz, S.A. (2009) Tobacco companies' use of developing countries' economic reliance on tobacco to lobby against global tobacco control: the case of Malawi. *American Journal of Public Health* 99, 1759–1771.
57. Groenewald, P., Vos, T., Norman, R., Laubscher, R., van Walbeek, C., Saloojee, Y., Sitas, F., Bradshaw, D. and the South African Comparative Risk Assessment Collaborating Group (2007) Estimating the burden of disease attributable to smoking in South Africa in 2000. *South African Medical Journal* 97, 674–681.

58. African Organization for Research and Training in Cancer (2013) *Cancer in Africa: Bridging Science and Humanity. The 9th International Conference of the African Organisation for Research and Training in Cancer*, 21–24 November 2013. AORTIC, Durban, South Africa.
59. Oxford Declaration (2009) *Prevention of Cervical Cancer in Africa: a Call to Action*. The Oxford Declaration, 27 March 2009.
60. de-Graft Aikins, A., Boynton, P. and Atanga, L.L. (2010) Developing effective chronic disease interventions in Africa: insights from Ghana and Cameroon. *Globalization and Health* 6, 6.
61. Mungal-Singh, V. (2011) United Nations High Level Meeting and NCD in South Africa. *Global Heart* 6, 215–217.
62. Parkin, D.M. (1994) Cancer in developing countries. *Cancer Surveys* 19–20, 519–561.
63. Anorlu, R.I. (2008) Cervical cancer: the sub-Saharan African perspective. *Reproductive Health Matters* 16, 41–49.
64. Parkin, D.M. (2006) The global health burden of infection-associated cancers in the year 2002. *International Journal of Cancer* 118, 3030–3044.

3 Chronic Non-communicable Diseases and Infectious Diseases

Tolu Oni[1]* and Nigel Unwin[2]

[1]*University of Cape Town, Cape Town, South Africa;* [2]*University of the West Indies, Cave Hill Campus, Barbados*

3.1 Introduction

The concept of the epidemiological transition was introduced by Omran [1] to capture interrelated changes in demography, disease patterns and economic development. Omran described how, with economic development, death rates from infectious diseases tend to fall, especially in infants and children, fertility declines, the population starts to age and chronic non-communicable diseases (NCDs) become the predominant health problems. In the classic epidemiological transition paradigm, as occurred for example in western Europe, this process took place over two to three centuries and was associated with the agricultural and industrial revolutions. In today's globalized world, however, many poorer countries are undergoing rapid changes that are associated with continuing high levels of certain infectious diseases, including human immunodeficiency virus (HIV), tuberculosis (TB), hepatitis and malaria, while concomitantly developing high rates of NCDs. For example, rapid urbanization, mechanization of the rural economy and the increasing activities of transnational food, drink and tobacco corporations are all associated with behavioural changes that increase the risk of NCDs. These changes include less healthy diets, lower physical activity, tobacco smoking and increased alcohol consumption. As a result, population health profiles and patterns are rapidly changing with an increase in cardiovascular and metabolic disorders.

The 2010 Global Burden of Disease study reported on 20-year trends in global and regional burdens of disease, risk factors and injuries. It demonstrated a shift towards NCDs. Burden of disease is measured in disability adjusted life years (DALYs), a measure that combines premature mortality and morbidity. The three leading risk factors for global burden of disease were high blood pressure, tobacco

*E-mail: tolullah.oni@uct.ac.za

smoking and household air pollution [2]. This distribution varied in different low- and middle-income country (LMIC) regions. In most of sub-Saharan Africa, the leading risk factors were childhood malnutrition and air pollution, while in southern Africa, eastern Europe and South America, alcohol use was the leading risk factor [2]. The prevalence of overweight/obesity, a risk factor for cardiovascular disease and type 2 diabetes mellitus (T2DM), has risen by 82% since 1990. Globally, a high body mass index is now a more important cause of morbidity than childhood malnutrition, and this is also the case in many LMICs (e.g. within southern Africa, Asia and Latin America) [3]. Furthermore, high blood pressure and tobacco smoking are ranked in the top five across most LMIC regions. Tables 3.1 and 3.2 demonstrate the heterogeneity of the top ten risk factors and disease burden across LMICs and within sub-Saharan Africa. Of note, in southern Africa, while HIV and TB rank first and fourth in the top ten causes of disease burden, respectively, 50% of the causes of disease burden are non-communicable.

As described above, DALYs are a combined measure of mortality and morbidity. When considering mortality alone, it is worth noting that 90% of persons dying under the age of 70 from NCDs live in LMICs [5]. Globally, NCDs already account for over 65% of deaths, and for 58% of deaths in LMICs. Sub-Saharan Africa is the only region where deaths from communicable disease still outnumber those from NCDs, and by more than two to one. In addition, the disease burden and deaths are occurring at younger ages than in high-income countries, resulting in a loss of economic output [6, 7] and increasing household expenditure associated with the management of chronic disease.

A good understanding of the burden of disease and risk factors is important because, in addition to these conditions, co-existing diseases, disease precursors and risk factors can also interact, influencing host susceptibility (e.g. T2DM increases the risk of TB, antiretroviral therapy (ART) can increase the risk of dysglycaemia), clinical manifestation and disease prognosis (e.g. chronic kidney disease (CKD) and the co-existence of HIV and hypertension), further impacting on population health. These interactions could potentially impede strategies in place to improve health and reduce poverty.

While acknowledging a wide range of infectious diseases and NCDs, the rest of this chapter will focus on diseases, disease precursors and risk factors that have a high prevalence in LMICs. In particular, we will focus on those conditions where interactions between them are known to be, or thought likely to be, of public health importance.

3.2 Disease-specific Interactions

This chapter reviews interactions between infectious diseases and NCDs. In discussing this overlap, it is important to acknowledge the limitation of classifying diseases into mutually exclusive infectious or non-communicable categories. Some NCDs have partially infectious causes, such as cervical cancer and human papilloma virus (see Adeloye and Grant, Chapter 2, this volume). Similarly, many infectious diseases are associated with NCD sequelae, e.g. Epstein–Barr virus and

Table 3.1. Risk factor rankings in different global regions based on their contribution to disease burden (DALYs). The risk factors are listed in order of global ranking. Shading indicates regions where these risk factors are in the region's top five. (Adapted from [3].)

Risk factor rankings	Southern Africa	Eastern Africa	Central Africa	Western Africa	North Africa/ Middle East	Southern Latin America	Tropical Latin America	Central Latin America	South-east Asia	South Asia	East Asia	Central Asia
High blood pressure	2	5	5	6	1	2	1	4	1	3	1	1
Tobacco smoking	5	7	12	10	3	3	4	5	2	2	2	2
Household air pollution	7	2	2	2	25	23	18	11	3	1	5	12
Diet low in fruits	8	8	11	13	6	6	6	7	4	5	3	4
Alcohol use	1	6	10	5	18	4	2	2	6	10	8	5
High body mass index	3	14	18	15	2	1	3	1	9	17	9	3
High fasting glucose	6	10	13	11	4	5	5	3	5	7	7	7
Childhood underweight	9	1	1	1	20	38	32	23	13	4	38	25
Ambient particulate matter pollution	25	16	14	7	7	24	27	19	11	6	4	10
Physical inactivity	11	15	15	16	5	7	8	6	8	11	10	9

Table 3.2. Rankings of diseases according to their contribution to DALYs in different global regions. Highlights indicate regions where these diseases are in the region's top five. (Adapted from [4].)

Risk factor rankings	Southern Africa	Eastern Africa	Central Africa	Western Africa	North Africa/ Middle East	Southern Latin America	Tropical Latin America	Central Latin America	South-east Asia	South Asia	East Asia	Central Asia
Ischaemic heart disease	14	21	19	20	1	1	1	2	3	4	2	1
Lower respiratory infections	2	3	4	2	5	6	7	6	4	1	15	2
Cerebrovascular disease	7	16	14	16	4	3	4	11	1	12	1	3
Diarrhoeal disease	3	4	2	3	11	44	26	14	8	3	49	18
HIV/AIDS	1	1	5	4	58	34	12	13	13	17	38	31
Malaria	20	2	1	1	66	166	145	154	22	44	169	162
COPD	9	20	20	22	13	7	10	16	9	5	3	11
Major depressive disorder	10	13	17	19	3	4	6	5	6	14	8	6
Tuberculosis	4	7	7	12	33	65	46	44	2	8	37	15
Diabetes	8	29	28	26	9	9	8	3	10	16	10	12

COPD, chronic obstructive pulmonary disease.

Burkitt's lymphoma; schistosomiasis and bladder cancer; and *Trypanosoma cruzi* and cardiomegaly.

There are extensive further examples of interactions between infectious diseases and NCDs, and these interactions are complex, often mediated by shared risk factors (Fig. 3.1). However the purpose of this chapter is not to be an exhaustive archive of all interactions but to focus on interactions associated with infectious diseases with the highest global burden. As such, we focus on HIV, TB and malaria and the most prevalent NCDs in LMICs: chronic obstructive pulmonary disease (COPD), T2DM, cardiovascular disease and metabolic syndrome, and CKD. Within each section, we will present available evidence on the prevalence of co-existence of diseases and risk factors, and describe the strength of association between the diseases and the impact of co-morbidity on clinical manifestation, diagnosis and prognosis of either condition.

3.2.1 TB

TB remains a leading cause of death globally, with an estimated 8.8 million new cases reported every year, threatening the goal of global TB elimination by 2050 [8]. Tackling this challenge will require not only improvements in diagnostic and treatment services but also identification and reduction of risk factors that

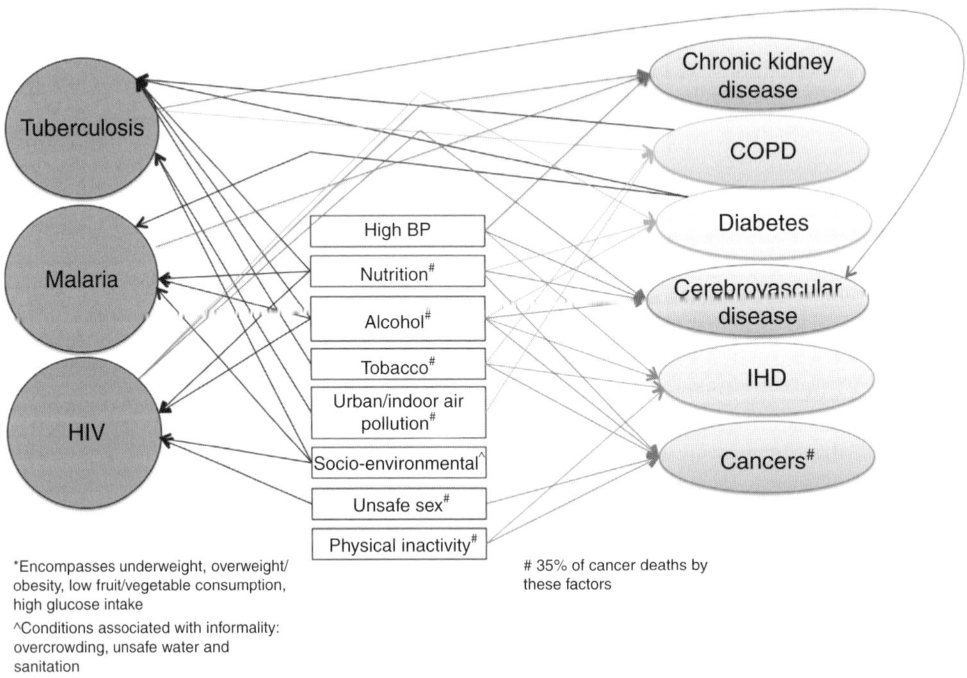

Fig. 3.1. Interaction between tuberculosis/malaria/human immunodeficiency virus (HIV), risk factors/disease precursors, and non-communicable diseases. BP, blood pressure; COPD, chronic obstructive pulmonary disease; IHD, ischaemic heart disease.

increase TB susceptibility. Diseases and risk factors that impair immune function, such as malnutrition, alcoholism or HIV co-infection, can increase the likelihood of infection or reactivation of latent TB.

TB and diabetes

Increasing evidence suggests that T2DM is a significant risk factor for TB and this emerging epidemic could therefore threaten TB control. In a recent systematic review, the relative risk for TB in diabetic patients was 3.1 in two cohort studies, with odds ratios that ranged from 1.16 to 7.83 in case–control studies [9]. The strength of this link was influenced by geographical/ethnic differences, and the relative risk was higher in younger than in older adults; in India, it is estimated that 15% of smear-positive pulmonary TB cases are attributable to DM [10]. However, these studies had a number of limitations. In particular, very few were carried out in low-income countries, with no sub-Saharan African studies included, raising uncertainty about the strength of the T2DM–TB association and the benefit of bidirectional screening for T2DM and TB in these settings (where not only is the prevalence of TB and HIV high but where the burden of T2DM is also predicted to increase most rapidly) [11]. None the less, the World Health Organization (WHO) has issued provisional recommendations that all TB patients be screened for T2DM and vice versa, while noting that evidence for the effectiveness and cost-effectiveness of integrated approaches is poor [12].

TB/T2DM co-morbidity influences the diagnostic accuracy of established algorithms for either condition, and there is a lack of knowledge of, or practical guidance on, the most appropriate screening methods, further impeding implementation of the WHO guidelines. WHO-approved approaches to the diagnosis of diabetes include the measurement of fasting glucose, an oral glucose tolerance test (which assesses blood glucose level after a standard glucose load) and, most recently, glycated haemoglobin (HBA1c, which reflects average blood glucose level over the preceding few weeks) [13, 14]. It is known that acute illness, such as TB, can result in a transient stress-induced hyperglycaemia, thus influencing the diagnostic reliability of these tests, especially the first two. HBA1c may be more reliable in TB given that it reflects average glucose levels over the preceding month or so. However, good data on the performance of diagnostic tests for diabetes in TB are lacking. Also lacking are good data on the potential importance in people with TB of levels of hyperglycaemia below the diabetes threshold, referred to as intermittent hyperglycaemia or pre-diabetes [13]. There are also presently insufficient data on which to base TB screening guidelines for diabetic patients.

In spite of these challenges, the importance of bidirectional screening for TB and T2DM is underscored by the impact of T2DM on TB outcomes and vice versa. The co-existence of T2DM in TB patients is associated with a longer duration of TB symptoms, more severe TB disease and poorer TB outcomes [15–20], with greater mortality reported among TB patients with T2DM compared with those without T2DM [21]. There is also some evidence to suggest further increased TB risk in persons with poor glycaemic control [22, 23]. TB can aggravate T2DM by worsening glycaemic control, complicating clinical management [24]. It has also been proposed that the metabolism of rifampicin could be affected by T2DM, making it less effective and predisposing patients to the acquisition of drug resistance [25, 26].

There is a paucity of data on whether T2DM is associated with a high prevalence of subclinical TB among patients attending diabetic clinics, as observed in HIV co-infected persons [27]. This has major importance when considering TB screening strategies, as symptom-based screening will not detect subclinical disease, with potential for amplification of transmission within diabetic clinics and also potentially serious consequences of false-negative TB screening.

TB and COPD

Figure 3.1 shows the bidirectional nature of the interaction between TB and COPD. Due to the similarity between TB and COPD symptoms, there is potential for delayed diagnosis of TB, further impacting outcomes. Persons with COPD have a two- to threefold higher risk of developing TB [28] and a twofold increased mortality compared with non-COPD patients [29]. The increased risk of TB associated with COPD is often attributed to smoking [30], but studies have also found an association between oral corticosteroid use in COPD patients and TB risk [28]. A systematic review confirmed that, although this association is independent of smoking [31], the risk of COPD is further increased by tobacco smoking and low socio-economic status, common risk factors for both COPD and TB.

The histopathological changes that occur in the lungs of TB patients can result in anatomical changes associated with both obstructive and restrictive patterns of impaired lung function of varying severity, which can persist after successful completion of TB treatment [32]. The prevalence of COPD after TB treatment completion varies from 28 to 68% [33], and is further increased in persons with multiple episodes of TB [34]. Childhood studies have also demonstrated this association, due to prolonged bronchial obstruction by enlarged lymph nodes during TB disease [35]. In LMICs, alongside a concomitant rise in the prevalence of tobacco smoking, TB is an important contributor to poor quality of life and DALYs lost due to COPD [36]. A study in South Africa reported that the strongest predictor of chronic bronchitis was a history of TB [37]. Early identification and management of chronic lung impairment is therefore crucial to minimize the long-term negative impact of TB.

3.2.2 HIV

Globally, HIV is the fifth and sixth leading cause of DALYs lost and mortality, respectively [4, 38]. In LMICs, particularly in sub-Saharan Africa, HIV ranks even higher. However, unlike the NCD trend, there are promising signs that the HIV pandemic is abating in high-burden settings, with declining incidence and mortality rates [39]. None the less, the rising NCD morbidity and mortality rates alongside an established HIV epidemic make it crucial to better understand the interactions that exist with emerging NCDs and disease precursors. These interactions can either be related to HIV infection directly or as a side effect of ART. LMICs bear a disproportionate burden of the HIV pandemic, with sub-Saharan Africa accounting for 70% of HIV cases. Improvements in access to ART have resulted in increased survival and an accompanying increased risk of developing NCDs associated with ageing and lifestyle. However, ART does not fully restore health in all individuals; HIV-infected adults on treatment have higher-than-expected risk of several non-AIDS disorders, including cardiovascular disease, kidney disease, liver disease, malignancy, dementia, neuropathies and musculoskeletal disorders. HIV has also been identified as an independent risk factor for stroke in urban and rural Tanzania [40], although there is a paucity of data on the nature and extent of this interaction in LMICs.

HIV and metabolic syndrome

Metabolic syndrome includes disturbances in glucose, lipid metabolism and insulin resistance and is a significant risk factor for cardiovascular disease and T2DM.

INSULIN RESISTANCE There is evidence that HIV infection is associated with abnormal glucose metabolism and hyperglycaemia independent of ART. The association of HIV infection and T2DM is poorly understood, and there is conflicting evidence of this association, independent of ART [41, 42]. The use of ART containing protease inhibitors (PIs) and nucleoside reverse transcriptase inhibitors (NRTIs) has been associated with insulin resistance [43, 44]. A Cape Town survey of HIV-infected persons on ART reported a 21.9% prevalence of newly detected hyperglycaemia and a significant association with the drug efavirenz [45]. This could contribute to the T2DM epidemic, as patients receive ART for longer periods.

DYSLIPIDAEMIA/LIPOATROPHY HIV-related hyperlipidaemia (particularly hypertriglyceridaemia), independent of ART, has been described [46]. However, the use of ART is also associated with dyslipidaemia, peripheral wasting and central fat accumulation. In particular, PIs and non-NRTI-based regimens have been associated with dyslipidaemia and atrophy. PI drugs are particularly associated with dyslipidaemia, a known risk factor for cardiovascular complications [47, 48]; patients with baseline elevated lipid levels have the greatest risk of developing hyperlipidaemia, especially hypertriglyceridaemia [47]. A study conducted in South Africa reported an association between ART use and increased central fat and reduced peripheral fat. This was partially improved by switching from a non-NRTI regimen to a PI-based regimen [49].

HIV and the heart

The burden of cardiovascular disorders is increasing in LMICs. The most commonly reported cardiac manifestation in HIV is pericardial disease, often due to TB [50]. HIV-related cardiomyopathy is also common, with a prevalence ranging between 18 and 43% in LMICs [51, 52], as is pulmonary hypertension. The prognosis of these conditions has historically been poor [53, 54]. Evidence from Africa on the prevalence of echocardiographic abnormalities in asymptomatic HIV-infected persons is limited, although it has been documented in other regions [55, 56]. There is also an increased risk of myocardial infarction in HIV-infected patients on ART, particularly in patients with metabolic syndrome [57].

HIV and CKD

CKD is an important cause of morbidity and mortality in HIV-infected persons, including HIV-associated nephropathy and membranoproliferative glomerulonephritis, particularly in the presence of hepatitis C virus co-infection [58]. The risk of CKD is further increased in the presence of other risk factors including older age, hypertension, diabetes and black ethnicity [59]. This is of particular concern, as the prevalence of T2DM and hypertension is rising within the same population with a high HIV prevalence. Although the incidence of CKD has been remarkably altered by widespread ART access, some ART regimens are associated with incident acute or chronic kidney disease; particularly with indinavir and tenofovir [60]. Studies of HIV-infected patients on ART in Taiwan and Vietnam reported a 7% prevalence of CKD, with older age, lower body weight and tenofovir use being independently associated with CKD [61, 62]. However, the benefits of tenofovir are considered to outweigh the nephrotoxic side effects, and tenofovir is recommended as the first-line ART regimen. The prevalence of proteinuria at baseline, with or without a raised serum creatinine level, is reported to be a sensitive predictor of the development of CKD [63], suggesting that this should be measured in all HIV-infected patients at diagnosis and at initiation of ART.

3.2.3 Malaria

Malaria is a parasitic infection that is responsible for at least half a million deaths per year (estimated to be 660,000 in 2010, uncertainty range of 490,000 to 836,000), and around 200 million clinical cases per year (219 million in 2010, uncertainty range of 154 million to 289 million) [64]. Eighty per cent of all deaths occur in just 14 countries, with 40% occurring in just two: Nigeria and the Democratic Republic of the Congo [64].

Malaria is caused by the protozoan *Plasmodium*, which is transmitted between humans by the *Anopheles* mosquito. There are four species of *Plasmodium* causing disease in humans, of which *Plasmodium vivax* and *Plasmodium falciparum* are the most common. *P. falciparum* is the most deadly because of its tendency to involve the brain (cerebral malaria). Roughly 30% of the world's population lives in areas where there is a risk of falciparum malaria [65]. Groups at high risk of severe and life-threatening infection are those with no immunity (e.g. children, and visitors from non-endemic areas) and those with impaired immunity (e.g. those with HIV/AIDS). However, immunity is relatively short lived, and those returning to endemic areas after several months or years are also at increased risk because of reduced or absent immunity [64].

Malaria is, of course, associated with the environmental conditions that favour the breeding of its mosquito vector. However, similar to the major NCDs, it is also associated with poor socio-economic conditions, and it has been suggested that economic development per se will reduce its impact [66]. Other shared risk factors with NCDs are less clear. The relationship between poor childhood nutrition – a risk factor for T2DM and cardiovascular disease – and the risk of malaria is unclear [67–70]. There is some evidence to suggest that the body odours associated with alcohol consumption, specifically beer, may attract *Anopheles* mosquitoes and thus increase the chance of being bitten [71].

Malaria and diabetes

There is evidence from a recent case–control study conducted in urban Ghana that people with T2DM are roughly 50% more likely to show evidence, based on testing for the DNA of the parasite, of infection with *P. falciparum* malaria [72]. It is important to note that participants in this study did not have clinical malaria. However, the findings do support the hypothesis that people with T2DM may be at increased risk of clinical malaria. It may also be the case that the increasing prevalence of T2DM in malaria endemic areas will provide a larger pool of infected individuals, thus making the control of transmission more difficult.

Clinical malaria in adults with T2DM must be relatively common in endemic areas that also have a high prevalence of T2DM, such as many urban centres in Africa and Asia. However, we could find no good evidence on whether people with T2DM who develop clinical malaria have poorer outcomes than people without T2DM. It would be expected that people who are physically less robust because of T2DM-related complications, particularly those of the renal and cardiovascular systems, are at greater risk of poorer outcomes. Indeed, as described in the next section, it is well known that malaria can cause renal damage, both acute and longer term. It is plausible, therefore, that people who already have some degree of diabetic renal disease are more susceptible to renal failure during a bout of malaria.

CKD and the risk of malaria

CKD was ranked as the 18th commonest cause of death in 2010, estimated to have caused 736,000 deaths (uncertainty range of 612,000 to 810,000) [73]. T2DM and hypertension are the two single most important risk factors for CKD [73], and as these increase in LMICs, so will CKD. The clinical end point of CKD is end-stage kidney disease, which can be defined by the requirement for life-saving dialysis or renal transplantation [74]. Worldwide, it is estimated that 1.9 million people are undergoing some form of renal replacement therapy, the vast majority of whom are in high-income countries [75]. In LMICs, only around a quarter of those who require renal replacement therapy receive it, resulting in an estimated 3.2 million premature deaths each year.

It is not known whether CKD increases the risk of clinical malaria. It is known, however, that renal transplantation in malarial areas is associated with a risk of malaria in the recipients, the infection being transmitted via the donor kidney [76]. Thus, it is recommended that renal transplant patients in malarial areas receive appropriate prophylaxis to eliminate the risk of this potentially life-threatening complication [76].

Finally, three of the drugs commonly used in malaria prophylaxis (malarone, proguanil and chloroquine) may be contraindicated in patients with CKD, depending on the level of renal impairment [77]. Therefore, specialist advice should be sought by people with CKD travelling to endemic areas.

Malaria as a cause of kidney disease

One form of malaria, caused by *Plasmodium malariae*, is associated with a risk of progressive renal damage (nephrotic syndrome), which, even after successful eradication of the infection, may progress to end-stage kidney disease and thus require renal replacement therapy for survival [76]. This condition occurs predominantly in children and young adults. While it is a well-recognized condition, good estimates of its incidence and its overall contribution to end-stage kidney disease are lacking. It is thought to occur in only a fraction of *P. malariae* infections but is described as one of the major causes of renal disease in children living in malarial areas [78].

It is estimated that *P. falciparum* malaria is associated with acute renal failure in 1–5% of cases occurring in local inhabitants in endemic areas, but that in non-immune visitors around a quarter suffer this complication [76]. Successful treatment of the infection normally leads to recovery of renal function within 2–6 weeks. However, during the acute phase, many patients (e.g. 40–70%) require dialysis if they are to survive [76].

3.3 Potential Targets for Intervention

In considering potential targets for primary, secondary and tertiary interventions, it is important to take the life course of the individual into account. The Barker hypothesis indicates foetal origins of adult chronic disease and risk factors, where factors operating *in utero* and in infancy are related to the risk of T2DM and cardiovascular disease in adulthood [79]. For example, adverse foetal exposures, such as those due to variations in the quality of maternal nutrition, during critical periods may permanently alter gene expression, leading to slowing of growth and sparing of brain development, to the detriment of the maturation of other organs, such as the liver and pancreas. Foetal programming of development associated with low birth weight has emerged as a risk factor for adult NCDs including cardiovascular disease, T2DM and adult obesity. The broader environment within which such adults reside in LMICs is also associated with a high prevalence of chronic infectious diseases such as those described in this chapter. This further propagates the dual epidemic and contributes to the increasing epidemic of multiple infectious diseases and NCDs in LMICs, occurring at younger ages than in developed countries. Using the example of malaria, risk factors such as low socio-economic status that increase the risk of childhood malaria also increase the risk of NCDs through adverse foetal and childhood exposures. Furthermore, malaria in pregnancy is associated with poorer foetal outcomes, including low birth weight, also leading to an increased risk of NCDs in adulthood [80].

The above considerations highlight the importance both of considering shared risk factors that influence the risk and outcomes of prevalent infectious diseases and NCDs, and of using a life-course approach (Fig. 3.2) when considering targets for intervention.

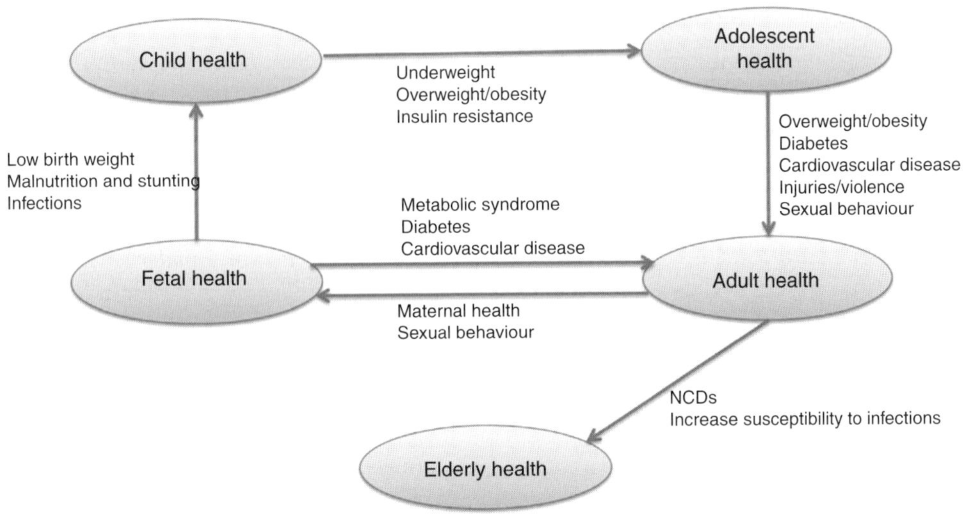

Fig. 3.2. Life-course approach to combined infectious disease and non-communicable disease prevention and control.

3.3.1 Childhood

The rising NCD epidemic in LMICs is occurring at younger ages than in developed countries. This is accompanied by a rise in NCD precursors and risk factors. It is relevant to note that there is evidence of negative interactions between factors in early life and later childhood, and in adolescence and adulthood. For example, a combination of low birth weight followed by obesity in later childhood or early adolescence has been shown to be associated with an almost doubling of the risk of cardiovascular disease as an adult [81]. By contrast, low-birth-weight infants who are normal-weight children or adolescents, or overweight children who were normal weight at birth, have relatively little increase in risk as an adult [81]. It is therefore of importance to note that the prevalence of childhood obesity is rising in LMICs, where there is a high prevalence of low birth weight. In addition, recurrent early-life infections and malnutrition are associated with stunting, which, when followed by the availability of excess calories in later life, is associated with an increased risk of obesity in children and adults. Furthermore, rapid urbanization is associated with environmental and nutritional changes with increased consumption of more unhealthy foods and decreased physical activity. Primary prevention of childhood obesity should be a priority and could be implemented in different settings. Schools serve as an ideal catchment area to target children for healthy lifestyle interventions including making unhealthy foods less available and increasing periods of physical activity. This should occur alongside more upstream legislative interventions with media campaigns and public policies that support these goals, including the banning of advertising 'junk foods' to children, and fiscal policies to increase their price (such as taxes on sugar-sweetened beverages). Policy measures are discussed in greater detail in Part III of this volume. Parents could also be targeted and encouraged to minimize sedentary behaviour, as well as offering healthy foods in appropriate portions. Lastly, infants and young children often have multiple visits to primary health facilities. Opportunistic screening could therefore be conducted to detect higher-than-normal growth rates and advice given to caregivers in this respect.

3.3.2 Adolescence/adulthood

In sub-Saharan Africa, 40% of DALYs lost are attributable to six risk factors: high blood pressure, high blood glucose, physical inactivity, overweight/obesity, high cholesterol, and low fruit and vegetable intake [82]. These are shared risk factors for infectious diseases and NCDs, and are therefore important targets in these settings. It is important to target the adult population in LMICs for interventions to prevent and limit the dual burden of infectious diseases and NCDs. Of note, male life expectancy is on average 3–5 years shorter than their female counterparts, partly due to higher rates of death from certain NCDs, especially cardiovascular diseases. However, women are disproportionally affected by certain NCD risk factors, particularly obesity and lower physical fitness and, in addition, show rising rates of smoking and alcohol consumption [5]. Given this fact, along with the impact of the state of maternal health (both infectious diseases, such as HIV, and NCDs, such as T2DM and obesity/malnutrition) on foetal and child health, and the likelihood of strongly influencing dietary household choices, female adolescents and adults represent an important population group for intervention. These interventions should ideally cover nutrition, physical activity, contraception, high-risk behaviour including high-risk sexual practices, smoking and alcohol consumption. This could involve mass media campaigns on the importance of female health even before pregnancy, and could target women of child-bearing age at schools, through community wellness centres, at primary healthcare facilities and at antenatal clinics, providing a holistic intervention to address prevalent infectious diseases and NCDs, and their shared risk factors. As noted above, policy measures, including legislative and fiscal approaches, are likely to be important and are discussed in a later chapter.

3.3.3 The elderly

The demographic transition occurring in many LMICs results in ageing and increasing life expectancy, and the populations in LMICs are ageing at a faster rate than in developed countries (see de-Graft Aikins *et al*., Chapter 4, this volume). A focus on healthy ageing will therefore be required in LMICs in response to this transition. It is well recognized that ageing is associated with increasing prevalence of NCDs such as cardiovascular disease and cancers. However, there is also an increased susceptibility to infectious diseases, so health threats due to infectious disease should not be overlooked. With increasing access to ART, there is increasing survival and ageing in HIV-infected persons. However, public health HIV control interventions often ignore this age group. Furthermore, immunocompromise associated with ageing increases the risk of other infectious diseases including TB (both primary infection and reactivation disease). Given the high prevalence of NCDs, older persons in LMICs are at a high risk of developing multimorbid infectious and non-communicable conditions [83]. This can result in disability, reduced quality of life and social isolation, limiting their ability to fulfil emotional, cultural and economic roles within families and society. Interventions that address isolation and promote social participation have been identified as potentially important in the elderly [84]. Primary prevention interventions including the promotion of physical activity and good nutrition are also of importance in this population. In implementing secondary and tertiary prevention, it is important to take a holistic interdisciplinary approach that includes taking into account the patient's social situation when addressing diagnosed conditions.

3.4 Implications for Policy and Research

The impact of NCDs on health systems and the importance of systems strengthening will be dealt with in detail later in this book (see, for example, Coast *et al.*, Chapter 6, and Mendis and Chestnov, Chapter 12, this volume). This section covers the specific health system policy and research implications related to the changing pattern of disease described in this chapter.

The current vertical chronic disease-specific health system model requires reconsideration in a setting of combined infectious disease and NCD epidemics. A better understanding of the epidemiology of these epidemics and accompanying appropriate programmes of monitoring and evaluation as well as quality improvement would assist population-based planning and resource allocation. There has been increasing discussion about the need to integrate service delivery for these conditions, although successful demonstration is limited. This is likely to facilitate continuity and coordination of care. In addition to service delivery, it is important to consider the integration of health promotion and prevention strategies as part of a more comprehensive well-being package of care.

The management of patients with co-morbid infectious diseases and NCDs is often associated with increasing complexity, with implications for the health provider's ability and capacity to manage these patients. This can lead to issues around role delineation between specialist and generalist doctors and nurses, and around how to coordinate care at the different levels of the health system. In these settings, teaching, training and mentoring of health professionals should be responsive to these population health changes, acknowledging the changing patterns of disease.

The change in disease patterns should be accompanied by changing research priorities. For example, a recent paper identified research priorities for the study of HIV, TB and T2DM [6]. Based on the diseases reviewed in this chapter, Box 3.1 summarizes a few identified research priorities to improve our understanding of the epidemiology of co-existing infectious diseases and NCDs in LMICs.

Chronic infectious disease and NCD programmes need to move beyond drug delivery and direct disease management to include NCD interventions. Such strategies include primary prevention, obesity management and smoking cessation interventions. It is crucial that patients and communities are activated and

Box 3.1 Infectious disease and NCD research priorities

Malaria: The impact of the presence of prevalent NCDs on malaria incidence and outcomes.

TB: The impact of screening for TB and T2DM in persons with either condition on improving TB and T2DM clinical outcomes and on interrupting TB transmission through earlier case detection.

HIV: A better understanding of the association between HIV and the risk of NCDs.

empowered by understanding the disease processes and susceptibilities in order to facilitate effective self-management of co-morbid conditions. However, taking into account the fact that some of these risk factors relate to life-course epidemiology and adverse *in utero*/childhood exposures, in order to significantly impact on population health, upstream factors and social determinants of health must be addressed. Many of these factors are global, and the determinants and influences often transcend geographical boundaries. The impact of these influences is experienced across all sectors of society and ultimately requires interventions beyond the health sector. It is common to hear reference to the 'unfinished agenda' of infectious diseases. What this chapter has shown is that, in many LMICs, the agendas for the prevention and control of infectious diseases and chronic diseases are inextricably linked and must be addressed together.

References

1. Omran, A.R. (2005) The epidemiologic transition: a theory of the epidemiology of population change. *Milbank Quarterly* 83, 731–757.
2. Bradshaw, D., Dorrington, R. and Laubscher, R. (2012) *Rapid Mortality Surveillance Report 2011*. Medical Research Council, South Africa.
3. Lim, S.S., Vos, T., Flaxman, A.D., Danaei, G., Shibuya, K., Adair-Rohani, H., Amann, M., Anderson, H.R., Andrews, K.G., Aryee, M. *et al.* (2012) A comparative risk assessment of burden of disease and injury attributable to 67 risk factors and risk factor clusters in 21 regions, 1990–2010: a systematic analysis for the Global Burden of Disease Study 2010. *Lancet* 380, 2224–2260.
4. Murray, C.J.L., Vos, T., Lozano, R., Naghavi, M., Flaxman, A.D., Michaud, C., Ezzati, M., Shibuya, K., Salomon, J.A., Abdalla, S. *et al.* (2012) Disability-adjusted life years (DALYs) for 291 diseases and injuries in 21 regions, 1990–2010: a systematic analysis for the Global Burden of Disease Study 2010. *Lancet* 380, 2197–2223.
5. WHO (2011) *Global Status Report on Noncommunicable Diseases*. World Health Organization, Geneva, Switzerland <http://whqlibdoc.who.int/publications/2011/9789240686458_eng.pdf>.
6. Oni, T., Stoever, K. and Wilkinson, R.J. (2013) Tuberculosis, HIV, and type 2 diabetes mellitus: a neglected priority. *Lancet Respiratory* 1, 356–358.
7. Boutayeb, A. (2006) The double burden of communicable and non-communicable diseases in developing countries. *Transactions of the Royal Society of Tropical Medicine and Hygiene* 100, 191–199.

8. WHO (2011) *Global Tuberculosis Control Report 2011*. World Health Organization, Geneva, Switzerland.
9. Jeon, C.Y. and Murray, M.B. (2008) Diabetes mellitus increases the risk of active tuberculosis: a systematic review of 13 observational studies. *PLoS Medicine* 5, e152.
10. Stevenson, C.R., Forouhi, N.G., Roglic, G., Williams, B.G., Lauer, J.A., Dye, C. and Unwin, N. (2007) Diabetes and tuberculosis: the impact of the diabetes epidemic on tuberculosis incidence. *BMC Public Health* 7, 234.
11. International Diabetes Federation (2013) *IDF Diabetes Atlas, 6th edn*. International Diabetes Federation, Brussels, Belgium <http://www.idf.org/diabetesatlas>.
12. WHO (2013) *TB Diabetes Report*. World Health Organization, Geneva, Switzerland.
13. WHO (2006) *Definition and Diagnosis of Diabetes Mellitus and Intermediate Hyperglycaemia*. World Health Organization, Geneva, Switzerland <http://www.who.int/diabetes/publications/Definition%20and%20diagnosis%20of%20diabetes_new.pdf>.
14. WHO (2011) *Use of Glycated Haemoglobin (HbA1c) in the Diagnosis of Diabetes Mellitus*. World Health Organization, Geneva, Switzerland <http://www.who.int/entity/diabetes/publications/report-hba1c_2011.pdf>.
15. Wang, C.S., Yang, C.J., Chen, H.C., Chuang, S.H., Chong, I.W., Hwang, J.J. and Huang, M.S. (2008) Impact of type 2 diabetes on manifestations and treatment outcome of pulmonary tuberculosis. *Epidemiology & Infection* 137, 203.
16. Chang, J.T., Dou, H.Y., Yen, C.L., Wu, Y.H., Huang, R.M., Lin, H.J., Su, I.J. and Shieh, C.C. (2011) Effect of type 2 diabetes mellitus on the clinical severity and treatment outcome in patients with pulmonary tuberculosis: a potential role in the emergence of multidrug-resistance. *Journal of the Formosan Medical Association* 110, 372–381.
17. Alisjahbana, B., Sahiratmadja, E., Nelwan, E.J., Purwa, A.M., Ahmad, Y., Ottenhoff, T.H., Nelwan, R.H., Parwati, I., van der Meer, J.W. and van Crevel, R. (2007) The effect of type 2 diabetes mellitus on the presentation and treatment response of pulmonary tuberculosis. *Clinical Infectious Diseases* 45, 428–435.
18. Baker, M.A., Harries, A.D., Jeon, C.Y., Hart, J.E., Kapur, A., Lönnroth, K., Ottmani, S.E., Goonesekera, S.D. and Murray, M.B. (2011) The impact of diabetes on tuberculosis treatment outcomes: a systematic review. *BMC Medicine* 9, 81.
19. Syed Suleiman, S.A., Ishaq Aweis, D.M., Mohamed, A.J., Razakmuttalif, A. and Moussa, M.A. (2012) Role of diabetes in the prognosis and therapeutic outcome of tuberculosis. *International Journal of Endocrinology* 2012, 645362.
20. Faurholt-Jepsen, D., Range, N., PrayGod, G., Kidola, J., Faurholt-Jepsen, M., Aabye, M.G., Changalucha, J., Christensen, D.L., Martinussen, T., Krarup, H., Witte, D.R., Andersen, Å.B. and Friis, H. (2012) The role of diabetes co-morbidity for tuberculosis treatment outcomes: a prospective cohort study from Mwanza, Tanzania. *BMC Infectious Diseases* 12, 165.
21. Faurholt-Jepsen, D., Range, N., PrayGod, G., Jeremiah, K., Faurholt-Jepsen, M., Aabye, M.G., Changalucha, J., Christensen, D.L., Grewal, H.M., Martinussen, T., Krarup, H., Witte, D.R., Andersen, A.B. and Friis, H. (2013) Diabetes is a strong predictor of mortality during tuberculosis treatment: a prospective cohort study among tuberculosis patients from Mwanza, Tanzania. *Tropical Medicine & International Health* 18, 822–829.
22. Leung, C.C., Lam, T.H., Chan, W.M., Yew, W.W., Ho, K.S., Leung, G.M., Law, W.S., Tam, C.M., Chan, C.K. and Chang, K.C. (2008) Diabetic control and risk of tuberculosis: a cohort study. *American Journal of Epidemiology* 167, 1486–1494.
23. Park, S.W., Shin, J.W., Kim, J.Y., Park, I.W., Choi, B.W., Choi, J.C. and Kim, Y.S. (2012) The effect of diabetic control status on the clinical features of pulmonary tuberculosis. *European Journal of Clinical Microbiology and Infectious Diseases* 31, 1305–1310.
24. Webb, E.A., Hesseling, A.C., Schaaf, H.S., Gie, R.P., Lombard, C.J., Spitaels, A., Delport, S., Marais, B.J., Donald, K., Hindmarsh, P., Beyers, N. (2009) High prevalence of *Mycobacterium*

tuberculosis infection and disease in children and adolescents with type 1 diabetes mellitus. *International Journal of Tuberculosis and Lung Disease* 13, 868–874.

25. Chang, J.T., Dou, H.Y., Yen, C.L., Wu, Y.H., Huang, R.M., Lin, H.J., Su, I.J. and Shieh, C.C. (2011) Effect of type 2 diabetes mellitus on the clinical severity and treatment outcome in patients with pulmonary tuberculosis: a potential role in the emergence of multidrug-resistance. *Journal of the Formosan Medical Association* 110, 372–381.
26. Restrepo, B.I. (2007) Convergence of the tuberculosis and diabetes epidemics: renewal of old acquaintances. *Clinical Infectious Diseases* 45, 436–438.
27. Oni, T., Burke, R., Tsekela, R., Bangani, N., Seldon, R., Gideon, H.P., Wood, K., Wilkinson, K.A., Ottenhoff, T.H. and Wilkinson, R.J. (2011) High prevalence of subclinical tuberculosis in HIV-1-infected persons without advanced immunodeficiency: implications for TB screening. *Thorax* 66, 669–673.
28. Lee, C.H., Lee, M.C., Shu, C.C., Lim, C.S., Wang, J.Y., Lee, L.N. and Chao, K.M. (2013) Risk factors for pulmonary tuberculosis in patients with chronic obstructive airway disease in Taiwan: a nationwide cohort study. *BMC Infectious Diseases* 13, 194.
29. Inghammar, M., Ekbom, A., Engström, G., Ljungberg, B., Romanus, V., Löfdahl, C.G. and Egesten, A. (2010) COPD and the risk of tuberculosis – a population-based cohort study. *PLoS One* 5, e10138.
30. Lin, H.H., Ezzati, M. and Murray, M. (2007) Tobacco smoke, indoor air pollution and tuberculosis: a systematic review and meta-analysis. *Plos Medicine* 4, e20.
31. Allwood, B.W., Myer, L. and Bateman, E.D. (2013) A systematic review of the association between pulmonary tuberculosis and the development of chronic airflow obstruction in adults. *Respiration* 86, 76–85.
32. Pasipanodya, J.G., Miller, T.L., Vecino, M., Munguia, G., Garmon, R., Bae, S., Drewyer, G. and Weis, S.E. (2007) Pulmonary impairment after tuberculosis. *Chest* 131, 1817–1824.
33. Willcox, P.A. and Ferguson, A.D. (1989) Chronic obstructive airways disease following treated pulmonary tuberculosis. *Respiratory Medicine* 83, 195–198.
34. Hnizdo, E., Singh, T. and Churchyard, G. (2000) Chronic pulmonary function impairment caused by initial and recurrent pulmonary tuberculosis following treatment. *Thorax* 55, 32–38.
35. Jordan, T.S., Spencer, E.M. and Davies, P. (2010) Tuberculosis, bronchiectasis and chronic airflow obstruction. *Respirology* 15, 623–628.
36. Maguire, G.P., Anstey, N.M., Ardian, M., Waramori, G., Tjitra, E., Kenangalem, E., Handojo, T. and Kelly, P.M. (2009) Pulmonary tuberculosis, impaired lung function, disability and quality of life in a high-burden setting. *International Journal of Tuberculosis and Lung Disease* 13, 1500–1506.
37. Ehrlich, R.I., White, N., Norman, R., Laubscher, R., Steyn, K., Lombard, C. and Bradshaw, D. (2004) Predictors of chronic bronchitis in South African adults. *International Journal of Tuberculosis and Lung Disease* 8, 369–376.
38. Lozano, R., Naghavi, M., Foreman, K., Lim, S., Shibuya, K., Aboyans, V., Abraham, J., Adair, T., Aggarwal, R., Ahn, S.Y. *et al.* (2012) Global and regional mortality from 235 causes of death for 20 age groups in 1990 and 2010: a systematic analysis for the Global Burden of Disease Study 2010. *Lancet* 380, 2095–2128.
39. WHO (2011) *Global HIV/AIDS Response*. World Health Organization, Geneva, Switzerland.
40. Walker, R.W., Jusabani, A., Aris, E., Gray, W.K., Unwin, N., Swai, M., Alberti G and Mugusi, F. (2013) Stroke risk factors in an incident population in urban and rural Tanzania: a prospective, community-based, case–control study. *Lancet Global Health* 1, e282–e288.
41. Butt, A.A., McGinnis, K., Rodriguez-Barradas, M.C., Crystal, S., Simberkoff, M., Goetz, M.B., Leaf, D., Justice, A.C. and the Veterans Aging Cohort Study (2009) HIV infection and the risk of diabetes mellitus. *AIDS* 23, 1227–1234.
42. Brown, T.T., Cole, S.R., Li, X., Kingsley, L.A., Palella, F.J., Riddler, S.A., Visscher, B.R., Margolick, J.B. and Dobs, A.S. (2005) Antiretroviral therapy and the prevalence and incidence of diabetes mellitus in the multicenter AIDS cohort study. *Archives of Internal Medicine* 165, 1179–1184.

43. De Wit, S., Sabin, C.A., Weber, R., Worm, S.W., Reiss, P., Cazanave, C., El-Sadr, W., D'Arminio Monforte, A., Fontas, E., Law, M.G., Friis-Møller, N., Phillips, A. and the Data Collection on Adverse Events of Anti-HIV Drugs (D:A:D) study (2008) Incidence and risk factors for new-onset diabetes in HIV-infected patients: the Data Collection on Adverse Events of Anti-HIV Drugs (D:A:D) study. *Diabetes Care* 31, 1224–1229.
44. Samaras, K. (2009) Prevalence and pathogenesis of diabetes mellitus in HIV-1 infection treated with combined antiretroviral therapy. *Journal of Acquired Immune Deficiency Syndromes* 50, 499–505.
45. Dave, J.A., Lambert, E.V., Badri, M., West, S., Maartens, G. and Levitt, N.S. (2011) Effect of non-nucleoside reverse transcriptase inhibitor-based antiretroviral therapy on dysglycemia and insulin sensitivity in South African HIV-infected patients. *Journal of Acquired Immune Deficiency Syndromes* 57, 284–289.
46. Grunfeld, C., Kotler, D.P., Hamadeh, R., Tierney, A., Wang, J. and Pierson, R.N. (1989) Hypertriglyceridemia in the acquired immunodeficiency syndrome. *American Journal of Medicine* 86, 27–31.
47. Montes, M.L., Pulido, F., Barros, C., Condes, E., Rubio, R., Cepeda, C., Dronda, F., Antela, A., Sanz, J., Navas, E., Miralles, P., Berenguer, J., Pérez, S., Zapata, A., González-García, J.J., Peña, J.M., Vázquez, J.J. and Arribas, J.R. (2005) Lipid disorders in antiretroviral-naive patients treated with lopinavir/ritonavir-based HAART: frequency, characterization and risk factors. *Journal of Antimicrobial Chemotherapy* 55, 800–804.
48. Anastos, K., Lu, D., Shi, Q., Tien, P.C., Kaplan, R.C., Hessol, N.A., Cole, S., Vigen, C., Cohen, M., Young, M. and Justman, J. (2007) Association of serum lipid levels with HIV serostatus, specific antiretroviral agents, and treatment regimens. *Journal of Acquired Immune Deficiency Syndromes* 45, 34–42.
49. Goedecke, J.H., Micklesfield, L.K., Levitt, N.S., Lambert, E.V., West, S., Maartens, G. and Dave, J.A. (2013) Effect of different antiretroviral drug regimens on body fat distribution of HIV-infected South African women. *AIDS Research and Human Retroviruses* 29, 557–563.
50. Thienemann, F., Sliwa, K. and Rockstroh, J.K. (2013) HIV and the heart: the impact of antiretroviral therapy: a global perspective. *European Heart Journal* 34, 3538–3546.
51. Twagirumukiza, M., Nkeramihigo, E., Seminega, B., Gasakure, E., Boccara, F. and Barbaro, G. (2007) Prevalence of dilated cardiomyopathy in HIV-infected African patients not receiving HAART: a multicenter, observational, prospective, cohort study in Rwanda. *Current HIV Research* 5, 129–137.
52. Luo, L., Ye, Y., Liu, Z., Zuo, L., Li, Y., Han, Y., Qiu, Z., Li, L., Zeng, Y. and Li, T.S. (2010) Assessment of cardiac diastolic dysfunction in HIV-infected people without cardiovascular symptoms in China. *International Journal of STD and AIDS* 21, 814–818.
53. Sliwa, K., Carrington, M.J., Becker, A., Thienemann, F., Ntsekhe, M. and Stewart, S. (2012) Contribution of the human immunodeficiency virus/acquired immunodeficiency syndrome epidemic to de novo presentations of heart disease in the Heart of Soweto Study cohort. *European Heart Journal* 33, 866–874.
54. Chillo, P., Bakari, M. and Lwakatare, J. (2012) Echocardiographic diagnoses in HIV-infected patients presenting with cardiac symptoms at Muhimbili National Hospital in Dar es Salaam, Tanzania. *Cardiovascular Journal of Africa* 23, 90–97.
55. Thöni, G.J., Schuster, I., Walther, G., Nottin, S., Vinet, A., Boccara, F., Mauboussin, J.M., Rouanet, I., Edérhy, S., Dauzat, M., Messner-Pellenc, P. and Obert, P. (2008) Silent cardiac dysfunction and exercise intolerance in HIV+ men receiving combined antiretroviral therapies. *AIDS* 22, 2537–2540.
56. Reinsch, N., Kahlert, P., Esser, S., Sundermeyer, A., Neuhaus, K., Brockmeyer, N., Potthoff, A., Erbel, R., Buck, T. and Neumann, T. (2011) Echocardiographic findings and abnormalities in HIV-infected patients: results from a large, prospective, multicenter HIV-heart study. *American Journal of Medicine* 1, 176–184.

57. Young, F., Critchley, J.A., Johnstone, L.K. and Unwin, N.C. (2009) A review of co-morbidity between infectious and chronic disease in Sub Saharan Africa: TB and diabetes mellitus, HIV and metabolic syndrome, and the impact of globalization. *Global Health* 5, 9.
58. Szczech, L.A., Gupta, S.K., Habash, R., Guasch, A., Kalayjian, R., Appel, R., Fields, T.A., Svetkey, L.P., Flanagan, K.H., Klotman, P.E. and Winston, J.A. (2004) The clinical epidemiology and course of the spectrum of renal diseases associated with HIV infection. *Kidney International* 66, 1145–1152.
59. Winston, J., Deray, G., Hawkins, T., Szczech, L., Wyatt, C. and Young, B. (2008) Kidney disease in patients with HIV infection and AIDS. *Clinical Infectious Diseases* 47, 1449–1457.
60. Berns, J.S. and Kasbekar, N. (2006) Highly active antiretroviral therapy and the kidney: an update on antiretroviral medications for nephrologists. *Clinical Journal of the American Society of Nephrology* 1, 117–129.
61. Hsieh, M.H., Lu, P.L., Kuo, M.C., Lin, W.R., Lin, C.Y., Lai, C.C., Tsai, J.J., Chen, T.C., Hwang, S.J., Chen, Y.H. (2013) Prevalence of and associated factors with chronic kidney disease in human immunodeficiency virus-infected patients in Taiwan. *Journal of Microbiology, Immunology, and Infection* 48, 256–262.
62. Mizushima, D., Tanuma, J., Kanaya, F., Nishijima, T., Gatanaga, H., Lam, N.T., Dung, N.T., Kinh, N.V., Kikuchi, Y. and Oka, S. (2013) WHO antiretroviral therapy guidelines 2010 and impact of tenofovir on chronic kidney disease in Vietnamese HIV-infected patients. *PLoS One* 8, e79885.
63. Gupta, S.K., Eustace, J.A., Winston, J.A., Boydstun, I.I., Ahuja, T.S., Rodriguez, R.A., Tashima, K.T., Roland, M., Franceschini, N., Palella, F.J., Lennox, J.L., Klotman, P.E., Nachman, S.A., Hall, S.D. and Szczech, L.A. (2005) Guidelines for the management of chronic kidney disease in HIV-infected patients: recommendations of the HIV Medicine Association of the Infectious Diseases Society of America. *Clinical and Infectious Diseases* 40, 1559–1585.
64. WHO (2013) *Malaria: Fact Sheet No. 94 2013*. World Health Organization, Geneva, Switzerland.
65. Gething, P.W., Patil, A.P., Smith, D.L., Guerra, C.A., Elyazar, I.R., Johnston, G.L., Tatem, A.J. and Hay, S.I. (2011) A new world malaria map: *Plasmodium falciparum* endemicity in 2010. *Malaria Journal* 10, 378.
66. Tusting, L.S., Willey, B., Lucas, H., Thompson, J., Kafy, H.T., Smith, R. and Lindsay, S.W. (2013) Socioeconomic development as an intervention against malaria: a systematic review and meta-analysis. *Lancet* 382, 963–972.
67. Perez-Escamilla, R., Dessalines, M., Finnigan, M., Pachon, H., Hromi-Fiedler, A. and Gupta, N. (2009) Household food insecurity is associated with childhood malaria in rural Haiti. *Journal of Nutrition* 139, 2132–2138.
68. Mitangala, P.N., D'Alessandro, U., Donnen, P., Hennart, P., Porignon, D., Bisimwa Balaluka, G., Zozo Nyarukweba, D., Cobohwa Mbiribindi, N. and Dramaix Wilmet, M. (2013) [Malaria infection and nutritional status: results from a cohort survey of children from 6–59 months old in the Kivu province, Democratic Republic of the Congo]. *Revue d'Epidémiologie et de Santé Publique* 61, 111–120 (in French).
69. Deribew, A., Alemseged, F., Tessema, F., Sena, L., Birhanu, Z., Zeynudin, A., Sudhakar, M., Abdo, N., Deribe, K. and Biadgilign, S. (2010) Malaria and under-nutrition: a community based study among under-five children at risk of malaria, south-west Ethiopia. *PLoS ONE* 5, e10775.
70. Crookston, B.T., Alder, S.C., Boakye, I., Merrill, R.M., Amuasi, J.H., Porucznik, C.A., Stanford, J.B., Dickerson, T.T., Dearden, K.A., Hale, D.C., Sylverken, J., Snow, B.S., Osei-Akoto, A. and Ansong, D. (2010) Exploring the relationship between chronic undernutrition and asymptomatic malaria in Ghanaian children. *Malaria Journal* 9, 39.
71. Lefevre, T., Gouagna, L.C., Dabiré, K.R., Elguero, E., Fontenille, D., Renaud, F., Costantini, C. and Thomas, F. (2010) Beer consumption increases human attractiveness to malaria mosquitoes. *PLoS One* 5, e9546.

72. Danquah, I., Bedu-Addo, G. and Mockenhaupt, F.P. (2010) Type 2 diabetes mellitus and increased risk for malaria infection. *Emerging Infectious Diseases* 16, 1601–1604.
73. Jha, V., Garcia-Garcia, G., Iseki, K., Li, Z., Naicker, S., Plattner, B., Saran, R., Wang, A.Y. and Yang, C.W. (2013) Chronic kidney disease: global dimension and perspectives. *Lancet* 382, 260–272.
74. White, S.L., Chadban, S.J., Jan, S., Chapman, J.R. and Cass, A. (2008) How can we achieve global equity in provision of renal replacement therapy? *Bulletin of the World Health Organization* 86, 229–237.
75. Anand, S., Bitton, A. and Gaziano, T. (2013) The gap between estimated incidence of end-stage renal disease and use of therapy. *PLoS One* 8, e72860.
76. Elsheikha, H.M. and Sheashaa, H.A. (2007) Epidemiology, pathophysiology, management and outcome of renal dysfunction associated with plasmodia infection. *Parasitology Research* 101, 1183–1190.
77. NICE (2013) *Malaria Prophylaxis*. Clinical Knowledge Summaries, 2012. National Institute for Health and Care Excellence, Manchester, UK.
78. Collins, W.E. and Jeffery, G.M. (2007) *Plasmodium malariae*: parasite and disease. *Clinical Microbiology Reviews* 20, 579–592.
79. Barker, D.J.P. (2012) Sir Richard Doll Lecture. Developmental origins of chronic disease. *Public Health* 126, 185–189.
80. Christensen, D.L., Kapur, A. and Bygbjerg, I.C. (2011) Physiological adaption to maternal malaria and other adverse exposure: low birth weight, functional capacity, and possible metabolic disease in adult life. *International Journal of Gynecology and Obstetrics* 115 (Suppl. 1), S16–S19.
81. Eriksson, J.G. (2007) Epidemiology, genes and the environment: lessons learned from the Helsinki Birth Cohort Study. *Journal of Internal Medicine* 261, 418–425.
82. WHO (2009) *Global Health Risks*. World Health Organization, Geneva, Switzerland.
83. WHO (2011) *Global Health and Aging*. World Health Organization, Geneva, Switzerland.
84. Holmes, W.R. and Joseph, J. (2011) Social participation and healthy ageing: a neglected, significant protective factor for chronic non communicable conditions. *Global Health* 7, 43.

4 Ageing and Neurodegenerative Diseases in Low- and Middle-income Countries

Ama de-Graft Aikins[1]*, Olutobi A. Sanuade[1] and Kofi A. Anie[2]

[1]*Regional Institute for Population Studies, University of Ghana, Legon, Ghana;* [2]*Imperial College London, London, UK*

4.1 Introduction

In 2013, the number of older persons (aged 60 years and above) was 841 million, representing an 11.7% share of the global population [1]. By 2050, this number is expected to more than double to 2 billion, representing a 21.1% share of the global population [1]. By this period, older persons will exceed the number of children for the first time. These trends have major implications for low- and middle-income countries (LMICs) in Africa, Asia and Latin America, as population ageing is occurring fastest in these regions due to complex modes of epidemiological transition (see Oni and Unwin, Chapter 3, this volume). Thus, while it took high-income countries like France more than 100 years for the share of the population aged 65 years or older to double from 7 to 14%, it is estimated that it will take LMICs such as Brazil and China less than 25 years to reach the same growth [2]. By 2050, 80% of the world's older population will be concentrated in LMIC regions.

The United Nations (UN) states that while population ageing 'is a triumph of development', it also 'presents social, economic and cultural challenges to individuals, families, societies and the global community'. The 2013 UN report on World Population Ageing [1] highlights a number of multifaceted challenges that face ageing populations globally, and LMICs specifically.

First, poverty rates of older persons tend to be higher than the population average in a number of countries. Poverty rates are likely to increase among the older populations, especially in countries with limited coverage of social security systems. Secondly, the prevalence of non-communicable diseases, neurodegenerative disorders and disability will rise among the older populations with implications for health systems and health and social care at the community and family

*E-mail: adaikins@ug.edu.gh

levels. Finally, the older population is predominantly female, as women have a higher life expectancy compared with men (this is true for both the 60+ years and 80+ years categories). However, the labour force participation of older persons is higher among men, with higher levels of participation in LMICs. This raises issues around gendered dimensions of social security, family and social care, both in terms of what older people contribute and what they receive. For example, the existing data suggest that older persons make 'net financial contributions to younger family members until rather advanced ages' [1]. 'Advanced ages' refers to those aged 80 years and above, or 'the oldest old' population.

In this chapter, we address one public health challenge of ageing in LMICs: the rising burden of neurodegenerative diseases among ageing populations and the implications for public health, social care and related policies. Neurodegenerative diseases are hereditary conditions characterized by progressive dysfunction of the nervous system. The dysfunction is caused by atrophy of the central or peripheral structures of the nervous system. Neurodegenerative diseases can also be pathological conditions affecting the brain. There are over 600 disorders that affect the nervous system and the brain. These include Alzheimer's disease (AD) and other dementias (which number over 100), brain cancer, degenerative nerve diseases, stroke, Parkinson's disease (PD), multiple sclerosis, amyotrophic lateral sclerosis (also known as Lou Gehrig's disease) and Huntington's disease [2, 3]. Research has shown that dementia and PD are the two most common types and together contribute significantly to the global burden of disease [2]. Between 1990 and 2010, the number of deaths attributed to PD more than doubled, and estimates of the number caused by AD and other dementias more than tripled. Furthermore, the years lived with disability attributed to these two disorders increased by more than 70% over the same period [4]. In high-income countries, there is more systematic information on neurodegenerative diseases because population ageing has been established for a number of decades and a strong body of research, interventions and policy has developed to address the complex dimensions [3, 5]. In contrast, research, practice and policy on neurodegenerative diseases are not well developed in LMICs because population ageing and its associated health outcomes are not priority issues [2, 5–7]. The 10/66 Dementia Research group, for example, is so named because it seeks to underscore the fact that while two-thirds (66%) of people living with dementia are located in LMICs, only 10% or less of population-based research has been carried out in these regions [6]. Population-based initiatives focusing on LMICs such as the World Health Organization Study on global AGEing and adult health (SAGE) and the International Network for the Demographic Evaluation of Populations and their Health (INDEPTH) have sought to redress the imbalance (see Kengne *et al.*, Chapter 7, this volume).

In this chapter, we limit attention to the two dominant types of neurodegenerative disease in LMICs – dementia and PD – and present current evidence on prevalence, morbidity, mortality and determinants. First, we describe the prevalence, mortality and morbidity of dementia and PD. Next, we discuss the determinants of dementia and PD. In the concluding section, we consider the key challenges for public health, social care and related policies for ageing populations in LMICs.

4.2 Dementia and PD Prevalence, Morbidity and Mortality

4.2.1 Dementia prevalence, morbidity and mortality

We identified dementia prevalence studies from 15 LMIC countries, the majority of which were cross-sectional community-based studies in Asian countries (Table 4.1). The most common type of dementia reported was AD. Focusing on community-based studies alone, the prevalence of dementia based on studies conducted on people aged 65 and older varied from 0.7% (in Taiwan) to 22.9% (in Turkey) [20, 25]. For the overall reviewed studies, the highest prevalence (85.0%) occurred in Cameroon based on a hospital study of human immunodeficiency virus (HIV)-positive patients aged 34–47 years [33].

There were some variations across regions. In Latin America, the prevalence of dementia ranged from 7.1 (in Brazil) [10] to 10.8% (in Cuba) [9]. The most common type of dementia was AD, followed by mixed dementia. The highest prevalence was recorded in Cuba from a prospective longitudinal study of 3015 adults aged 65 years and above in municipalities of Havana city and Matanzas provinces [9]. Research has shown that Cuba exhibits health indictors that are similar to those of the high-income countries. The population is ageing rapidly, and by 2020, about 21.6% of the population will be 60 years and above, making it the country with the highest proportion of elderly people in Latin America.

In Africa, the prevalence of dementia varied from 2.01% (in Egypt [30]) to 85.0% (in Cameroon [33]). AD was more common than vascular dementia. The highest overall prevalence (85%) occurred among HIV patients in Cameroon, and the highest prevalence from community studies was 21.6% and this occurred in Tanzania [28].

Dementia was associated with behavioural and psychiatric complications (Table 4.2). A community study of 1271 people living with dementia in China showed that sleep disturbance was the most common symptom associated with dementia and this was present in more than one-fifth (21.9%) of this population [34]. The other forms of complications associated with dementia included irritability, apathy, depression and aberrant motor behaviour. In Taiwan, a hospital study of 142 people showed that more than half had at least one form of delusion, as well as hallucinations, aggressiveness, affective disturbances, anxiety and phobia [35].

Dementia mortality ranged from 0.9% (in a cross-sectional study in China [37]) to 66.4% (in a prospective study in China [38]). The predictors of dementia mortality included: advancement in age [37, 38, 40], severe dementia [38], substantial disability [38], co-morbidity [38], living in urban areas [37], physical illness at the time of diagnosis [41], living with cardiovascular disease [42] and depression [40]. There were mixed results regarding low levels of education [40] or high levels of education [37] as a predictor of dementia mortality. There were also mixed results on gender and dementia mortality. A cross-sectional community study in China showed that females had higher odds of dementia mortality, and dementia mortality was higher for AD than for vascular dementia [37]. Another 5-year longitudinal study of 91 people living with dementia in China showed that 51 people (37.2%) died during this period and the death rates were higher among males [38].

Table 4.1. Prevalence, risk factors and types of dementia in LMICs.

Country	Reference	Study design	Setting	Sample size	Prevalence	Determinants	Types
Cuba	Llibre *et al.*, 2009 [8]	Cross-sectional	Community based	18,351	The prevalence of dementia was 8.2% and was similar among males and females (8.3 and 8.1%, respectively)	Advancement in age, history of stroke, hypertension, depression, skull-brain trauma, family history, low education	AD was the most common
Cuba	Llibre *et al.*, 2011 [9]	Prospective	Community based	3,015	The prevalence of dementia was 10.8%		
Brazil	Herrera *et al.*, 2002 [10]	Cross-sectional	Census	1,656	The prevalence of dementia was 7.1%	Illiteracy	
Brazil	Lopes *et al.*, 2012 [11]	Cross-sectional	Community based	1,145	The prevalence of dementia was 12.5%	Advancement in age, low education, stroke, absence of arthritis and not reading books	AD accounted for 60.3%
China	Guo *et al.*, 2012 [12]	Cross-sectional	Hospital based	264	The prevalence of dementia was 36.7%	Advancement in age, being female, low education and living in a nursing home	
China	Chen *et al.*, 2012 [13]		Community based	6,244	The prevalence of dementia was 9.2% for women and 7.3% for men	Being female, living in rural areas, advancement in age, lower education, larger waist circumference and lower income	
China	Zhou *et al.*, 2006 [14]	Cross-sectional	Community based	16,095	The prevalence of dementia was 5.3%	Advancement in age and lower level of education	AD accounted for 80.5%

continued

Table 4.1. *continued.*

Country	Reference	Study design	Setting	Sample size	Prevalence	Determinants	Types
China	Zhang *et al.*, 2005 [15]	Cross-sectional	Community based	34,807	The prevalence of dementia was 3.0%	AD was higher for women, while VaD was higher for men	AD accounted for 71.3% and VaD 38.7%
China	Li *et al.*, 2007 [16]	Cross-sectional	Community based	1,593	The prevalence of dementia was 2.5%	Advancement in age, illiteracy and low income	The prevalence was higher for AD
China	Wu *et al.*, 2011 [17]	Cross-sectional	Community based	2,788	The prevalence of dementia was 6.1%		
Turkey	Arslantas *et al.*, 2009 [18]		Community based	3,100	The prevalence of dementia was 8.4%	Being female, low level of education, living in rural areas, family history of dementia and advancement in age	VaD accounted for 51.1% and AD for 48.8%
Turkey	Gurvit *et al.*, 2008 [19]	Prospective	Community based	1,019	The prevalence rate was 20%	Advancement in age and being female	The prevalence of AD was 11.0%
Turkey	Keskinoglu *et al.*, 2006 [20]	Cross-sectional	Community based	204	The prevalence of dementia was 22.9%	Advancement in age, being female, having bad health status, no occupation and high level of depressive symptoms	
Sri Lanka	de Silva *et al.*, 2003 [21]		Community based	703	The crude prevalence rate of dementia was 3.98%	Advancement in age	AD, 71.4%; VaD, 14.3%; mix of AD and VaD, 7.1%

Lebanon	Chahine *et al.*, 2006 [22]	Cross-sectional	Hospital based	117	The prevalence of dementia was 59.8%	Being female	Mild dementia, 27.9%; moderate dementia, 22.9%; severe dementia, 49.2%
India	Shaji *et al.*, 2005 [23]	Cross-sectional	Community based	1,934	The prevalence of dementia was 33.6 per 1000 of the population	Family history and history of hypertension and being male	AD, 54%; VaD, 39%; infection, tumour and trauma, 7%
Taiwan	Chien *et al.*, 2008 [24]	Prospective	Community based	22,118	The annual prevalence rate of dementia increased from 0.71 to 1.92% from 1996 to 2003		
Taiwan	Su *et al.*, 2012 [25]	Longitudinal quasi-experimental	Sanatorium	129	The prevalence of dementia among the leprosy patients was 45.7–50.4%		
Central Africa	Guerchet *et al.*, 2013 [26]		Community based	244	The prevalence of dementia was 8.0%	Peripheral arterial disease	AD, 75.7%; VaD, 24.3%
South Africa	Ramlall *et al.*, 2013 [27]	Cross-sectional	Elderly home	140	The prevalence of dementia was 7.9%	Advancement in age, high blood pressure, age, years of education, blackouts, not engaging in physical activities	
Tanzania	Paddick *et al.*, 2013 [28]	Cross-sectional	Community based	296	The age-standardized prevalent rate of dementia was 21.6%		

continued

Table 4.1. *continued.*

Country	Reference	Study design	Setting	Sample size	Prevalence	Determinants	Types
Nigeria	Yusuf *et al.*, 2013 [29]	Cross-sectional	Hospital based	121	The prevalence of dementia was 9.1%	Advancement in age and enuresis	
Egypt	El Tallawy *et al.*, 2014 [30]	Cross-sectional	Community based	4,329	The prevalence among those who were 50+ years was 2.01%	Illiteracy and advancement in age	AD, 48.3%
Senegal	Toure *et al.*, 2012 [31]	Cross-sectional	Hospital based	507	The prevalence of dementia was 8.87%	Advancement in age, illiteracy, epilepsy and family history	
Tanzania	Longdon *et al.*, 2012 [32]	Cross-sectional	Community based	1,198	The age-adjusted prevalence rate was 6.4%	Advancement in age	
Cameroon	Atashili *et al.*, 2013 [33]	Cross-sectional	Hospital	400	The prevalence among HIV patients was 85.0%	Low education, being formerly married and having HIV symptoms	

AD, Alzheimer's disease; VaD, vascular dementia.

Table 4.2. Mortality and morbidity of dementia.

Country	Reference	Study design	Setting	Sample size	Key findings
China	Haibo *et al.*, 2013 [34]	Cross-sectional	Community based	1271	50.1% of the patients experienced at least one form of behavioural and psychiatric symptoms of dementia. The most common symptoms were sleep disturbance, irritability, apathy, depression and aberrant motor behaviour
Malaysia	Eshkoor *et al.*, 2013 [35]	Cross-sectional	Community based	1210	41% of the patients had sleep disturbance and this was higher among those who were single, female, those with no education, those who were isolated and those in the Malay ethnic group.
Taiwan	Liu *et al.*, 2007 [36]	Prospective	Hospital based	142	50.7% experienced delusion with the most common type being delusion of theft, 24.6% experienced hallucinations and 40.1% experienced activity disturbances; aggressiveness was found in 27.5%, diurnal rhythm disturbance in 29.5%, affective disturbances in 30.3% and anxiety and phobia in 50%. Men had higher scores on aggression, while women had higher affective scores
China	Wen *et al.*, 2011 [37]	Cross-sectional	Community based	3885	The mortality rate of dementia was 0.9% and this increased with age and was higher among females. Other predictors of low mortality were higher levels of education, living in urban areas and being married. The age-standardized mortality rate for AD among 65+ was 0.42% and that of VaD was 0.36%. The mortality in both AD and VaD patients increased with age and was higher among females
China	Wang *et al.*, 2010 [38]	Prospective	Community based	137	The mortality rate of dementia was 66.4% during the 5-year period. The median time of survival was 4.2 years. Those with severe dementia, substantial disability, co-morbid conditions and a higher age had a shortened survival time. There was no sex difference
Tanzania	Mushi *et al.*, 2014 [39]	Cross-sectional	Community based	41 PWD and caregivers	Knowledge about dementia and its causes was low. Both PWD and their caregivers had pluralistic health-seeking behaviour. Dementia was accepted as a problem of old age. It had a huge impact on the social and economic life of families. The majority of PWD were poor and economically inactive

AD, Alzheimer's disease; VaD, vascular dementia; PWD, people with dementia.

4.2.2 PD prevalence, morbidity and mortality

The lowest and highest prevalence of PD occurred in Latin America and ranged from 50.2 per 100,000 of the population (in Bolivia) [43] to 3300 per 100,000 of the population (in Brazil) [44] (Table 4.3). The mean age of PD onset was between 54 years in Pakistan [58] and 61.5 in Nigeria [61]. In terms of morbidity, Asian studies reported associations between PD and physical problems (higher rate of hip fracture) and mental health disorders (dyskinesias, and depression) [13, 59, 63] (Table 4.4). In Africa, hypertension and diabetes were co-morbid conditions for PD [61]. Tanzanians living with PD also experienced other neurological symptoms such as dyskinesias [60].

4.3 Determinants of Dementia and PD

4.3.1 Determinants of dementia

Determinants of dementia in LMICs included socio-economic factors, socio-demographic characteristics, a history of cardiovascular diseases, depression, poor health condition, lifestyles and a family history of dementia. The key dimensions of socio-economic status, highlighted in studies from Latin America, Asia and Africa, included low levels of education, illiteracy, a low income, unemployment and living in rural areas.

For instance, a cross-sectional study of 1656 people aged 65 years and above in an urban area in Brazil showed that the prevalence of dementia ranged from 3.5% in people with eight or more years of schooling to 12% among those who were illiterate [10]. A hospital study of 264 elderly people in China showed that a low level of education was associated with a higher dementia risk [12]. Other community-based studies in China and Turkey showed that those who live in rural areas had higher risks of dementia compared with those who live in urban areas [12, 18]. A hospital study of 400 patients attending the Bamenda Regional Hospital AIDS-treatment Centre in Cameroon showed that, after adjusting for other confounding factors, those with a higher level of education had a lower risk of dementia compared with those with only primary education or less [33].

Advancement in age was a major risk factor of dementia. However, the associations between other socio-demographic characteristics and dementia were not so clear cut. There were contradictory findings with respect to sex. Asian studies reported contradictory findings relating to sex, while studies in Latin America and Africa showed that the risk of dementia was the same for men and women (Table 4.2).

A history of cardiovascular diseases like stroke, hypertension and peripheral artery disease was also shown to be associated with dementia. For instance, a community-based study in Cuba showed that a history of stroke and hypertension was associated with dementia. Those who had a history of stroke were about six times more likely to develop dementia than those without a history of stroke [8].

Other determinants of dementia included depression and a family history of dementia. A community study of elderly residents in Havana Municipality, Cuba,

Table 4.3. Prevalence of Parkinson's disease in LMICs.

Country	Reference	Study design	Setting	Sample size	Key findings
Brazil	Barbosa *et al.*, 2006 [44]	Cross-sectional	Community based	1,186	The prevalence rate of PD was 3.3 per 1000 of the population and the rates for men and women were not statistically different
Bolivia	Nicoletti *et al.*, 2003 [43]	Cross-sectional	Community based	9,955	The crude prevalence rate of PD was 50.2 per 100,000 and 286 per 100,000 of the population among those aged 40+. The prevalence increased with age and was higher among women for those aged 40+
Argentina	Bauso *et al.*, 2012 [45]	Cross-sectional	Hospital based	140,000	The prevalence of PD was 394 per 100,000 of the population aged 40+
Argentina	Melcon *et al.*, 1997 [46]	Cross-sectional	Community based	7,765	The prevalence of PD was 656.8 per 100,000 of the population and was higher in men
Cuba	Giroud Benitez *et al.*, 2000 [47]	Cross-sectional	Community based	17,784	The prevalence of PD was 135 per 100,000 of the population. About 12.5% of patients with PD showed a family history of the disease
Colombia	Sánchez *et al.*, 2004 [48]	Case–control	Hospital based		The prevalence of PD was 176.4 per 100,000 of the population of people aged 50+
Ecuador	Del Brutto *et al.*, 2013 [49]	Cross-sectional	Community based	642	The prevalence of PD among those who were 40+ was 312 per 100,000 and 671 per 100,000 of the population among those who were 60+
Thailand	Bhidavasiri *et al.*, 2011 [50]	Cross-sectional	Hospital based	60,565	The age-adjusted prevalence of PD was 424.57 per 100,000 of the population. It was higher in urban areas compared with rural areas (126.83 per 100,000 vs 90.82 per 100,000). The rate was highest in areas with a high level of pesticide use
Jordan	Alrefai *et al.*, 2009 [51]	Cross-sectional	Hospital based	102	The crude prevalence rate of PD was 59 per 100,000 person-years. About 10.9% of those with PD had a family history of the disease
Thailand	Lolekha *et al.*, 2010 [52]	Cross-sectional	Hospital based	704	The crude prevalence rate of PD among boxers was 710 per 100,000 and 980 per 100,000 of the population for those aged 50+; this increased with age, and the number of boxing fights (>100) was also associated with PD
China	Zhang *et al.*, 2005 [53]	Cross-sectional	Community based	16,488	The age-sex adjusted prevalence rate of PD was 522 per 100,000 of the population
China	Woo *et al.*, 2004 [54]	Cross-sectional	Community based	415	The prevalence of PD among those 55+ was 480 per 100,000 of the population

continued

Table 4.3. *continued.*

Country	Reference	Study design	Setting	Sample size	Key findings
China	Zhang *et al.*, 2005 [55]	Cross-sectional	Community based	29,454	The prevalence rate of PD for those 65+ was 1700 per 100,000 of the population and was higher for men
China	Zhang *et al.*, 2003 [56]		Community based	5,952	The prevalence of PD was 1% (100 per 100,000 of the population) and increased with age. There was no gender difference. However, in urban areas, the rate was higher for men at older ages and higher for women in rural areas at older ages
Taiwan	Chen *et al.*, 2012 [57]	Case–control	Hospital based	3,940	Those with PD had a significantly higher rate of hip fracture than those without PD (10.4 vs 4.1%). Those with PD had a significantly higher rate of hypertension, hyperlipidaemia and osteoporosis
Pakistan	Khealani and Baig, 2006 [58]		Hospital based	80	The prevalence of PD was higher among men. The mean age of onset was 54 years. PD was associated with rigidity, bradykinesia (slow movement), tremors, hypomimia, primitive reflexes, difficulty in performing fine work and difficulty in walking
China	Wen *et al.*, 2012 [59]	Cross-sectional	Hospital based	901	Dyskinesias and depression were associated with PD pain
Tanzania	Dotchin *et al.*, 2008 [60]	Cross-sectional	Community based	308	The age-standardized prevalence of PD to the UK population was 40 per 100,000 of the population (64 per 100,000 for males and 20 per 100,000 for females)
Nigeria	Okubadejo *et al.*, 2010 [61]	Cross-sectional	Hospital based	1,360	Out of 124 people with parkinsonism, 79% had PD while 21% had secondary parkinsonism. Males had a higher risk of PD and the incidence of PD was higher among the older age group. Hypertension and diabetes were co-morbid conditions for PD. The mean age at onset was 61.5 (standard deviation 10). Males were more than females
Egypt	Khedr *et al.*, 2012 [62]	Cross-sectional	Community based	5,920	The crude prevalence rate of PD was 57 per 100,000 of the population. It accounted for more than 80% of parkinsonism (84.6%).There was no significant difference between males and females. It was highest among those aged 70–79 years, rural residents and those who were illiterate

Table 4.4. Morbidity and mortality of PD.

Country	Reference	Study design	Setting	Sample size	Key findings
Taiwan	Chen *et al.*, 2012 [57]	Case–control	Hospital based	3940	Those with PD had a significantly higher rate of hip fracture than those without PD (10.4 vs 4.1%). Those with PD had a significantly higher rate of hypertension, hyperlipidaemia and osteoporosis
China	Wen *et al.*, 2012 [59]	Cross-sectional	Hospital based	901	Dyskinesias and depression were associated with PD pain

showed that the risk of dementia was two times higher for those who had a history of depression [8]. The study also showed that the risk of dementia was higher for those who had a family history of dementia. Another study of 204 elderly people aged 64 years and above in Turkey showed that those who had higher depressive symptoms had higher odds of developing dementia [20].

4.3.2 Determinants of PD

The determinants of PD include socio-economic and demographic factors, hereditary factors, environmental factors and health status including having high haemoglobin levels and living with diabetes (Table 4.3). With the exception of the strong association between advancement in age and PD, the findings on socio-economic and demographic determinants of PD were contradictory. For example, while a study in Thailand showed that the rate of PD was higher among people living in urban areas [64], a community-based study in Egypt showed that PD was higher in rural areas [62]. Also, while some studies showed that the PD risk was higher among males, others showed a higher risk among females and some showed no sex difference in PD prevalence. This inconclusiveness of the effect of sex on risk of PD was shown in all three regions (Latin America, Asia and Africa). One study in Thailand linked PD risk to environmental factors and showed that PD was higher in urban areas with a high level of pesticide use [64]. Other determinants of PD included hypertension, hyperlipidaemia, osteoporosis (in Taiwan) [13] and a family history of PD (in Jordan) [51].

4.4 Ageing and Neurodegenerative Diseases: Future Challenges for Public Health, Social Care and Related Policies

People living with dementia and PD require long-term sustained care because of the progressive debilitating nature of these conditions. In LMICs, these care needs are complex because of the characteristics of the elderly populations at risk and the characteristics of the systems of formal healthcare and informal health and social care. We discuss these complex care needs and highlight three major challenges for public health and social care.

The first challenge is the quality of and access to healthcare. Healthcare for neurological conditions should ideally be provided through an optimal mix of primary, secondary and tertiary care [2]. Primary care focuses on health promotion, prevention and treatment offered at the level of the community and by primary care professionals. For neurological disorders, this represents the first point of entry for diagnosis and treatment and the opportunity for delivering better clinical outcomes, and should ideally be managed by trained primary care professionals. Secondary care focuses on more sophisticated management and treatment of severe cases, often provided at the level of district or regional health facilities, and requires advanced human and technical resources. Individuals with severe or advanced cases of neurological disorders need access to specialist professionals who can offer expert care, well-equipped health facilities with diagnostic equipment such as electroencephalography and computerized tomography, and other resources such as specialist beds to provide intensive care and respite care. The tertiary care level offers the most specialized package of diagnostic, treatment and rehabilitation interventions, usually at the level of the teaching hospital. Tertiary care facilities ideally constitute a repository of evidence-based care, drawing on epidemiological and clinical research, providing training and educational support, and providing referral services including liaising with community-based support services. The majority of LMIC health systems are not structured to provide the kind of long-term treatment, management and rehabilitative care required for neurodegenerative diseases because they face multiple health crises and lack the optimal mix of trained health professionals, infrastructure and financial resources [65] (see also Coast *et al.*, Chapter 6, this volume).

For those that offer some services for neurological conditions, the cost of care is prohibitive. Globally, the direct and indirect cost of managing dementia and PD is estimated to be very high [66, 67]. In 2003, the worldwide direct costs of dementia – including medical consultations, investigations, pharmaceuticals, provision of personal and nursing care, and residential care in the later stages of dementia – was estimated to be US$156 billion [66]. This was based on a worldwide prevalence estimate of 27.7 million people with dementia. In 2010, based on a worldwide estimate of 36 million people with dementia, the global cost of dementia had almost quadrupled to US$604 billion [68]. In the USA, a study that followed 20,016 people living with PD for an average of 853 days showed that the total annual direct costs were US$23,101 per person with PD [69]. In India, a study of 175 people living with PD showed that the annual income of nearly half of these individuals was less than US$1,148.63 and they spent 16–41.7% of their annual income on medicines [70]. In LMICs, a significant proportion of people pay for healthcare out of their own pocket [71]. Our review suggests that the majority of elderly individuals living with PD or dementia are likely to be of low socio-economic status. This presents major challenges in terms of access and affordability of formal healthcare services. For many individuals living with neurodegenerative diseases, care tends to be provided by family members or community-based carers, and the high cost of care raises the risk of poverty for affected families [2]. An important new trend is the growth of support groups for people living with dementia across LMICs (see de-Graft Aikins *et al.*, Chapter 9, this volume). However the impact of dementia support groups on quality and continuity of care is yet to be evaluated, and there remains a need for support groups for other neurological disorders.

The second challenge is ensuring the quality and sustainability of social care and social support. Social care and support also raise the burden of chronic physical and mental health risks within families, as caregivers are likely to experience caregiver stress and associated problems. Much of the research on caregiver stress has come from high-income countries, and the research suggests that in addition to the financial burden of care, caregivers experience physical and mental health problems [72–75]. The type and level of stress depends on the kind of condition the recipient of care has and the level of disability arising from the condition. This has implications for caring for elderly individuals with neurodegenerative conditions who are likely to live with other chronic physical conditions (e.g. hypertension, diabetes, heart disease). The combination of financial strain and caregiver stress can lead to family and social tensions that may affect the quality and sustainability of care and support.

Finally, the evidence from studies on ageing in LMICs suggests that the aged are themselves providers of care and support to young family members [1]. In Africa, for example, HIV/AIDS morbidity and mortality among the productive adult African population has created insecure conditions for older people who, in most affected countries like South Africa, now live in 'missing generation households' [76] or 'skip generation households' [77] and have to take on caregiving responsibilities for grandchildren. In some communities in South Africa, 76% of older people are the sole providers of household necessities, and they care for the sick in their families and for their grandchildren [77]. Within these contexts, elderly caregivers who develop neurodegenerative diseases might experience social isolation if they lack access to broader social networks beyond their households.

Neurodegenerative conditions constitute a ticking public health time bomb for LMICs because their prevalence is rising, they affect a rapidly rising demographic in many countries and their impact is interlinked with major challenges in health financing, social security and social care for the aged. It is important that health systems are strengthened to address the current double burden of infectious and chronic non-communicable diseases affecting LMIC populations. However, the response to the public health challenge of neurodegenerative diseases must go beyond strengthening of health systems to tackle the broader social, structural and public policy dimensions of ageing. The response must also be context specific because of the unique social, cultural and policy dynamics operating across countries. At present, the evidence has been generated from research conducted in a limited number of countries. The African region, for example, is poorly represented. Yet current evidence suggests that the socio-economic and cultural challenges resulting from population ageing are likely to be disproportionately experienced in sub-Saharan Africa. Help Age International [78] released its 2014 Global AgeWatch Index, which ranked 96 high-, middle- and low-income countries (representing 91% of people over 60) in terms of social and economic wellbeing. The indicators included income security, health status, capability and enabling environment. Most LMICs scored poorly on income security, with only one in four people aged 65 and above having access to pensions. However, African countries (Ghana, Morocco, Nigeria, Rwanda, Zambia, Uganda, Tanzania, Malawi and Mozambique) occupied the lowest quarter and within this quarter made up 'half of those with low security rankings and poor health results' [78]. Researchers observed that rapid urbanization, the breakdown in family and community structures, and rising costs of living and healthcare deepen the vulnerabilities experienced by elderly Africans [79, 80].

Interventions targeting the rising burden of neurodegenerative diseases must be developed with a focus on the broader health and socio-economic challenges facing elderly populations in LMICs. As the 10/66 Dementia Research Group [6] suggest, key issues will include improving access to good-quality age-appropriate healthcare, addressing the problem of disability and strengthening social protection for the most vulnerable groups.

References

1. United Nations (2013) *World Population Ageing 2013*. New York: United Nations <http://www.un.org/en/development/desa/population/publications/pdf/ageing/WorldPopulationAgeing2013.pdf>.
2. WHO (2006) *Neurological Disorders: Public Health Challenges*. World Health Organization. Geneva, Switzerland.
3. European Commission (2008) Major and Chronic Diseases, Report 2007. European Commission, Brussels <http://ec.europa.eu/health/archive/ph_threats/non_com/docs/mcd_report_en.pdf>.
4. Horton, R. (2012) GBD 2010: understanding disease, injury, and risk. *Lancet* 380, 2053–2054.
5. Fratiglioni, L., De Ronchi, D. and Aguero-Torres, H. (1999) Worldwide prevalence and incidence of dementia. *Drugs & Aging* 15, 365–375.
6. Prince, M., Acosta, D., Albanese, E., Ariaga, R., Ferri, C.P., Guerra, M., Huang, Y., Jacob, K.S. Jimenez-Velazquez, I.Z., Rodriguez, J.L., Salas, A., Sosa, A.L., Sousa, R., Uwakwe, R., van der Poel, R., Williams, J. and Wortmann, M. (2008) Ageing and dementia in low and middle income countries – using research to engage with public and policy makers. *International Review of Psychiatry* 20, 332–343.
7. Strong, K., Mathers, C., Leeder, S. and Beaglehole, R. (2005) Preventing chronic diseases: how many lives can we save? *Lancet* 366, 1578–1582.
8. Llibre, J.D.J., Fernández, Y., Marcheco, B., Contreras, N. and López, A.M. (2009) Prevalence of dementia and Alzheimer's disease in a Havana municipality: a community-based study among elderly residents. *MEDICC Review* 11, 29–35.
9. Llibre, J.D.J., Valhuerdi, A., Calvo, M., García, R. M., Guerra, M., Laucerique, T. and Moreno, C. (2011) Dementia and other chronic diseases in older adults in Havana and Matanzas: the 10/66 study in Cuba. *MEDICC Review* 13, 30–37.
10. Herrera, E. Jr, Caramelli, P., Silveira, A.S. and Nitrini, R. (2002) Epidemiologic survey of dementia in a community-dwelling Brazilian population. *Alzheimer Disease and Associated Disorders* 16, 103–108.
11. Lopes, M.A., Ferrioli, E., Nakano, E.Y., Litvoc, J. and Bottino, C.M. (2012) High prevalence of dementia in a community-based survey of older people from Brazil: association with intellectual activity rather than education. *Journal of Alzheimer's Disease* 32, 307–316.

12. Guo, M., Gao, L., Zhang, G., Li, Y., Xu, S., Wang, Z., Qu, Q. and Guo, F. (2012) Prevalence of dementia and mild cognitive impairment in the elderly living in nursing and veteran care homes in Xi'an, China. *Journal of the Neurological Sciences* 312, 39–44.
13. Chen, R., Ma, Y., Wilson, K., Hu, Z., Sallah, D., Wang, J., Fan, L., Chen, R.L. and Copeland, J.R. (2012) A multicentre community-based study of dementia cases and subcases in older people in China – the GMS-AGECAT prevalence and socio-economic correlates. *International Journal of Geriatric Psychiatry* 27, 692–702.
14. Zhou, D.F., Wu, C.S., Qi, H., Fan, J.H., Sun, X.D., Como, P., Qiao, Y.L., Zhang, L. and Kieburtz, K. (2006) Prevalence of dementia in rural China: impact of age, gender and education. *Acta Neurologica Scandinavica* 114, 273–280.
15. Zhang, Z.X., Zahner, G.E., Román, G.C., Liu, J., Hong, Z., Qu, Q.M., Liu, X.H., Zhang, X.J., Zhou, B., Wu, C.B., Tang, M.N., Hong, X. and Li, H. (2005) Dementia subtypes in China: prevalence in Beijing, Xian, Shanghai, and Chengdu. *Archives of Neurology* 62, 447–453.
16. Li, S., Yan F., Li, G., Chen, C., Zhang, W., Liu, J., Jia, X. and Shen, Y. (2007) Is the dementia rate increasing in Beijing? Prevalence and incidence of dementia 10 years later in an urban elderly population. *Acta Psychiatrica Scandinavica* 115, 73–79.
17. Wu, X.G., Tang, Z., Fang, X.H., Guan, S.C., Liu, H.J., Diao, L.J. and Sun, F. (2011) [A cohort study on mortality and risk of death among population diagnosis as dementia, at base-line survey, in Beijing]. *Zhonghua Liu Xing Bing Xue Za Zhi* 32, 973–977 (in Chinese).
18. Arslantas, D., Ozbabalik, D., Metintas, S., Ozkan, S., Kalyoncu, C., Ozdemir, G. and Arslantas, A. (2009) Prevalence of dementia and associated risk factors in Middle Anatolia, Turkey. *Journal of the Neurological Sciences* 16, 1455–1459.
19. Gurvit, H., Emre, M., Tinaz, S., Bilgic, B., Hanagasi, H., Sahin, H., Gurol, E., Kvaloy, J.T. and Harmanci, H. (2008) The prevalence of dementia in an urban Turkish population. *American Journal of Alzheimer's Disease and Other Dementias* 23, 67–76.
20. Keskinoglu, P., Giray, H. Picakciefe, M., Bilgic, N. and Ucku, R. (2006) The prevalence and risk factors of dementia in the elderly population in a low socio-economic region of Izmir, Turkey. *Archives of Gerontology and Geriatrics* 43, 93–100.
21. de Silva, H.A., Gunatilake, S.B. and Smith, A.D. (2003) Prevalence of dementia in a semi-urban population in Sri Lanka: report from a regional survey. *International Journal of Geriatric Psychiatry* 18, 711–715.
22. Chahine, L.M., Bijlsma, A., Hospers, A.P. and Chemali, Z. (2007) Dementia and depression among nursing home residents in Lebanon: a pilot study. *International Journal of Geriatric Psychiatry* 22, 283–285.
23. Shaji, S., Bose, S. and Verghese, A. (2005) Prevalence of dementia in an urban population in Kerala, India. *British Journal of Psychiatry* 186, 136–140.
24. Chien, I.C., Lin, Y.C., Chou, Y.J., Lin, C.H., Bih, S.H., Lee, C.H. and Chou, P. (2008) Treated prevalence and incidence of dementia among National Health Insurance enrollees in Taiwan, 1996–2003. *Journal of Geriatric Psychiatry and Neurology* 21, 142–148.
25. Su T W., Wu, L.L. and Lin, C.P. (2012) The prevalence of dementia and depression in Taiwanese institutionalized leprosy patients, and the effectiveness evaluation of reminiscence therapy – a longitudinal, single-blind, randomized control study. *International Journal of Geriatric Psychiatry* 27, 187–196.
26. Guerchet, M., Banzouzi-Ndamba, B., Mbelesso, P., Pilleron, S., Clement, J.-P., Dartigues, J.-F. and Preux, P.-M. (2013) Prevalence of dementia in two countries of Central Africa: comparison or rural and urban areas in the EPIDEMCA study. In: *3rd International Congree on Neurology and Epidemiology*, Abstract 363. *Neuroepidemiology* 41, 223–316.
27. Ramlall, S., Chipps, J., Pillay, B.J. and Bhigjee, A.L. (2013) Mild cognitive impairment and dementia in a heterogeneous elderly population: prevalence and risk profile. *African Journal of Psychiatry* 16, 456–465.

28. Paddick, S.M., Longdon, A.R., Kisoli, A., Dotchin, C., Gray, W.K., Dewhurst, F., Chaote, P., Kalaria, R., Jusabani, A.M. and Walker, R. (2013) Dementia prevalence estimates in sub-Saharan Africa: comparison of two diagnostic criteria. *Global Health Action* 6, 1–7.
29. Yusuf, A.J., Maitama, H.Y., Amedu, M.A., Sheikh, T.L., Ahmed, M. and Mbibu, H.N. (2013) Male urinary incontinence and dementia in Zaria, Nigeria. *West African Journal of Medicine* 32, 263–266.
30. El Tallawy, H.N., Farghly, W.M., Badry, R., Rageh, T.A., Shehata, G., Hakeem, N.A., Abd El Hamed, M., Sayd, M.A., Hamed, Y. and Kandil, M.R. (2014) Prevalence of dementia in Al-Quseir city, Red Sea Governorate, Egypt. *Clinical Interventions in Aging* 9, 129–134.
31. Toure, T., Coume, M., Ndiaye, M., Zunzunegui, M.V., Bacher, Y., Diop, A.G. and Ndiaye, M. (2012) Risk factors for dementia in a Senegalese elderly population aged 65 years and over. *Dementia and Geriatric Cognitive Disorders Extra* 2, 160–168.
32. Longdon, A.R., Paddick, S.M., Kisoli, A., Dotchin, C., Gray, W.K., Dewhurst, F., Chaote, P., Teodorczuk, A., Dewhurst, M., Jusabani, A.M. and Walker, R. (2013) The prevalence of dementia in rural Tanzania: a cross-sectional community-based study. *International Journal of Geriatric Psychiatry* 28, 728–737.
33. Atashili, J., Gaynes, B.N., Pence, B.W., Tayong, G., Kats D., O'Donell, J.K., Ndumbe, P.M. and Njamnshi, A.K. (2013) Prevalence, characteristics and correlates of a positive-dementia screen in patients on antiretroviral therapy in Bamenda, Cameroon: a cross-sectional study. *BMC Neurology* 13, 86.
34. Haibo, X. and Shifu, X. (2013) Prevalence and severity of behavioral and psychological symptoms of dementia (BPSD) in community dwelling Chinese: findings from the Shanghai three districts study. *Aging and Mental Health* 17, 37–41.
35. Eshkoor, S.A., Hamid, T.A., Nudin, S.S. and Mun, C.Y. (2013) The effects of sleep quality, physical activity, and environmental quality on the risk of falls in dementia. *American Journal of Alzheimer's Disease and Other Dementias* 28, 403–407.
36. Liu, C., Wang, P., Lin, K. and Liu, H. (2007) Behavioural and psychological symptoms in Taiwanese patients with Alzheimer's disease. *International Psychogeriatrics* 19, 605–613.
37. Wen, H., Zhang, Z.X., Huang, J.B., Duan, L.L. and Wang, Q.H. (2011) Mortality of dementia and its major subtypes in urban and rural communities of Beijing. *Biomedical and Environmental Sciences* 24, 483–490.
38. Wang, Y., Huang, Y., Liu, Z., Zhuo, C., Li, S. and Prince, M. (2010) A five-year community-based longitudinal survival study of dementia in Beijing, China: a 10/66 Dementia Research Group population-based study. *International Psychogeriatrics* 22, 761–768.
39. Mushi, D., Rongai, A., Paddick, S.M., Dotchin, C., Mtuya, C. and Walker, R. (2014) Social representation and practices related to dementia in Hai District of Tanzania. *BMC Public Health* 14, 260.
40. Cho, M.J., Kim, J.K. and Suh, G. (2003) Community study of dementia in the older Korean rural population. *Australian and New Zealand Journal of Psychiatry* 37, 600–612.
41. Ueki, A., Shinjo, H., Shimode, H., Nakajima, T. and Morita, Y. (2001) Factors associated with mortality in patients with early-onset Alzheimer's disease: a five-year longitudinal study. *International Journal of Geriatric Psychiatry* 16, 810–815.
42. Meguro, K., Chubaci, R.Y.S., Meguro, M., Kawamorida, K., Goto, N. and Caramelli, P. (2011) Incidence of dementia and cause of death in elderly Japanese emigrants to Brazil before World War II. *Archives of Gerontology and Geriatrics* 52, 75–78.
43. Nicoletti, A., Sofia, V., Bartoloni, A., Bartalesi, F., Gamboa Barahon, H., Giuffrida, S. and Reggio, A. (2003) Prevalence of Parkinson's disease: a door-to-door survey in rural Bolivia. *Parkinsonism and Related Disorders* 10, 19–21.
44. Barbosa, M.T., Caramelli, P., Maia, D.P., Cunningham, M.C.Q., Guerra, H.L., Lima-Costa, M.F. and Cardoso, F. (2006) Parkinsonism and Parkinson's disease in the elderly: a community-based survey in Brazil (the Bambuí study). *Movement Disorders* 21, 800–808.

45. Bauso, D.J., Tartari, J.P., Stefani, C.V., Rojas, J.I., Giunta, D.H. and Cristiano, E. (2012) Incidence and prevalence of Parkinson's disease in Buenos Aires City, Argentina. *European Journal of Neurology* 19, 1108–1113.
46. Melcon, M.O., Anderson, D.W., Vergara, R.H. and Rocca, W.A. (1997) Prevalence of Parkinson's disease in Junín, Buenos Aires Province, Argentina. *Movement Disorders* 12, 197–205.
47. Giroud Benítez, J.L., Collado-Mesa, F. and Esteban, E.M. (2000) [Prevalence of Parkinson disease in an urban area of the Ciudad de La Habana province, Cuba. Door-to-door population study]. *Neurologia* 15, 269–273 (in Spanish).
48. Sánchez, J.L., Buriticá, O., Pineda, D., Uribe, C.S. and Palacio, L.G. (2004) Prevalence of Parkinson's disease and parkinsonism in a Colombian population using the capture-recapture method. *International Journal of Neuroscience* 114, 175–182.
49. Del Brutto, O.H., Santibáñez, R. and Santamaría, M. (2013) Prevalence of Parkinson's disease in a rural village of coastal Ecuador. A two-phase door-to-door survey. *Acta Neurologica Belgica* 113, 253–256.
50. Bhidayasiri, R., Wannachai, N., Limpabandhu, S., Choeytim, S., Suchonwanich, Y., Tananyakul, S., Tharathep, C., Panjapiyakul, P., Srismith, R., Chimabutra, K., Phanthumchinda, K. and Asawavichienjinda, T. (2011) A national registry to determine the distribution and prevalence of Parkinson's disease in Thailand: implications of urbanization and pesticides as risk factors for Parkinson's disease. *Neuroepidemiology* 37, 222–230.
51. Alrefai, A., Habahbih, M., Alkhawajah, M., Darwish, M., Batayha, W., Khader, Y. and El-Salem, K. (2009) Prevalence of Parkinson's disease in Northern Jordan. *Clinical Neurology and Neurosurgery* 111, 812–815.
52. Lolekha, P., Phanthumchinda, K. and Bhidayasiri, R. (2010) Prevalence and risk factors of Parkinson's disease in retired Thai traditional boxers. *Movement Disorders* 25, 1895–1901.
53. Zhang, L., Nie, Z.Y., Liu, Y., Chen, W., Xin, S.M., Sun, X.D., Fan, J.H., Liu, Y.H., Gao, X.H., Lu, L.Q., Como, P., McDermott, M.P., Qiao, Y.L. and Kieburtz, K. (2005) The prevalence of PD in a nutritionally deficient rural population in China. *Acta Neurologica Scandinavica* 112, 29–35.
54. Woo, J., Lau, E., Ziea, E. and Chan, D.K. (2004) Prevalence of Parkinson's disease in a Chinese population. *Acta Neurologica Scandinavica* 109, 228–231.
55. Zhang, Z.X., Roman, G.C., Hong, Z., Wu, C.B., Qu, Q.M., Huang, J.B., Zhou, B., Geng, Z.P., Wu, J.X., Wen, H.B., Zhao, H. and Zahner, G.E. (2005) Parkinson's disease in China: prevalence in Beijing, Xian, and Shanghai. *Lancet* 365, 595–597.
56. Zhang, Z., Anderson, D.W., Huang, J., Li, H., Hing, X., Wei, J., Yang, E. and Maraganore, D.M. (2003) Prevalence of Parkinson's Disease and related disorders in the elderly population of greater Beijing, China. Movement Disorders 18(7), 764–772.
57. Chen, Y.Y., Cheng, P.Y., Wu, S.L. and Lai, C.H. (2012) Parkinson's disease and risk of hip fracture: an 8-year follow-up study in Taiwan. *Parkinsonism and Related Disorders* 18, 506–509.
58. Khealani, B.A. and Baig, S.M. (2006) Clinical spectrum of Parkinson's disease from Pakistan. *Singapore Medical Journal* 47, 1075–1079.
59. Wen, H., Zhang, Z., Wang, H., Li, L., Chen, H., Liu, Y., Zhang, B. and Xu, Q. (2012) Epidemiology and clinical phenomenology for Parkinson's disease with pain and fatigue. *Parkinsonism and Related Disorders* 18, 222–225.
60. Dotchin, C., Msuya, O., Kissima, J., Massawe, J., Mhina, A., Moshy, A., Aris, E., Jusabani, A., Whiting, D., Masuki, G. and Walker, R. (2008) The prevalence of Parkinson's disease in rural Tanzania. *Movement Disorders* 23, 1567–1672.
61. Okubadejo, N.U., Ojo, O.O. and Oshinaike, O.O. (2010) Clinical profile of Parkinsonism and Parkinson's disease in Lagos, Southwestern Nigeria. *BMC Neurology* 10, 1.
62. Khedr, E.M., Al Attar, G.S., Kandil, M.R., Kamel, N.F., Abo Elfetoh, N. and Ahmed, M.A. (2012) Epidemiological study and clinical profile of Parkinson's disease in the Assiut Governorate, Egypt: a community-based study. *Neuroepidemiology* 38, 154–163.

63. Suzuki, K., Miyamoto, T., Miyamoto, M., Okuma, Y., Hattori, N., Kamel, S., Yoshii, F., Utsumi, H., Iwasaki, Y., Iijima, M. and Hirata, K. (2008) Excessive daytime sleepiness and sleep episodes in Japanese patients with Parkinson's disease. *Journal of the Neurological Sciences* 271, 47–52.
64. Bhidayasiri, R., Wannachai, N., Limpabandhu, S., Choeytim, S., Suchonwanich, Y., Tananyakul, S., Tharathep, C., Panjapiyakul, P., Srismith, R., Chimabutra, K., Phanthumchinda, K. and Asawavichienjinda, T. (2011) A national registry to determine the distribution and prevalence of Parkinson's disease in Thailand: implications of urbanization and pesticides as risk factors for Parkinson's disease. *Neuroepidemiology* 37, 222–230.
65. Allotey, P., Davey, T. and Reidpath, D.D. (2014) NCDs in low and middle-income countries-assessing the capacity of health systems to respond to population needs. *BMC Public Health* 14, 1–3.
66. Wimo, A., Jonsson, L. and Winblad, B. (2006) An estimate of the worldwide prevalence and direct costs of dementia in 2003. *Dementia and Geriatric Cognitive Disorders* 21, 175–181.
67. Alzheimer's Association (2007) *Alzheimer's Disease Facts and Figures*. Alzheimer's Association, Chicago, Illinois <http://www.alznyc.org/news/March/2007/alzFS.asp>.
68. Batsch, N.L. and Mittelman, M.S. (2012) World Alzheimer's Report 2012. Overcoming the stigma of dementia. Alzheimer's Disease International, London, UK <http://www.alz.org/documents_custom/world_report_2012_final.pdf>.
69. Huse, D.M., Schulman, K., Orsini, L., Castelli-Haley, J., Kennedy, S. and Lenhart, G. (2005) Burden of illness in Parkinson's disease. *Movement Disorders* 20, 1449–1454.
70. Ragothaman, M., Govindappa, S.T., Rattihalli, R., Subbakrishna, D.K. and Muthane, U.B. (2006) Direct cost of managing Parkinson's disease in India: concerns in a developing country. *Movement Disorders* 21, 1755–1758.
71. Tanner, C.M., Brandabur, M. and Dorsey, E.R. (2008) Parkinson disease: a global view. *Parkinson Report* Spring 2008, 9–11.
72. Lai, D.W.L. (2012) Effect of financial costs on caregiving burden of family caregivers of older adults. *SAGE Open* 1–14.
73. Beeson, R.A. (2003) Loneliness and depression in spousal caregivers of those with Alzheimer's disease versus non-caregiving spouses. *Archives of Psychiatric Nursing* 17, 135–143.
74. Parrish, M.M., Satariano, W.A., Freisthler, B., Feinberg, L.F. and Adams, S. (2005) Older women with breast cancer: caregiving and the risk of depression: an exploratory analysis. *Social Work in Health Care* 40, 41–59.
75. Yajima, Y., Tsutsui, T., Nakajima, K., Li, H.Y., Takigawa, T., Wang, D.H. and Ogino, K. (2007) The effects of caregiving resources on the incidence of depression over one year in family caregivers of disabled elderly. *Acta Medica Okayama* 61, 71–80.
76. Kautz, T., Bendavid, E., Bhattacharya, J. and Miller, G. (2010) AIDS and declining support for dependent elderly people in Africa: a retrospective analysis using demographic and health surveys. *British Medical Journal* 340, c2841.
77. Kimuna, S.R. and Makiwane, M. (2007) Older people as resources in South Africa. *Journal of Aging and Social Policy* 19, 97–114.
78. HelpAge International (2014) A global movement for the rights of older people; 2014 <http://www.helpage.org>.
79. Apt, N.A. (2005) 30 Years of African research on ageing: history, achievements and challenges for the future generations. *Review* 15, 4–6.
80. Parmar, D., Williams, G., Dkhimi, F., Ndiaye, A., Asante, F., Arhinful, D.K. and Mladovsky, P. (2014) Enrolment of older people in social health protection programs in West Africa – does social exclusion play a part? *Social Science and Medicine* 119, 36–44.

5 Chronic Non-communicable Diseases and Mental Health in Africa

Keng-Yen Huang[1]*, Sabrina Cheng[1], Rajni Gathibandhe[2], Besa H. Bauta[3] and Dickens H. Akena[4]

[1]*Department of Population Health, New York University Langone Medical Center, New York University, New York, USA;* [2]*NYU Global Institute of Public Health, New York University, New York, USA;* [3]*Center for Evidence Based Implementation and Research (CEBIR), NYU Silver School of Social Work, New York University, New York, USA;* [4]*College of Health Sciences, Makerere University, Uganda*

5.1 Introduction

Non-communicable diseases (NCDs) are the leading cause of mortality in the world [1]. The majority of deaths can be attributed to cardiovascular disease (CVD), diabetes, cancer and chronic respiratory disease [1]. NCDs and chronic health conditions have an enormous impact on mental health and well-being, not just for patients but also for their families and caregivers. The co-occurrence of NCDs and mental disorders is well recognized, and there have been increasing calls to expand the NCD umbrella to include common mental disorders, such as depression, anxiety, schizophrenia and bipolar disorder [2]. About three-quarters of NCD deaths occur in low- and middle-income countries (LMICs) [1]. However, most of the research into NCDs and mental disorders is conducted in high-income countries. Few epidemiological and prevention/intervention studies for co-morbidity of NCDs and mental disorders have been carried out in Africa. In addition, most NCDs and mental health studies worldwide have been carried out separately and independently [3]. Given their shared risk factors, pathways and co-morbidity with mental disorders [4, 5], as well as country variations in environmental and system contexts, studying the aetiology of NCDs and mental health poses a unique challenge. Therefore, it is critical to examine the epidemiological mechanisms and prevention/intervention approaches separately by country or region.

*E-mail: huangk01@nyumc.org

In this chapter, we provide a summary of the recent publications in basic science, practice and policy research related to mental health and NCDs in African settings. First, we present the prevalence and epidemiological research on the co-occurrence of NCDs and mental disorders. Then we outline the global agenda for mental health and NCD prevention and control, mental health resources/systems/policy in Africa, and challenges in integrating mental health and NCD care in African settings. Lastly, we outline frameworks and strategies to address the co-occurrence of NCDs and mental disorders in LMIC settings, and offer suggestions and recommendations for future studies.

5.2 Mental Health and Non-communicable Diseases

5.2.1 Mental disorder prevalence among NCDs

The burden of mental, neurological and substance (MNS) disorders accounts for 10–14% of the global burden of disease [6, 7], and this has grown over the past 20 years. This rise is expected to continue, in part due to the ongoing epidemiological transition from communicable diseases to NCDs, and co-morbidity between mental disorders, human immunodeficiency virus (HIV) infection and other chronic health conditions [8–10]. Worldwide, MNS disorders account for a larger percentage of lost disability-adjusted life years (DALYs) than CVD or cancer [11]. It is expected that by 2020, unipolar depressive disorders will be the second leading cause of disability [12].

The majority of studies that have investigated the prevalence of MNS disorders have been conducted in high-income countries, with less work having been done in LMICs or sub-Saharan African countries. For 64% of the world's population, there is a paucity of information on the prevalence of common mental disorders (e.g. depression and anxiety) [13]. Most of this information is missing from LMIC countries, and data from sub-Saharan Africa are particularly lacking. Sub-Saharan African countries make up the greatest proportion of the least-developed countries in the world [13]. Empirical evidence on national prevalence of MNS disorders in African countries is limited [14]. Most research in Africa has used small, specialized populations including people living in urban settings and hospitalized patients [15]. Because of the high rates of poverty and the physical health burden and inadequate mental health systems, it is reasonable to assume that the burden of MNS disorders in African countries might be greater than in high-income countries [16]. Some evidence has supported these findings, and has reported a higher prevalence of post-traumatic stress disorder, anxiety and depression (20–60%) in sub-Saharan African countries [17, 18] than in high-income countries (19–27%) [19, 20].

NCDs are often considered diseases of the middle-aged and elderly, and often exist with other co-morbidities. Examples of these co-morbidities include mental disorders, cognitive impairment and other NCDs, including renal, endocrine, neurological, gastroenterological, musculoskeletal, skin and oral diseases, disabilities and genetic disorders [21]. Although the co-morbidities of MNS disorders and NCDs are well recognized [5, 22–24], most studies have focused on the co-morbidity of 'depression' (one major MNS disorder) and chronic physical diseases. Also, fewer studies have focused on ethnic/country differences in the co-morbidity of NCDs and MNS disorders [25]. Several studies, including one based on the World Health Organization (WHO) World Health Survey (data collected from 26 European, 15 African, six American, four eastern Mediterranean, five South-east Asian and four western Pacific countries), have provided estimates for the prevalence of depression and NCDs. These studies reported that the prevalence of major depression is lower for individuals without NCDs (2–15%) [26, 27] than for individuals with NCDs, and is 29% for individuals with hypertension [27], 22% for individuals with myocardial infarction [27], 19–27% for individuals with diabetes [28–31], 33% for individuals with cancer [29] and 25% for individuals with co-morbidity of two or more chronic physical conditions [27]. Some studies have also suggested that the co-occurrence of NCD and MNS disorders might be higher in Africa or LMICs because of a lower socio-economic status [27, 32]. For example, one study conducted in Uganda found that the prevalence of depression among patients with diabetes was 35%, and was associated with being more impoverished, unemployed and having a poorer overall quality of life [32].

5.2.2 Mechanisms of co-occurrence

The co-occurrence of NCDs and MNS disorders plays an integral role in the development, progression and response to the treatment of major NCDs. Understanding the mechanisms of co-occurrence has critical implications for developing better-integrated prevention and/or intervention strategies to address population health needs. Despite the importance of aetiology research, little research is conducted in sub-Saharan African, and most research has focused on developed countries.

Current evidence suggests that several mechanisms may explain the high co-occurrence of NCDs and MNS disorders. The co-occurrence can be explained by shared important pathways to disease and a bidirectional mechanism. It is well established that MNS disorders affect, and are affected by, other NCDs. Individuals with a mental disorder are more likely to develop a medical condition, while individuals with NCDs are at increased risk for a mental disorder such as depression or anxiety. MNS disorders can be a precursor or a consequence of NCDs; the co-occurrence can also be the result of interactive effects [33–35].

Among studies that examined the causal pathway from MNS disorders to NCDs, several review studies supported the role that anxiety and depression play as independent risk factors for incident of coronary heart disease, cardiac death, myocardial infarction and diabetes [21, 33, 34]. Schizophrenia-spectrum disorders and bipolar disorder are also key independent risk factors for NCDs (e.g. diabetes, dyslipidaemia, hypertension) [36]. For example, patients with anxiety or depression are 1.26–1.48 times more likely to develop NCDs than patients without such mental disorders, and such findings are independent of demographic variables, biological risk factors and health behaviours [33]. Furthermore, individuals with schizophrenia-spectrum disorders and bipolar disorder are

1.5–2 times more likely to develop diabetes, dyslipidaemia, hypertension and obesity than the general population [36].

The increased risk for developing NCDs among MNS patients (or the causal link from MNS disorders to NCDs) can be explained by biological and social–behavioural mechanisms. It has been found that MNS disorders (i.e. anxiety and depression) are associated with progression of atherosclerosis, decreased heart rate variability, risk of ventricular arrhythmias and adverse medical outcomes, which increase the risk for acute coronary syndrome and coronary heart disease [33, 35]. From a social–behavioural perspective, MNS disorders were found to be associated with poor health behaviours (e.g. poor medication adherence, physical activities, eating style and self-care), higher stress (e.g. family, social/cultural stress, financial stress) [37–40] and higher rates of hospitalization [21, 39]. These negative health behaviours and stress worsen health outcomes and exacerbate NCD conditions [39].

In examining a reverse causal pathway from NCDs to MNS disorders, substantial evidence in the literature suggests that NCDs are a risk factor for the development of MNS disorders [21]. Patients with physical NCDs (e.g. heart disease) are 1.4–2.2 times more likely to develop MNS disorders (e.g. depression, anxiety, alcohol abuse/dependence) than those without physical NCDs [27, 28, 30, 41]. Similar patterns have also been found across high-, low- and middle-income countries [42]. The increased risk for developing MNS among NCDs patients can be attributed to stress (e.g. psychological or financial stress, harmful coping behaviours) or stress-induced harmful health behaviour. It is likely that NCD-related complications and disability (such as an amputation, blindness or paralysis) place significant demands and stress on individual and family social welfare, which impacts on the social interaction, productivity, financial status and health behaviours of the families [21]. Such explanations/mechanisms are similar to the pathway from MNS disorder to NCDs (described above). For individuals with either an NCD or an MNS disorder, this can impact on their health behaviours and stress, and these shared consequences may explain the development of other disorders.

Despite the strong connections between NCDs and MNS disorders and substantial research investigating the bidirectional mechanism, the pathways leading to co-morbidity are complex. One major gap in the literature is a lack of research examining moderation effects. Whether the prevalence of co-morbidity is moderated by country/race/ethnicity, family/community characteristics, individual characteristics or disease characteristics (e.g. severity or number of diseases co-occurrences) is not well understood [25, 43–45]. Because different country/ethnic groups have different cultural values, social norms, economic status, health practices and social determinants, it is likely that the mechanisms for co-occurrence of NCDs and MNS disorders vary by ethnicity/country. In LMICs and Africa, the co-occurrence of NCDs and MNS disorders is likely to be higher because of the combination of poorer social determinants [46–48], a higher burden of physical and mental health problems, and multiple intersecting causes, such as genetic/epigenetic factors, higher poverty and stress, reduced access to preventative health services, worse health education, limited culturally competent healthcare, predisposing neighbourhood factors, and structural and financial limitation on positive health behaviours [21, 25, 49]. In addition, different family/community contexts (e.g. economical, emotional, support available, community resources, community views regarding illness, neighbourhood support/safety) and individual characteristics (e.g. age, gender) may influence disease development processes, and result in different rates of co-occurrence of NCDs and MNS disorders. It is critical for future research to systematically examine the moderation effect and dynamic processes in order to be more effective in minimizing the burden of NCDs and MNS disorders.

5.3 Global Agenda for Mental Health and Non-communicable Disease Prevention and Control

Many factors contribute to the rising prevalence of NCDs and MNS disorders and the high co-morbidity of both disorders. To address these population health burdens, a comprehensive agenda and integrated approach will be required [21]. In recent years, there has been a push to integrate mental health into the broader NCD agenda, not just as chronic health conditions but also as precursors to other NCDs [50]. Several international lead agencies, such as the WHO and the US Centers for Disease Control and Prevention (CDC), have proposed action plans to prevent and control the burden of mental health and NCDs. Table 5.1 summarizes the objectives from three action plans – the CDC Public Health Action Plan to Integrate Mental Health Promotion and Mental Illness Prevention with Chronic Diseases Prevention 2011–2015 [51], the WHO Global Action Plan for the Prevention and Control of NCDs 2013–2020 [21] and the WHO Comprehensive Mental Health Action Plan 2013–2020 [10].

The CDC Public Health Action Plan to Integrate Mental Health Promotion and Mental Illness Prevention with Chronic Diseases Prevention 2011–2015, developed in 2011, aims to integrate mental health promotion and mental illness prevention with chronic disease prevention [51]. The action plan includes three overarching objectives: improving the science of NCDs and MNS research, effective dissemination of scientific information, and translating information into actions to improve NCDs and mental health (see Table 5.1 for details). The WHO issued NCD and mental health action plans in 2013. The WHO Global Action Plan for the Prevention and Control of NCDs 2013–2020 includes six overall objectives (Table 5.1). It provides a road map to address nine global NCD targets, including a reduction in risk of premature mortality from NCDs, harmful use of alcohol, prevalence of insufficient physical activity, mean population intake of salt/sodium, prevalence of current tobacco use, prevalence of raised blood pressure, prevalence of diabetes and obesity, and an increase in the number of people receiving drug therapy and counselling to prevent heart attacks and strokes [21]. Similarly, the WHO Comprehensive Mental Health Action Plan 2013–2020 recognizes the essential role of mental health in achieving health for all people. The plan includes four objectives (Table 5.1); it aims to achieve equity in mental health through universal health coverage, and stresses the importance of prevention [10].

Table 5.1. CDC and WHO action plans for the prevention and control of NCDs and mental disorders.

CDC Public Health Action Plan to Integrate Mental Health Promotion and Mental Illness Prevention with Chronic Diseases Prevention 2011–2015 [51]					
Objective 1 To obtain better scientific information through surveillance, epidemiology and prevention research (e.g. examine the relationships between MNS and NCDs; improve mental health promotion and prevention research)	*Objective 2* To disseminate scientific information to appropriate audiences though communication and education	*Objective 3* To translate this information into action through programmes, policies and systems			
WHO Global Action Plan for the Prevention and Control of NCDs 2013–2020 [21]					
Objective 1 To strengthen international cooperation and advocacy and to raise the priority accorded to prevention and control of NCDs in global, regional and national agendas	*Objective 2* To strengthen national capacity, leadership, governance, multi-sectoral action and partnerships to accelerate country response for the prevention and control of NCDs (e.g. consider strategies to deal with underlying social determinants of health)	*Objective 3* To promote interventions to reduce the main shared modifiable risk factors for NCDs and address underlying social determinants through creation of health-promoting environments (e.g. developing supportive environment that promote healthy behaviours)	*Objective 4* To strengthen and orient health systems to address NCDs and the underlying social determinants though people-centred primary healthcare and universal health coverage	*Objective 5* To promote and support national capacity for high-quality research and development for the prevention and control of NCDs	*Objective 6* To monitor the trends and determinants of NCDs and evaluate progress

WHO Comprehensive Mental Health Action Plan 2013–2020 [10]			
Objective 1	*Objective 2*	*Objective 3*	*Objective 4*
To strengthen effective leadership and governance for mental health (e.g. develop and strengthen policy and law; resource planning stakeholder collaboration)	To provide comprehensive, integrated and responsive mental health and social care services in community-based settings (e.g. service reorganization and expended coverage; integrated and responsive care; resources planning; address disparities)	To implement strategies for promotion and prevention in mental health (e.g. addressing a range of social and economic determinants; promote mental health and prevent suicide)	To strengthen information systems, evidence and research for mental health (e.g. integrate mental health into the routine health information system; improve evidence and research)

Although the three action plans were developed independently, there are overlapping objectives and strategies across the plans, such as increasing epidemiological and prevention/intervention research, and obtaining better scientific information to inform better-integrated intervention strategies and policy decisions. The two WHO action plans for NCDs and mental health were developed at the same time, which allowed both plans to be linked to each other in a conceptually and strategically consistent way. For example, both action plans consider the following: strengthening effective leadership and governance in mental health and NCDs; promoting interventions to reduce the main underlying shared modifiable risk factors (including addressing social determinants of health and promoting healthy behaviours); strengthening information systems and research evidence; and providing comprehensive, integrated and responsive services in community-based settings that coordinate service delivery for the prevention and control of NCDs and MNS disorders. Addressing underlying social determinants and promoting healthy behaviours (e.g. physical activity, a healthy diet, a reduction in tobacco use and harmful use of alcohol), both plans include social and mental health benefits.

In line with the two WHO action plans, other global health scholars have also proposed similar strategies to address existing NCD and mental health research and service gaps. For example, Ngo *et al.* [4] and Collins *et al.* [2] suggested a need to develop collaborative care models, where NCD care and mental healthcare are integrated and provided in the primary care settings, to effectively address patients' needs, strengthen healthcare systems and reduce healthcare costs. Developing such collaborative care approaches requires investment in human resources, services and additional research (e.g. testing integrated evidence-based interventions). It must also take into account differences in social, political, cultural and health system parameters, and must consider intersectoral collaboration and health system-wide strategies [2, 4].

5.4 Mental Health Resources, Systems and Policies in Africa

The mental health burden presents an enormous challenge for health systems at every level of development [52]. The review thus far suggests that global action plans for NCD-related development targets post-2015 require consideration of the increased burden of disability associated with MNS disorders and other comorbid conditions. To develop effective strategies to address the co-morbidities of NCDs and MNS disorders in African settings requires consideration of the system capacity and service contexts. In this section, we focus on the mental health policy and system capacity in African countries, because most African countries have systems in place to address NCDs, but their mental health systems tend to be underdeveloped and underfunded (see also Coast *et al.*, Chapter 6, this volume). It has been reported that 90% of countries have a unit/branch/department in the Ministry of Health with a responsibility for dealing with NCDs and ensuring that there is funding for NCD treatment and control; NCD prevention and health promotion activities are also generally available in most countries [1] (see also Mendis and Chestnov, Chapter 12, this volume). In contrast, mental health policies/plans/legislation in African or sub-Saharan African countries are not always developed. A lack of capacity in mental health research and service can pose a tremendous barrier for implementing the action plans. In this section, we review the mental health system in the African region and 12 selected sub-Saharan African countries to provide a better sense of the scope of the challenges.

To understand the mental health system, we utilized data from the WHO Global Health Observatory Data Repository [53] and Mental Health Atlas 2011 [54]. The Observatory Data Repository provides indicators on priority health topics and health system information (i.e. health workforce, service delivery, health financing). The Mental Health Atlas provides additional country-specific information and provides a more in-depth understanding of mental health systems based on the domains of the WHO Assessment Instrument for Mental Health Systems (WHO-AIMS). WHO-AIMS was designed to gather information on six specific components/domains of a country's mental health system and its infrastructure in order to provide a standardized database for cross-country comparisons and useful information to promote the development of mental health policies. The six domains evaluated comprise: (i) policy and legislative framework; (ii) mental health services; (iii) mental health in primary care; (iv) human resources; (v) education of the public at large; and (vi) monitoring and research [55]. In addition to these WHO data, recent publications related to mental health system reviews in LMICs or African countries were also utilized to provide comparative views about mental health systems in LMICs [56–58]. Table 5.2 summarizes the mental health policies, services and human resources across the African region and for the 12 selected African countries.

Our review shows that the overall mental health system is weak in the African region. In the domains of 'mental health policy' and 'mental health legislation' (under WHO-AIMS), only 44% of countries have mental health policy or legislation. Most country policies/plans/legislation (e.g. Zambia, Uganda, Ghana, South Africa) offer protection (e.g. decriminalizing, taking into consideration international or human rights standards) for patients with mental disorders, and provide some guidance on how mental health services and resources should be provided/allocated (such as providing guidelines for decentralizing services and moving from an institutional model to community-based facilities, or integrating mental health services into primary care) [54, 59–62].

In the domain of 'mental health services', most African countries spend a very low percentage (less than 3%) of government health expenditure on mental health, and most mental health expenditure (average 71%) is consumed by mental hospitals. The funding is much lower than the WHO recommendation, which suggests a minimum of 15% of total health budget to run an effective and efficient mental health service system for a resource-constrained country [29]. There are also limited financial resources allocated to outpatient care in community or primary care settings. Therefore, mental health outpatient, day treatment and community residential facilities are inadequate in most countries (fewer than 0.5 beds per 100,000 population), with the exception of South Africa (with 6.85 beds per 100,000 population). The majority of services are provided through dedicated psychiatric hospitals, psychiatric units and clinics. The private healthcare sector plays a limited role in provision of mental health services, and many people turn to spiritual or

Table 5.2. Mental health capacity in the African region and for 12 selected African countries. Data are derived from the WHO Global Health Observatory Data Repository [53] and Mental Health Atlas 2011 [54]. African regions data for 45 countries were analysed. The availability of country level data varied as indicated, with less country-provided data on government expenditure.

	African region		Benin	Congo	Ethiopia	Ghana	Kenya	Nigeria	Rwanda	Sierra Leone	South Africa	Tanzania	Uganda	Zambia
WHO-AIMS domains (policy, services, human resources)	% or mean (SD)	Range	% or mean (SD)	% or mean (SD)	% or mean (SD)	% or mean (SD)	% or mean (SD)	% or mean (SD)	% or mean (SD)	% or mean (SD)	% or mean (SD)	% or mean (SD)	% or mean (SD)	% or mean (SD)
Mental health policy	44%		No	No	No	Yes (1996)	No	Yes (1991)	Yes (revised 2010)	Yes (2010)	Yes (reviewed 1997)	Yes (2006)	No (draft in 2005)	Yes (2005)
Mental health plan	67%		No	No	No	Yes (2007)	Yes (1994)	Yes (1991)	Yes (2007)	Yes (2010)	Yes (2009)	Yes (2005)	Yes (2010)	Yes (2007)
Mental health legislation	44%		No	No	No	Yes (revised 2012)	Yes (1991)	Yes (1958)	No	No	Yes (2002)	Yes (2008)	Yes (reviewed 2012)	Yes (reviewed 2011)
Government expenditure on mental health as a percentage of total government expenditures on health (%)*	1.60%	0.01–7.37%	–	–	–	2.00%	–	–	–	–	–	2.40%	–	–
Government expenditure on mental hospitals as a percentage of total government expenditures on mental health (%)*	71%	33–100%	–	–	85%	–	–	–	–	–	–	33%	–	–

Psychiatrists working in mental health sector+	0.24 (0.49)	0–2.36	0.14	0.03	0.04	0.07	0.19	0.06	0.05	0.02	0.27	0.04	0.09	0.03
Nurses working in mental health sector+	5.73 (22.81)	0.02–146.28	0.22	0.45	0.59	2.47	–	0.19	1.30	0.09	9.72	–	0.76	1.36
Social workers working in mental health sector+	0.12 (0.22)	0–1.18	0.01	0.03	0	0.02	0.01	0.02	0.12	0	0.39	0.01	–	0.15
Psychologists working in mental health sector+	0.39 (0.93)	0–4.26	0.02	0.11	0.02	0.04	–	0.02	0.07	0	0.31	0.01	0.02	0.02
Mental health outpatient facilities+	0.50 (1.27)	0–6.85	0.16	0	0.07	0.16	–	0.03	0.01	0	6.85	0.28	0.08	0.54
Mental health day treatment facilities+	0.07 (0.18)	0–0.83	0	–	0	0.01	–	–	0.01	0	0.16	0	0	0.01
Community residential facilities+	0.01 (0.03)	0–0.12	0.04	–	0	0.01	–	–	0.01	0	0.12	–	0	0.03
Mental hospitals+	0.06 (0.20)	0–1.18	0.02	0	0	0.02	–	0.01	0.01	0.02	0.12	0	0	0.01

A '*' indicates that the mental health expenditure data for the African region were computed from a small number of countries (7–11 out of 45) because of unavailability. A '+' indicates the mean (±standard deviation (SD)) value of beds provided in units per 100,000 population. A '–' indicates that information was not available.

traditional healers for assistance [58, 63]. Furthermore, few non-governmental organizations work directly on mental health or co-occurrence of NCDs and MNS disorders, but a large number provide mental health services as part of other infectious disease programmes, such as counselling in HIV programmes [7].

In the domain of 'human resources', most African countries have a limited number of mental health workers, with fewer than one psychiatrist, nurse or social worker per 100,000 population in most countries, compared with between 10 and 60 in developed countries [53, 64]. In the domain of 'mental health in primary care', most countries (i.e. Ghana, South Africa, Uganda and Zambia) have mental health policies/plans/legislation defined to integrate mental healthcare with primary healthcare. Consistent with the policy, most countries have included trained doctors in primary care who are authorized by the Department of Health to prescribe psychotherapeutic medicine. In some countries, such as Uganda and Zambia, primary healthcare nurses are also authorized to prescribe and treat mental disorders and provide management and treatment of MNS disorders. Although efforts have been made to increase the integration of mental health services in primary care settings, resources remain limited in sub-Saharan African countries to support primary care staff and patients to provide adequate and quality services [54, 59–62].

In the domain of 'public education and links with other sectors', the mental health legislation in African countries does not provide a framework to support or organize public education campaigns for mental health, and implementation of public education varies by country. In some countries (i.e. Ghana and South Africa), the education is coordinated by the Department of Health or Mental Health Association. In other countries (i.e. Uganda and Zambia), public education and mental health awareness campaigns are voluntarily conducted by national mental hospitals and other non-governmental organizations [54, 59–62].

In the domain of 'mental health monitoring and research', most sub-Saharan African countries continue to have challenges in these areas. Mental health research is limited because resources have been allocated for epidemiological or population-based surveillance research, and there are few trained research personnel to support monitoring and research. However, progress has been made in some countries. For example, in Ghana, as part of the Mental Health and Poverty Project, the country is setting up a partially computerized Mental Health Information System at three state psychiatric hospitals. These systems, along with improved data collection techniques, are expected to provide additional useful mental health-related indicators for the health department [65]. In South Africa, the Department of Health has instituted a policy that prescribes standards for data collection. Progress continues to be made in processing and analysing data and disseminating findings [60].

5.5 Challenges in Integrating Mental Health and Non-communicable Disease Care

Results from our review suggest that African countries share a similar profile of service and research capacity in response to the growing co-occurrence of NCDs and MNS disorders. Most African countries have funding support and a designated unit/branch/department in the Ministry of Health that is responsible for NCD prevention/intervention and health promotion [1]. However, there are insufficient financial and human resources for mental health services and research. This includes limited financial investment, low numbers and few types of workers who are trained and supervised in mental healthcare, and inequitable mental health service distribution. The lack of human resources in healthcare facilities also limits the capacity for appropriate diagnosis and management of common MNS disorders and co-morbidity of NCDs and MNS disorders at the primary care level.

Poor mental health resources and services can primarily be attributed to weak implementation of mental health policies/plans/legislation [66]. Although several sub-Saharan African countries have developed mental health policies/plans/legislation to guide the development of human resources and integrated community-based physical and mental health services, many gaps remain in supporting their implementation [58, 63]. Barriers to mental health policies/plans/legislation implementation include the low priority and lack of political commitment, the frequent scarcity of public health perspectives in mental health leadership, a lack of intersectoral collaboration and consultation, inadequate policy dissemination and an absence of research-based evidence to inform mental health policies [66].

To overcome NCD and mental health research and service gaps in African countries, it is important to consider improving political will and financial investment in human resources, capacity building (both in research and service), better education of key stakeholders, effective dissemination of research information, improved intersectoral collaboration and integrated primary care [3]. To ensure service sustainment in primary care, investment should be preceded or accompanied by the development of community mental health services, to allow training, supervision and continuous support for primary care workers to provide comprehensive care. Mobilization and recognition of non-formal resources in the community must also be increased, and community members without formal professional training and people impacted by NCDs and MNS disorders need to partake in advocacy and service delivery [67].

5.6 Emerging Frameworks and Strategies

There is a critical need to close the gap between the epidemic growth of MNS disorders and NCDs. As mentioned above, the burden of MNS disorders and NCDs might be greater in African countries because of disadvantages in multiple domains of social determinants of health (SDH) [46]. Addressing the rising burden of NCDs and MNS disorders in African countries will require the elimination of inequality in social determinants. According to the WHO Commission on Social Determinants of Health, a comprehensive SDH approach of addressing health disparities should include three areas of research: (i) identification of the social determinants that contribute to inequities in health; (ii) clarification of the mechanisms by which social determinants generate these inequities; and

(iii) documentation of the specific levels of intervention and policy entry points for action on SDH [68]. Guided by these suggestions, a comprehensive SDH approach of addressing rising NCDs and the mental health burden in African countries will require identification of social determinants (e.g. common environmental risks for MNS disorders and NCDs, the health system, services gaps), understanding the mechanisms involved in the impact of SDH on NCDs and mental health disparities, and applying the findings to develop policy or service actions to improve NCDs and mental health-related SDH.

Consistent with the SDH perspective, the global action plans for NCDs and MNS disorders (described above) were generally developed based on this framework. Most strategies proposed under these action plans were intended to improve social determinants (e.g. eliminating knowledge, intervention/services, mental health policy gaps) in the African region. In the following sections, we provide some emerging strategies that have been developed and tested in African contexts.

5.6.1 Emerging strategies for addressing policy gaps

It is recognized that more than half of the countries in the African region do not have a mental health policy or legislation, and for those with a policy or legislation, most are poorly implemented. Lack of a policy/legislation or poor implementation of policies/legislation has consequences for the performance of a health system and the distribution and quality of service. Therefore, to strengthen health research and services, an important step would be to strengthen the effective leadership and governance to increase the development and implementation of effective policies/plans/legislation. The Mental Health Leadership and Advocacy Program (mhLAP) and the Mental Health and Poverty Project (MHaPP) are two examples based on this leadership and governance strengthening approach.

The mhLAP [69] was developed by the University of Ibadan, Nigeria, in partnership with the University of Melbourne, Australia, and was launched in 2010. The aims of the mhLAP are to provide and enhance the acquisition of skills in mental health leadership, service development, advocacy and policy planning, and to build partnerships for action. It helps participating countries to build capacity for mental health leadership and advocacy, and develop stakeholder groups with the ability to identify and pursue country-specific mental health service development needs and targets. The training course is targeted at mental health leaders, senior and mid-level government officials, policy makers, leaders of civil society and service provider organizations. The objective is to create a critical mass of informed and empowered opinion leaders who can generate action for positive change in their communities. The programme was first implemented in Gambia, Ghana, Liberia, Nigeria and Sierra Leone, which share similar mental health country profiles, with low policy priority for mental health, poor funding, inadequate human resources for mental health, widespread misconceptions about mental health issues, stigmatization and human rights abuses [67, 69]. The programme was later expanded to nine African countries (for details, see [69]). The evaluation of the programme has shown improvement in the establishment of a broad coalition of service user groups, non-governmental organizations, media practitioners and mental health professionals in each participating country to implement concerted mental health advocacy efforts that are focused on country-specific priorities [69–71]. The mhLAP is a successful example that considers strengthening effective leadership and governance to influence policy processes, which have implications in addressing both mental health capacity and NCD needs.

The MHaPP [72] was initiated by the Consortium Coordinator (University of Cape Town) and was launched between 2005 and 2010. The aim of the MHaPP was to strengthen multi-sectoral research–policy partnership (e.g. Ministry of Health decision makers and researchers) to promote mental health policy/law development or implementation to break the cycle of poverty. The MHaPP was implemented by a consortium of institutions from Africa and Europe, including Ministry of Health representatives from Ghana, South Africa, Uganda and Zambia. The MHaPP research included two phases: phase 1, situational analysis, which aimed to understand the context and identify priority areas in each country; and phase 2, implementation and evaluation of the following country-specific interventions: mental health policy and legislation (all countries except Zambia), mental health information systems (Ghana and South Africa) and strengthening district mental health service delivery (all countries). The study identified several contextual factors that have an impact on the quality of the policy research partnership. It has contributed to a better understanding of the processes of research–policy partnerships to improve policy change and impacts [72].

5.6.2 Emerging strategies for addressing intervention and service gaps

The growing burden of NCDs and MNS disorders demands new ways of organizing health systems and clinical practices to deal with new challenges. In Africa, most countries also have limited human resources, particularly mental health human resources, to provide the needed NCD and mental health services. Two viable, interconnected and potentially cost-effective strategies for mitigating systems-level barriers and optimizing the management of NCDs and MNS disorders in African countries are: (i) the integration of mental health treatments into primary care services; and (ii) task-shifting of primary care duties from physicians to non-physician healthcare providers for the management of chronic diseases [2, 4, 73].

Integration of mental health treatment into primary care services

Management of NCDs relies on the assessment and early detection of risk factors, early disease symptoms, combined pharmacological and psychosocial intervention, and long-term follow-up with regular monitoring and promotion of adherence to treatment [4]. Integration of healthcare models (sometimes called collaborative care models) that address multiple service needs is potentially more cost-efficient and has the potential to reduce the burden of managing NCDs.

Two approaches for integrating services have been developed and applied in African countries. The *integrated approach* can either: (i) include a team-based approach and have different skilled professionals (e.g. nurses) that see patients with a specific chronic disorder within the primary care clinic (i.e. having patients with mental disorders or NCDs seen by different skilled professionals but within the same clinic); or (ii) include trained professionals to assess and treat both mental and physical health problems simultaneously. In the latter model (treatment of co-morbid disorders by the same health professional), the co-morbid problems of a patient are treated holistically by a health professional, and MNS disorders are managed as additional NCDs [73]. The *partnership approach* includes basic services provided by in-house health staff and specialty services provided by external health staff on a support-needed basis [73]. For example, general primary care nurses can provide basic mental health services and treat patients with uncomplicated MNS disorders in the primary care clinic setting, while specialist mental health professionals can visit the clinic to provide consultation and manage complex cases.

Empirical evidence has supported positive impacts using the integrated/partnership service models. For example, studies based on high income countries (including a review of 12 studies) found that integrated care intervention for depression and chronic medical conditions improved outcomes for depression, behavioural outcomes (e.g. diet, physical activity) and quality of life in primary care patients with varying medical conditions [74, 75]. In South Africa, integrated and partnership approaches have also been applied in selected districts. Significant improvement was found in providing mental healthcare in a primary care setting (from almost no mental health service delivered to 50–80% mental health service delivered in the primary clinic) [73]. Similar evidence was also found in Uganda, which applied the integrated approach. In the Sembabule District, primary care workers identify mental health problems, treat patients with uncomplicated mental disorders, manage emergencies and refer patients who require changes in medication or hospitalization. The inclusion of the integrated service model has improved access, produced better health outcomes and minimized disruption to people's lives compared with the previous institutional care model [73]. The integrated service model in Uganda is consistent with its National Health Policy and Health Sector Strategic Plan (initiated in 1995/1996), which is defined in the Uganda Minimum Health Care Package (UMHCP). The UMHCP was intended to be the cardinal reference in determining the allocation of public funds and other essential inputs. The UMHCP includes the control of communicable diseases (e.g. malaria, HIV/AIDS, tuberculosis), the integrated management of childhood illnesses, sexual and reproductive health and rights, public health intervention (e.g. immunization, school health, health education and promotion), epidemics and disaster prevention, and strengthening of mental health services and essential clinical care [73].

Despite the progress made in treating co-morbidities of NCDs and MNS disorders, there are many challenges that remain in integrating mental health into primary care. Many patients with MNS disorders prefer seeking services from a religious leader and/or traditional healers. Most general health workers also had negative attitudes towards MNS disorders, and most primary care staff's pre-service training had not equipped them to provide mental health services. Furthermore, access to medicines remains difficult. Psychotropic medications are frequently unavailable at health centres in sub-Saharan African countries; therefore, many people with NCDs discontinued their treatment [76].

Task-shifting NCD and mental healthcare into primary care

Given the limited number of health professionals in African countries, it is not feasible to rely on such professionals to manage health needs when trying to address the growing burden of NCDs and MNS disorders. Task-shifting, endorsed by the WHO, offers a solution to overcome this human resource barrier. Task-shifting involves redistributing tasks from professionally trained workers to those with less training and fewer qualifications [77, 78]. Under the right conditions (e.g. political support, community embeddedness, appropriate training and coaching, remuneration and incentive systems), this approach can lead to significant health gains [79, 80].

In the context of NCDs and co-morbid chronic disease management, task-shifting will require shifting of primary care duties (including physical and mental health) from physicians to non-physician healthcare providers (NPHPs). Successful task-shifting for co-occurrence of NCDs and MNS disorders will involve: (i) modifying and integrating NCDs and mental health interventions to be delivered by NPHPs; (ii) training the NPHPs in either or both NCD and mental health preventation/intervention; and (iii) providing adequate consultation and support so that the NPHPs implement the interventions with fidelity. Adapting existing efficacious programmes to African or sub-Saharan African countries using task-shifting also requires thoughtful consideration of individual- and system-level factors (e.g. leadership support, organization climate, NPHP characteristics) that may influence the effectiveness of task-shifting or programme implementation outcomes [79, 81–84].

Most task-shifting of mental healthcare focuses on task-shifting from mental health specialists (e.g. psychiatrists, psychologists) to physicians and nurses. A well-established body of research exists on implementation of evidence-based practices by primary care providers in high-income countries, including interpersonal therapy and cognitive behavioural therapy for depressive conditions, and motivational interviewing for alcohol use disorders. There is also a small but growing number of studies in the literature suggesting that lay health workers (with limited health training) can be effectively trained to provide screening, psychoeducation, and brief behavioural interventions [4]. Task-shifting mental healthcare to primary care settings is relatively new in LMICs and African countries but has recently received increased attention. For example, several trials have been conducted to integrate depression treatment into chronic disease management (e.g. primary care, HIV clinics) in LMICs, such as Uganda and Vietnam [85, 86]. Although some preliminary outcomes suggest such approaches to be acceptable, feasible and effective in reducing depression outcomes, cultural and health system barriers (e.g. relatively low levels of psychological mindedness useful for understanding of psychological interventions, lack of mental health specialists, overburdened health providers unfamiliar with behavioural interventions) require further attention in future task-shifting approaches of mental healthcare [86].

5.6.3 Emerging strategies for addressing epidemiological research gaps

From our review, many epidemiological, intervention, service and policy research gaps have been identified in Africa. To overcome research barriers, several strategies have been developed by researchers. These include: (i) training and capacity development both in research and services research through regional or international partnerships [87, 88]; (ii) designing systematic large-scale basic scientific and practice-based research, which can include accurate and thorough assessment of the prevalence and mechanisms of co-occurrence of NCDs and MNS disorders in adult populations in different African countries, and systematic evaluation of a range of specific interventions or packages of interventions that target co-morbidity and are tailored to the local context; (iii) developing and testing better dissemination strategies to disseminate mental health information to the general public and policy makers to reduce stigma, treatment and policy barriers; (iv) a well-articulated research plan to address the barriers to the implementation of mental health policy/legislation; and (v) widening of consultation and multi-disciplinary research collaboration [11, 66].

5.7 Conclusions

This chapter summarized the current state of knowledge of and practices on the co-occurrence of NCDs and mental health disorders in African settings. Co-morbidity of NCDs and MNS disorders involves complex physiological, social and contextual factors. Epidemiological research based on African populations remains limited, and mechanisms of co-morbidity of NCDs and MNS disorders with interaction of social determinants remain understudied. Although several global action plans, based on the SDH framework, have been proposed to guide the actions for addressing the growing burden of NCDs and MNS disorders, attention needs to be paid to the mental health policy, policy implementation and primary healthcare resource issues mentioned in this chapter. These are among the biggest challenges in current research and practice.

Our review also shows some encouraging signs in addressing the double burden of NCDs and MNS disorders. Several policies, services/interventions and research strategies have been proposed and tested, with some encouraging evidence showing improvements in changing policy, capacity development, service provision, patient impacts and research partnerships. Future research should continue to monitor the disease trajectory of the co-occurrence of NCDs and MNS disorders, investigate mechanisms of co-morbidities of NCDs and MNS disorders using representative African populations, systematically test the integrated/partnership approaches of using task-shifting interventions and implementation in primary settings, and expand on research–policy partnerships to revise and further develop effective country-specific action plans to improve services and to reduce population health risks.

References

1. WHO (2014) *Global Status Report on Noncommunicable Diseases 2014*. World Health Organization, Geneva, Switzerland.
2. Collins, P.Y., Insel, T.R., Chockalingam, A., Daar, A. and Maddox, Y.T. (2013) Grand challenges in global mental health: integration in research, policy, and practice. *PLoS Medicine* 10, e1001434.
3. O'Neil, A., Jacka, F.N., Cocker, F., Taylor, C.B., Odldenburg, B. and Berk, M. (2015) A shared framework for the common mental disorders and non-communicable disease: key considerations for disease prevention and control. BMC Psychiatry 15, 15.
4. Ngo, V.K., Rubinstein, A., Ganju, V., Kanellis, P., Loza, N. and Rabadan-Diehl, C. (2013) Grand challenges: integrating mental health care into the non-communicable disease agenda. *PLoS Medicine* 10, e1001443.
5. Prince, M., Patel, V., Saxena, S., Maj, M., Maselko, J. and Phillips, M.R. (2007) No health without mental health. *Lancet* 370, 859–877.
6. Murray, C.J., Vos, T., Lozano, R., Naghavi, M., Flaxman, A.D., Michaud, C., Ezzati, M., Shibuya, K., Salomon, J.A., Abdalla, S. *et al.* (2013) Disability-adjusted life years (DALYs) for 291 diseases and injuries in 21 regions, 1990–2010: a systematic analysis for the Global Burden of Disease Study 2010. *Lancet* 380, 2197–2223.
7. Omar, M.A., Green, A.T., Bird, P.K., Mirzoev, T., Flisher, A.J., Kigozi, F., Lund, C., Mwanza, J., Ofori-Atta, A.L. and the Mental Health and Poverty Research Programme Consortium (MHaPP) (2010) Mental health policy process: a comparative study of Ghana, South Africa, Uganda and Zambia. *International Journal of Mental Health Systems* 4, 24.
8. WHO (2001) *World Health Report 2001: Mental Health: New Understanding, New Hope*. World Health Organization, Geneva, Switzerland.
9. WHO (2005) *Project ATLAS: Resources for Mental Health and Neurological Disorders*. World Health Organization, Geneva, Switzerland.
10. WHO (2013) *Mental Health Action Plan 2013–2020*. World Health Organization, Geneva, Switzerland.
11. Jack, H., Wagner, R.G., Petersen, I., Thom, R., Newton, C.R., Stein, A., Kahn, K., Tollman, S. and Hofman, K.J. (2014) Closing the mental health treatment gap in South Africa: a review of costs and cost-effectiveness. *Global Health Action* 7, 23431.
12. Mathers, C. and Loncar, D. (2006) Projections of global mortalitiy and burden of disease from 2002 to 2030. *PLoS Medicine* 3, e442.
13. Charlson, F.J., Stapelberg, N.J.C., Baxter, A.J. and Whiteford, H.A. (2011) Should global burden of disease estimates include depression as a risk factor for coronary heart disease? *BMC Medicine* 9, 47.
14. Baxter, A.J., Patton, G., Scott, K.M., Degenhardt, L. and Whiteford, H.A. (2013) Global epidemiology of mental disorders: what are we missing? *PLoS One* 8, e65514.
15. Sipsma, H., Ofori-Atta, A., Canavan, M., Osei-Akoto, I., Udry, C. and Bradley, E.H. (2013) Poor mental health in Ghana: who is at risk? *BMC Public Health* 13, 288.
16. Saxena, S., Sharan, P., Cumbrera, M. and Saracento, B. (2006) World Health Organization's mental health Atlas 2005: implications for policy development. *World Psychiatry* 5, 179–184.
17. Jamison, D.T. (2006) *Disease and mortality in sub-Saharan Africa*, 2nd edn.World Bank Publications, Washington, DC.
18. Ssanyu, R. (2007) *Mental Illness and Exclusion: Putting Mental Health on the Development Agenda in Uganda*. Policy brief 2. Chronic Poverty Research Centre, Kampala, Uganda.
19. Substance Abuse and Mental Health Services Administration (2012) *Results from the 2010 National Survey on Drug Use and Health*. Mental Health Findings, Rockville, Maryland.

20. Wittchen, H.-U. and Jacobi, F. (2005) Size and burden of mental disorders in Europe – a critical review and appraisal of 27 studies. *European Neuropsychopharmacology* 15, 357–376.
21. WHO (2013) *Global Action Plan for the Prevention and Control of Noncommunicable Diseases 2013–2020.* World Health Organization, Geneva, Switzerland.
22. Lett, H.S., Blumenthal, J.A., Babyak, M.A., Sherwood, A., Strauman, T., Robins, C. and Newman, M.F. (2004) Depression as a risk factor for coronary artery disease: evidence, mechanisms, and treatment. *Psychosomatic Medicine* 66, 305–315.
23. Goldston, K. and Baillie, A.J. (2008) Depression and coronary heart disease: a review of the epidemiological evidence, explanatory mechanisms and management approaches. *Clinical Psychology Review* 28, 288–306.
24. Rugulies, R. (2002) Depression as a predictor for coronary heart disease: a review and meta-analysis. *American Journal of Preventive Medicine* 23, 51–61.
25. Carliner, H., Collins, P.Y., Cabassa, L.J., McNallen, A., Joestl, S.S., and Lewis-Fernandez, R. (2014) Prevalence of cardiovascular risk factors among racial and ethnic minorities with schizophrenia spectrum and bipolar disorders: a critical literature review. *Comprehensive Psychiatry* 55, 233–247.
26. Ustun, T.B., Ayuso-Mateos, J.L., Chatterji, S., Mathers, C. and Murray, C.J. (2004) Global burden of depressive disorders in the year 2000. *British Journal of Psychiatry* 184, 386–392.
27. Moussavi, S., Chatterji, S., Verdes, E., Tandon, A., Patel, V. and Ustun, B. (2007) Depression, chronic diseases, and decrements in health: results from the World Health Surveys. *Lancet* 370, 851–858.
28. Rotella, F. and Mannucci, E. (2013) Diabetes mellitus as a risk factor for depression. A meta-analysis of longitudinal studies. *Diabetes Research and Clinical Practice* 99, 98–104.
29. World Health Organization (2003) *Investing in Mental Health.* World Health Organization, Geneva, Switzerland.
30. Kagee, A. (2008) Symptoms of depression and anxiety among a sample of South African patients living with a chronic illness. *Journal of Health Psychology* 13, 547–555.
31. Agbir, T., Audu, M., Adebowale, T. and Goar, S. (2010) Depression among medical outpatients with diabetes: a cross-sectional study at Jos University Teaching Hospital, Jos, Nigeria. *Annals of African Medicine* 9, 5–10.
32. Akena, D., Kadama, P., Ashaba, S., Akello, C., Kwesiga, B., Rejani, L., Okello, J., Mwesiga, E.K. and Obuku, E.A. (2015) The association between depression, quality of life, and the health care expenditure of patients with diabetes mellitus in Uganda. *Journal of Affective Disorders* 174, 7–12.
33. Roest, A.M., Martens, E.J., de Jonge, P. and Denollet, J. (2010) Anxiety and risk of incident coronary heart disease: a meta-analysis. *Journal of the American College of Cardiology* 56, 38–46.
34. Rotella, F. and Mannucci, E. (2013) Depression as a risk factor for diabetes: a meta-analysis of longitudinal studies. *Journal of Clinical Psychiatry* 74, 31–37.
35. Lichtman, J.H., Froelicher, E.S., Blumenthal, J.A., Carney, R.M., Doering, L.V. and Frasure-Smith, N. (2014) Depression as a risk factor for poor prognosis among patients with acute coronary syndrome: systematic review and recommendations: a scientific statement from the American Heart Association. *Circulation* 129, 1350–1369.
36. Newcomer, J.W. and Hennekens, C.H. (2007) Severe mental illness and risk of cardiovascular disease. *Journal of the American Medical Association* 298, 1794–1796.
37. Gonzalez, J.S., Safren, S.A., Delahanty, L.M., Cagliero, E., Wexler, D.J., Meigs, J.B. and Grant, R.W. (2008) Symptoms of depression prospectively predict poorer self-care in patients with type 2 diabetes. *Diabetic Medicine* 25, 1102–1107.
38. Gonzalez, J.S., Peyrot, M., McCarl, L.A., Collins, E.M., Serpa, L., Mimiaga, M.J. and Safren, S.A. (2008) Depression and diabetes treatment nonadherence: a meta-analysis. *Diabetes Care* 31, 2398–2403.

39. Strine, T.W., Mokdad, A.H., Dube, S.R., Balluz, L.S., Gonzalez, O. and Berry, J.T. (2008) The association of depression and anxiety with obesity and unhealthy behaviors among community-dwelling US adults. *General Hospital Psychiatry* 30, 127–137.
40. DiMatteo, M., Lepper, H.S. and Croghan, T.W. (2000) Depression is a risk factor for noncompliance with medical treatment: meta-analysis of the effects of anxiety and depression on patient adherence. *Archives of Internal Medicine* 160, 2101–2107.
41. Huffman, J.C., Celano, C.M., Beach, S.R., Motiwala, S.R. and Januzzi, J.L. (2013) Depression and cardiac disease: epidemiology, mechanisms, and diagnosis. *Cardiovascular Psychiatry and Neurology* 2013, 695925.
42. Ormel, J., Von Korff, M., Burger, H., Scott, K., Demyttenaere, K., Huang, Y.Q., Posada-Villa, J., Pierre Lepine, J., Angermeyer, M.C., Levinson, D., de Girolamo, G., Kawakami, N., Karam, E., Medina-Mora, M.E., Gureje, O., Williams, D., Haro, J.M., Bromet, E.J., Alonso, J. and Kessler, R. (2007) Mental disorders among persons with heart disease – results from World Mental Health surveys. *General Hospital Psychiatry* 29, 325–334.
43. Bronfenbrenner, U. (1986) Ecology of the family as a context for human development: research perspectives. *Developmental Psychology* 22, 723–742.
44. Bronfenbrenner, U. and Morris, P.A. (1998) The ecology of developmental processes. In: Damon, W. (ed.) *Handbook of Child Psychology*, 4th edn. Wiley, New York.
45. Huang, K.Y., Bruzzese, J.-M., Kane, K. and Cheng, S. (2010) Child health and development: a longitudinal perspective conceptual model. In: Fiedler, A. and Kuester, I. (eds) *Child Development and Child Poverty*. Nova Science Publishers Hauppauge, New York.
46. Satcher, D. (2010) Include a social determinants of health approach to reduce health inequities. *Public Health Reports* 125, 6–7.
47. WHO (2009) *Reducing Health Inequities through Action on the Social Determinants of Health*. World Health Organization, Geneva, Switzerland.
48. Wilkinson, R. and Marmot, M. (2003) *Social Determinants of Health: the Solid Facts*. World Health Organization, Geneva, Switzerland.
49. CDC (2010) *Establishing a Holistic Framework to Reduce Inequities in HIV, Viral Hepatitis, STDs, and Tuberculosis in the United States*. US Department of Health and Human Services, Centers for Disease Control and Prevention, Atlanta, Georgia.
50. Armstrong, K. and Henshall, S. (2013) Mental health, NCDs and the post-2015 development goals. *Commonwealth Health Partnerships* 2013, 33–38.
51. CDC (2011) Public health action plan to integrate mental health promotion and mental illness prevention with chronic disease prevention, 2011–2015. Department of Health and Human Services, Centers for Disease Control and Prevention, Atlanta, Georgia.
52. Whiteford, H.A., Degenhardt, L., Rehm, J., Baxter, A.J., Ferrari, A.J., Erskine, H.E., Charlson, F.J., Norman, R.E., Flaxman, A.D., Johns, N., Burstein, R., Murray, C.J. and Vos, T. (2013) Global burden of disease attributable to mental and substance use disorders: findings from the Global Burden of Disease Study 2010. *Lancet* 382, 1575–1586.
53. WHO (2014) *Global Health Observatory Data Repository: Health Systems*. World Health Organization, Geneva, Switzerland.
54. WHO (2011) *Mental Health Atlas 2011 Country Profiles*. World Health Organization, Geneva, Switzerland.
55. WHO (2005) *World Health Organization Assessment Instrument for Mental Health Systems (WHO-AIMS)*, version 2.2. World Health Organization, Geneva, Switzerland.
56. Jacob, K.S., Sharan, P., Mirza, I., Garrido-Gumbrera, M., Seedat, S., Mari, J.J., Sreenivas, V. and Saxena, S. (2007) Mental health systems in countries: where are we now? *Lancet* 370, 1061–1077.
57. Saxena, S., Lora, A., Morris, J., Berrino, A., Esparza, P., Barrett, T., van Ommeren, M. and Saraceno, B. (2011) Mental health services in 42 low and middle-income countries: a WHO-AIMS crosss-national analysis. *Psychiatric Services* 65, 123–125.

58. Roberts, M., Mogan, C. and Asare, J.B. (2014) An overview of Ghana's mental health system: results from an assessment using the World Health Organization's Assessment Instrument for Mental Health Systems (WHO-AIMS). *International Journal of Mental Health Systems* 8, 16.
59. WHO (2011). *Ghana. Mental Health Atlas 2011*. World Health Organization, Geneva, Switzerland.
60. Ministry of Health South Africa and WHO (2007) *WHO-AIMS Report on Mental Health System in South Africa 2007*. World Health Organization, Geneva, Switzerland.
61. WHO (2011) *Uganda. Mental Health Atlas 2011*. World Health Organization, Geneva, Switzerland.
62. WHO (2011) *Zambia. Mental Health Atlas 2011*. World Health Organization, Geneva, Switzerland.
63. Doku, V.C.K., Wusu-Takyi, A. and Awakame, J. (2012) Implementing the mental health act in Ghana: any challenges ahead? *Ghana Medical Journal* 46, 241–250.
64. Kigozi, F., Ssebunnya, J., Kizza, D., Cooper, S., Ndyanabangi, S. and the Mental Health and Poverty Project (2010) An overview of Uganda's mental health care system: results from an assessment using the World Health Organization's assessment instrument for mental health system (WHO-AIMS). *International Journal of Mental Health System* 4, 1–9.
65. Ofori-Atta, A.L.C. and Mirzoev, T. (2010) *Mental Health Information System – Ghana*. University of Ghana Medical School/Ministry of Health Partner, Ghana.
66. Awenva, A.D., Read, U.M., Ofori-Attah, A., Doku, V.C.K., Akpalu, B., Osei, A., Flisher, A.J. and the MHaPP Research Programme Consortium (2010) From mental health policy development in Ghana to implementation: what are the barriers? *African Journal of Psychiatry* 13, 184–191.
67. Saraceno, B., van Ommeren, M., Batniji, R., Cohen, A., Gureje, O., Mahoney, J., Sridhar, D. and Underhill, C. (2007) Barriers to improvement of mental health services in low-income and middle-income countries. *Lancet* 370, 1164–1174.
68. WHO (2007) *A Conceptual Framework for Action on the Social Determinants of Health*. World Health Organization, Geneva, Switzerland.
69. Abdulmalik, J., Fadahunsi, W., Kola, L., Nwefoh, E., Minas, H., Eaton, J. and Gureje, O. (2014) The mental health leadership and advocacy program (nhLAP): a pioneering response to the neglect of mental health in Anglophone West Africa. *International Journal of Mental Health Systems* 8, 5.
70. Roberts, M., Asare, J.B., Mogan, C., Adjase, E.T. and Osei, A. (2013) *The Mental Health System in Ghana*. Ministry of Health, Republic of Ghana, Accra, Ghana.
71. WHO (2012) proMIND: *Profiles on Mental Health in Development for Sierra Leone*. World Health Organization, Geneva, Switzerland.
72. Mirzoev, T.N., Omar, M.A., Green, A.T., Bird, P.K., Lund, C., Ofori-Atta, A. and Doku, V. (2012) Research-policy partnership – experiences of the Mental Health and Poverty Project in Ghana, South Africa, Uganda and Zambia. *Health Research and Policy and Systems* 10, 30.
73. WHO (2008) *Integrating Mental Health into Primary Care: a Global Perspective*. World Health Organization, Geneva, Switzerland.
74. Watson, L.C., Amick, H.R., Gaynes, B.N., Brownley, K.A., Thaker, S., Viswanathan, M. and Jonas, D.E. (2013) Practice-based intervnetions addressing concomitant depression and chronic medical conditions in the primary care settings: a systematic review and meta-analysis. *Journal of Primary Care and Community Health* 4, 294–306.
75. Rosenberg, D., Lin, E., Peterson, D., Ludman, E., Von Korff, M. and Katon, W. (2014) Integrated medical care management and behavioral risk factor reduction for multicondition patients: behavioral outcomes of the TEAMcare trial. *General Hospital Psychiatry* 36, 129–134.
76. World Bank (2007) *Early Education for Poor and Indigenous Communities of Nicaragua*. The World Bank, Washington, DC.
77. PEPFAR and UNAIDS (2007) *Task shifting – Global Recommendations and Guidelines*. World Health Organization, Geneva, Switzerland.

78. WHO (2007) *Task Shifting to Tackle Health Worker Shortages*. World Health Organization, Geneva, Switzerland.
79. Health Resources and Services Administration (2007) *Community Health Worker National Workforce Study*. US Department of Health and Human Services Health Resources and Services Administration, Bureau of Health Professions, Rockville, Maryland.
80. WHO (2006) *Treat, Train, Retain. The AIDS and Health Workforce Plan*. Report on the Consultation on AIDS and Human Resources for Health. World Health Organization, Geneva, Switzerland.
81. Wittkowski, A., Gardner, P.L., Bunton, P. and Edge, D. (2014) Culturally determined risk factors for postnatal depression in sub-Saharan Africa: a mixed method systematic review. *Journal of Affective Disorders* 163, 115–124.
82. Damschroder, L.J. and Lowery, J.C. (2013) Evaluation of a large-scale weight management program using the consolidated framework for implemenation research (CFIR). *Implementation Science* 8, 2–17.
83. Kisia, J., Nelima, F., Otieno, D.O., Emmanuel, W., Sohani, S., Siekmans, K., Nyandigisi, A. and Akhwale, W. (2012) Factors associated with utilization of community health workers in improving access to malaria treament among children in Kenya. *Malaria Journal* 11, 1–7.
84. Sengwana, M.J. and Puoane, T. (2004) Knowledge, beliefs and attitudes of community health workers about hypertension in the Cape Peninsula, South Africa. *Curationis* 27, 65–71.
85. Wagner, G.J., Ngo, V., Glick, P., Obuku, E.A., Musisi, S. and Akena, D. (2014) INtegration of DEPression Treatment into HIV Care in Uganda (INDEPTH-Uganda): study protocol for a randomized controlled trial. *Trials* 15, 248.
86. Ngo, V.K., Weiss, B., Lam, T., Dang, T., Nguyen, T. and Nguyen, M.H. (2014) The Vietnam Multicomponent Collaborative Care for Depression Program: development of depression care for low- and middle-income nations. *Journal of Cognitive Psychotherapy* 28, 156–167.
87. Masseli, D., Lys, J.-A. and Schmid, J. (2005) *Improving Impacts of Research Partnerships*. Swiss Commission for Research Partnerships with Developing Countries (KFPE), Bern, Switzerland.
88. de-Graft Aikins, A., Arhinful, D.K., Pitchforth, E., Ogedegbe, O., Allotey, P. and Agyemang, C. (2012) Establishing and sustaining research partnerships in Africa: a case study of the UK–Africa Academic Partnership on Chronic Disease. *Globalization and Health* 8, 29.

6 Health Systems and Chronic Non-communicable Diseases in Low- and Middle-income Countries

Ernestina Coast[1]*, Eleanor Hukin[2] and Nahid Kamal[3,4]

[1]*London School of Economics and Political Science, London, UK ;* [2]*Options Consultancy Services, UK;* [3]*International Centre for Diarrhoeal Disease Research, Bangladesh (icddr,b), Dhaka, Bangladesh;* [4]*University of North Carolina at Chapel Hill, North Carolina, USA*

6.1 What is a Health System?

A health system, at its broadest, includes everything that influences health. The goal of a health system (also known as a healthcare system) is to improve and preserve the health of individuals and populations. This aim is achieved through a combination of promotive, preventative, curative and rehabilitative services. A health system therefore includes all of the people, resources, organizations and institutions needed to improve health: funding, the workforce, supplies, transport, communications, management and service delivery. Without an understanding of the complex links and interactions among these different components of a health system, it is difficult to understand whether, and how, to change a health system to improve health outcomes.

There are many ways of conceptualizing health systems such as the frameworks of the United States Agency for International Development (USAID) or the European Observatory on Health Systems and Policies [1], and critiques of these ways of conceptualizing health systems [2]. In their article on future health systems, Bloom and Standing [3] were critical of the limiting way that debates about health systems in low- and middle-income countries (LMICs) revolve around how to adapt models from high-income countries to LMICs, and made a radical call for new ways of thinking about health system development, taking into account past failures and successes, and the dynamics of institutional development in specific contexts.

*E-mail: e.coast@lse.ac.uk

Here, we use the World Health Organization (WHO) definition of a health system [4], which:

> . . . consists of all organizations, people and actions whose *primary intent* is to promote, restore or maintain health. This includes efforts to influence determinants of health as well as more direct health-improving activities. A health system is therefore more than the pyramid of publicly owned facilities that deliver personal health services. It includes, for example, a mother caring for a sick child at home; private providers; behaviour change programmes; vector-control campaigns; health insurance organizations; occupational health and safety legislation. It includes inter-sectoral action by health staff, for example, encouraging the ministry of education to promote female education, a well-known determinant of better health.

WHO uses the concept of building blocks to break down the components of the health system. These constituents include: service delivery, the health workforce, the health information system, medical supplies, technology and vaccines, the health financing system, and leadership and governance [4].

Health systems are context specific – as are the needs of the populations that they serve – and health systems in LMICs can be characterized by a combination of under-resourcing, high disease burdens, political instability and inadequate human resources – operating against a background of poverty. The quick turnover rate of administrative regimes coupled with political upheavals in many LMICs disrupt continuity and act as a deterrent to establishing a strong, evolved health system [5]. Health systems in LMICs are characterized as weak and fragmented. They tend to be oriented towards dealing with single episodes of ill health, or acute infectious disease prevention and treatment [6, 7].

6.2 Why Do Health Systems Matter for Non-communicable Diseases?

A well-functioning health system means that a father gets a message to his mobile phone reminding him that his adolescent son with diabetes is due for a check-up; a person with asthma gets an inhaler, smoking cessation counselling and regular check-ups at an affordable clinic; a person with depression is able to access cognitive behavioural therapy at a therapy centre because of a government-sponsored mental health project; they are all benefiting from a health system that is dealing with chronic non-communicable diseases (NCDs). In many LMICs, however, NCDs remain a low priority, with poor resources allocated to them, and there is low NCD literacy – both in governments and in the populations they serve.

Population growth and ageing will lead to a substantial increase in the morbidity and mortality attributable to NCDs in LMICs, and much of the mortality will occur at younger ages compared with high-income countries [8]. This means that NCDs will increasingly dominate healthcare needs in most LMICs in the near future [9]. NCDs therefore represent a major brake on development in settings where health systems, and the resources they have, are already overstretched [10]. In most settings, NCDs are the diseases of poor people, those least likely to be able to cope with the financial implications of a chronic condition. The way in which health systems approach (or ignore) NCDs therefore plays a critical role in shaping the future of population health and well-being in LMICs.

Health systems are already trying to cope with substantial demands from patients with NCDs [11]. NCDs require long-term and sustained effort by multiple components of health systems – from the intensive use of technology and pharmaceuticals to community engagement in order to improve patient self-care and access to services. Health systems need to cope not only with the multiple and long-term need for contact with the health system, for conditions that are of long duration and often have slow progression, but also with acute episodes. The absolute and relative numbers of individuals with multiple chronic disorders will increase, and co-morbidity is likely to affect the poorest disproportionately (see also Oni and Unwin, Chapter 3, de-Graft Aikins *et al.*, Chapter 4 and Huang *et al.*, Chapter 5, this volume). For example, as increasing numbers of people living with HIV/AIDS in LMICs manage HIV/AIDS as a chronic condition, the co-morbidity of HIV/AIDS and NCDs will increase [12].

The NCD epidemic is driven by demographic ageing, rapid unplanned urbanization, the globalization of unhealthy lifestyles, environmental degradation and consumption of adulterated food [10]. The shared risk factors for these diseases are the same across countries and are spreading rapidly: tobacco use; foods high in saturated and *trans*-fats, salt and sugar; physical inactivity and alcohol consumption [13]. NCDs are largely preventable, and can be controlled and treated, but the task is beyond the scope of public health authorities alone [10]. As well as strong healthcare systems, non-health sectors need to be engaged within government, civil society and the private sector [10]. Taxation of tobacco and alcohol, for example, has been shown to reduce consumption [14].

The chronic nature of NCDs, which often progress slowly and have a long duration, and the scale of the epidemiological transition towards higher rates of NCDs, requires health systems to be reoriented as well as strengthened [15, 16]. As population ageing increases, health systems will have to cope not only with the changing burden of disease patterns but also with increases in multi-morbidity, which disproportionately affects the poorest in society [7]. The challenge for health systems in LMICs is to deal with co-morbidities that combine NCDs with infectious diseases [7]. The long-term nature of many NCDs has implications for patient self-care and self-management – and the need for health systems to understand how they can support individuals and communities to take on that role. However, the evidence base for what works in LMICs is small compared with that of high-income countries [17, 18]. There are cost pressures from the increase in NCDs due to the epidemiological transition and demographic change in LMICs. Health systems can help to reduce the burden of NCDs in young and middle-aged populations – for example through tobacco control – but overall population ageing means that NCD burdens will increase.

The boundary of what is meant by a health system is particularly important when considering NCDs. It must be conceptualized as being beyond the biomedical public and private systems of clinics and hospitals so that it includes not only healthcare but also broader aspects of lifestyle such as diet and exercise (important, for example, in diabetes) [19]. Five priority interventions were identified by the Lancet NCD Action Group and the NCD Alliance: (i) tobacco control;

(ii) salt reduction; (iii) improved diets and physical activity; (iv) reduction in hazardous alcohol intake; and (v) essential drugs and technologies [13]. Evidence based on modelling of public health interventions in 23 LMICs showed that two costed strategies (salt intake reduction and tobacco use control) had the potential to reduce mortality and prevent and control chronic diseases [20]. The authors of these analyses suggested that such interventions are highly cost-effective because they are relatively easy (compared with basic health services) to introduce and maintain, and do not incur individual-level health expenditure. Given the shortage of primary care doctors in many LMICs, how can health systems involve non-physicians in the prevention and management of chronic diseases [21]?

The growing burden of NCDs requires innovative ways of organizing health systems in order to meet these needs, and there are many attempts to achieve this. For example, the Collaborative Care Model [22], which involves a team-based approach to NCD management, including task shifting to primary and community healthcare workers with support from specialists, is one approach that has been shown to be effective in high-income countries – although the evidence base for LMICs is emergent and limited. There is an urgent need to better understand which efficacious interventions can be scaled up, and to what extent they need to be adapted to local social, political and cultural health system settings.

The ability of LMIC health systems to recognize, and cope with, the burden of NCDs has been central to much recent global attention paid to NCDs [4, 15, 23–26]. Developing and maintaining health systems that are responsive to the challenge of NCDs – both prevention and treatment – is a priority in most countries [7]. Data that describe the epidemiology of chronic diseases in LMICs have become more available, although many countries lack good population data on both the risk factors and specific diseases, especially neglected NCDs (e.g. mental illnesses, liver and renal diseases and conditions caused by environmental factors such as pollution and arsenic poisoning – arsenic in drinking water increases the risk of respiratory infections [27]). Healthcare systems in LMICs have to deal with the growing burden of NCDs against a background of persistent diseases of poverty (e.g. tuberculosis) and poorly understood interactions between infectious and NCDs [16].

Health systems in most LMICs can be described as fragmented and weak – often structured to deal with the prevention and control of infectious diseases or single episodes of care – rather than the changing care needs of people with (multiple) chronic conditions. In settings with highly constrained resources, competition between infectious diseases and NCDs can lead to 'counterproductive competition' [28]. Until very recently, most global health partnerships had focused on communicable diseases (e.g. HIV, tuberculosis and malaria) and maternal, neonatal and child health rather than NCD diseases.

Multiple barriers to scaling up or establishing NCD health services include: production of locally relevant evidence (including cost-effectiveness) to inform policy/decision making, securing resources (fiscal and human), establishment and support of services (including training), and capacity development of health system leadership and governance. In addition, numerous actors must be considered, not just national governments but also bilateral aid agencies, multi-lateral aid agencies, non-governmental organizations (NGOs), international NGOs and civil society (including community-, patient- and faith-based organizations). The large informal sector operating in LMICs can be harnessed by providing training to non-certified health providers on screening for NCDs. This is often the first point of contact for patients with NCDs in South Asian countries [29].

6.2.1 LMIC health systems and selected NCDs

In order to situate the experiences of health systems dealing with NCDs in LMICs, we will briefly review some recent country examples of experiences with four NCDs: diabetes, chronic cardiovascular diseases (CVDs), cancer and mental health.

Overall, 85% of all undiagnosed people with diabetes are estimated to be living in LMICs where resources and political will are often lacking for screening and treatment [30], with India and China representing the largest numbers of people with diabetes [31]. The prevalence of diabetes is surprisingly high in many LMICs. A study of diabetes prevalence in a rural and a semi-urban region of Cambodia revealed that the prevalence was much higher than expected – 5 and 11%, respectively, although Cambodians have relatively traditional lifestyles and are not obese by international standards [32]. A cross-sectional study of consenting adults aged 30 and over from a middle-income neighbourhood in Dhaka, Bangladesh, showed that 35% of the participants had type 2 diabetes, while 45% had metabolic syndrome. Insulin resistance was significantly associated with older age, the female sex, obesity, high wealth index and a family history of diabetes [33]. The prevalence of diabetes in rural areas has risen dramatically, where 55% of the total population of LMICs are rural [34]. The urgent need for greater public awareness and strengthening of health services for diabetes cannot be overemphasized. The Diabetes Community Lifestyle Improvement Program is an ongoing randomized control trial in India aiming to evaluate the cost-effectiveness and sustainability of a culturally appropriate low-cost intervention for prevention of type 2 diabetes mellitus that could be replicated as a model for prevention of chronic diseases in LMICs [35].

The Iranian rural primary healthcare system, the Behvarz system, showcases how strengthening the building blocks of the health system or making optimal use of available resources can effectively address NCDs and risk factors at the population level. As interventions at the primary healthcare level are constrained by the cost of physicians and health facilities, the Behvarz system used community health workers with 2 years of training to identify individuals in rural Iran who were at high risk of diabetes and hypertension. Those identified as high risk were referred to physicians at community health centres for diabetes testing and treatment with subsidized drugs. The community health workers made monthly visits to monitor drug adherence, in addition to holding sessions on healthy diet and lifestyle at the community level. As a result of this intervention, the treatment of diabetes was found to be more effective in rural Iran, despite greater coverage and access in urban areas. However, the urban–rural differential in prevalence of hypertension was not as pronounced, plausibly because, unlike the National Diabetes Control and Prevention Program outlining specific roles of Behvarz workers, the national hypertension programme was limited in its scope. The success of the Behvarz system in rural Iran highlights a number of factors – that worker density matters, monitoring of drug adherence plays a determining role in diabetes treatment and, most importantly, a national framework and defined guidelines are integral in tackling chronic diseases [36].

Four out of five cases of the global burden of CVDs occur in LMICs [37]. Although HIV/AIDS is the leading cause of death in sub-Saharan Africa, CVDs – predominantly stroke – are the most common cause of death among young adults aged 30 or older [38]. India has experienced CVD morbidity and mortality at an accelerated rate with as many as 32 million estimated to be living with ischaemic heart disease [39]. Effective community-based interventions aimed at reducing the risk factors for CVDs in LMICs have been limited to the urban poor [40].

The Heart of Soweto study in South Africa is a broad programme that was adapted to suit local needs. The programme included community-based screening for cardiovascular risk factors, clinical registry of tertiary cases of CVDs, secondary prevention programmes and extension to primary care clinics. The multi-drug regimen, polypill approach, may not have worked here as lipid disorder is not a major problem in urban African communities [37]. Targeting high-risk individuals with the polypill appears to work in some settings but not in others [38]. Advocates of this cost-effective multi-drug regimen, which is administered through primary healthcare centres, acknowledge that country-specific agenda and donor involvement are needed for addressing chronic CVDs in LMICs [41]. A population-based strategy for primary prevention to reduce risk factors through public promotion, legislative changes and government support will help to meet the challenges posed by the increasing burden of CVDs as well as other chronic diseases.

Health systems in LMICs are not well prepared to deal with cancer, despite the majority of the disease burden occurring in these countries [42, 43] (see also Adeloye and Grant, Chapter 2, this volume). Priority setting within health systems needs to be based on knowledge of the local cancer burden and mix of cancer types, and such data are still unavailable in large parts of the world [44]. The International Agency for Research on Cancer (IARC) estimated that over half of the 12.4 million incident cases and two-thirds of the 7.6 million cancer deaths arise in LMICs [44]. The types of cancer differ between high-income countries and LMICs, with stomach, liver, oral cavity and cervical cancer dominating the latter group. However, those cancers common in high-income countries – lung, breast, prostate and colorectal cancers – are rapidly increasing elsewhere [44]. Breast cancer is now the most, or second most, common cancer in women in all regions of the world [45]. Lung cancer, extremely rare at the start of the 20th century, is now one of the most common forms and is growing rapidly. In LMICs, the proportion of cancers attributable to chronic infection is 25%, while 12% is caused by tobacco. However, as the prevalence of tobacco smoking is rapidly increasing in LMICs, the delay – of around 40 years – between changes in smoking prevalence and disease rates means that the peak of smoking-related cancers is yet to occur in LMICs [44]. Priorities in LMICs for cancer control are 'tobacco control and (low-tech) screening for down-staging, with treatment frequently aimed at palliation'. [44]. Vaccinations against cervical and liver cancers and tobacco control can and should be implemented [46].

The absence of cancer specialists is frequently cited as a reason why the scale-up of cancer control cannot be expanded in low-income countries. One approach to overcoming this has been an international partnership, including Harvard Medical School, to provide support and training to physicians in rural Malawi, Rwanda and Haiti [43]. Physicians and nurses in these countries are now successfully delivering cancer care including chemotherapy, supported by remote consultants. Currently, this is a pilot project, and funding constraints prevent scale-up; however, it shows the potential for innovative solutions.

Finally, mental health remains a low priority for public financing in health systems globally, and for LMICs in particular [47], reflecting the stigma associated with mental ill health, with substantial proportions of costs being met by out-of-pocket payments (see also Huang *et al.*, Chapter 5, this volume). However, mental health has received increasing international attention in the last decade [48]. A recent review of the English-speaking Caribbean has demonstrated that – in those countries with well-developed primary healthcare systems – it is possible to improve mental health policies, funding, services and systems [49]. However, the authors note that mental health legislation often lags behind, even in those countries where substantial proportions of health budgets are committed to mental health (e.g. Jamaica, a middle-income country, where 6% of health budget expenditure is on mental health). In many LMICs, mental health services are not community based but remain in large, centrally located mental hospitals, especially in Africa [50]. Limited evidence from mental health professionals suggests that there is a preference for community-based mental healthcare, but that community primary healthcare workers would require substantial training and support in order to deliver such a model [50].

6.3 Health Systems: Building Blocks and NCDs

There are multiple ways of describing the functional components of a health system. The WHO uses a six 'building blocks' model (service delivery, workforce, information, technology, finance and governance) – albeit configured dependent upon local context conditions [4]. These six components represent the functions that a health system has to deliver if it is going to achieve its goals, and this model is probably the most widely used framework globally. We use these building blocks in order to examine the ways in which they are, or should, cope with NCDs.

6.3.1 Service delivery

Service delivery refers to the availability and distribution of health services. Service provision is the ultimate end result of the inputs that go into the health system in the form of stewardship and human/financial resources. Among the useful measures of health service delivery are access, availability, utilization and coverage [4]. The services must reach the target population they are intended for in a safe, timely, practical and culturally acceptable manner with minimum waste of resources. Quality of care is another dimension of service delivery.

Most LMICs have weak service delivery systems, which compounds the challenges of addressing the growing burden of NCDs. Chronic diseases require early detection, extended periods of care, sophisticated treatment for diseases like cancer, often monitoring of treatment adherence and palliative care. Tackling the growing burden of NCDs requires a strong primary healthcare system, which is compromised in most LMICs in terms of quality, weak structure, coverage and utilization [51]. Primary healthcare is the first point of contact between a patient and the healthcare system, which needs to be strengthened for continuity of care [5]. A study of care-seeking behaviour for fatal NCDs among women of reproductive age in a rural area in Bangladesh revealed that women delayed seeking treatment for chronic diseases due to the cost of services, the distance to health facilities, established contact with non-certified health providers and a lack of recognition of the severity of the problem [29]. Thus, many people in need of treatment are far removed or insulated, be it due to physical inaccessibility, cost or cultural reasons, from the formal health service delivery infrastructure. The utilization rate of basic health services is low in Bangladesh; the health success in the country has been achieved through innovative, context-specific interventions, in particular the strategy of taking high-priority services to households by fieldworkers [52, 53]. Much of the provision of health services in LMICs to date has been hospital or clinic based, for example the treatment of HIV/AIDS, which is increasingly viewed as a chronic disease.

There is a pressing need to extend the provision of health services to rural settings where health infrastructure for service delivery is lacking [21]. Among those with type 1 diabetes, insulin is essential for survival. Many afflicted with the condition do not have access to insulin, which then leads to deaths that could have been avoided [54]. Outreach services like satellite clinics and door step delivery among high-risk clusters are alternative means that could be explored; this approach has been successful in Bangladesh, in the Indian state of Tamil Nadu [55] and in rural Iran [36].

The INTERHEART and INTERSTROKE studies suggest that, globally, the risk factors for ischaemic heart disease and for stroke are similar – smoking, obesity, hypertension, dyslipidaemia, diabetes and inadequate consumption of fruits and vegetables [39]. A multi-drug combination is advocated to treat those who have been identified in primary care as being at high risk of CVDs, or for patients who have already had a clinical event [41]. A pre-requisite for this approach to work is utilization of health services; people need to be using health facilities in order to be identified as being high risk and therefore eligible for the intervention. An alternative strategy is a population-based approach for primary reduction of risks in the community to combat CVDs through public promotion and legislative changes [37].

The infrastructure for diagnosis and management of chronic respiratory diseases is either not available or is given low priority [56]. National priorities should determine whether countries adopt standardized management programmes for asthma and/or chronic obstructive pulmonary disease [57].

In low-income countries, cancer treatments and therapies are not universally available [44] (see also Adeloye and Grant, Chapter 2, this volume). Middle-income countries have treatment and diagnosis capacities but low resources for upgrading equipment, purchasing new drugs and training specialized health workers [44]. The concept of cancer control involves dealing with cancer at each stage of its development: primary prevention involves determining risk determinants and reducing exposure to them; secondary prevention involves detecting early-stage cancers through screening and then treating them; and tertiary prevention involves treating cancers that are more advanced [44]. Radiotherapy is an essential part of curative and palliative cancer treatment; however, there is a global shortage of radiotherapy machines, with over 30 countries in Africa and Asia having no services [44]. The strides that have been made in reducing cancer mortalities in high-income countries are not mirrored in other regions, as interventions for early detection and treatment are unavailable [43]. The Global Task Force on Expanded Access to Cancer Care and Control in Developing Countries (GTF.CCC) has called for expansion of 'coverage of existing vaccines, early detection and treatment of cancers for which cure or major improvements in life expectancy can be achieved, and palliation to reduce suffering and pain'. [43].

The WHO's six building blocks of a health system do not operate in a vacuum but re-enforce one another. A good health service delivery model is the result of committed governance and stewardship, which can successfully mobilize the human, financial and technological resources to meet the pressing health needs of the country. Health systems in LMICs are largely influenced by global policies and politics [18]. The alternating focus of the international health community between vertical and horizontal/integrated approaches to health service delivery since the 1960s at least partly explains why health systems in low-income countries have not evolved and strengthened over time [2].

Farmer *et al.* [43] called for a diagonal approach to meeting the challenge to health systems faced by cancer. Moving beyond the debates on the merits of vertical programmes – 'focused, proactive, disease-specific interventions on a massive scale' – versus horizontal programmes – 'more integrated, demand driven, resource-sharing health services' – a diagonal approach acknowledges the need for both to coexist [58]. Such an approach entails 'the proactive, supply-driven provision of a set of highly cost-effective interventions on a large scale that bridges health clinics and homes' [58]. This means health system strengthening simultaneously with disease focus: 'Strategies include: awareness building and services for prevention; management of infections and adverse drug reactions; community-based care and support; education to combat stigma; provision of pathological testing for accurate and timely diagnoses; and surgical support where indicated.'[43]. A diagonal approach would help to link and integrate cancer care and control with other health services, reinforcing human resources and physical infrastructure, while avoiding parallel structures in service delivery [43].

There are recent examples of innovative methods of health system strengthening and integration for the effective delivery of health services. Ethiopia and Malawi have used funding for HIV/AIDS to strengthen primary healthcare centres that can be used as a platform for providing services for NCD prevention and treatment. In South-east Asian countries such as Thailand, Vietnam, Cambodia and Burma, instead of introducing separate vertical programmes for diabetes and hypertension, these have been integrated with HIV/AIDs service delivery [7].

6.3.2 Health workforce

Task shifting has been suggested by the WHO as an innovation for scaling-up provision of chronic HIV treatment, and the same should be considered for chronic NCD treatment. Essential activities, such as detection and monitoring of risk factors, initiation and monitoring of treatments, can be moved from physicians to nurses or other health or community workers [21]. Holistic responses to staff shortages have been seen in Cambodia, Ethiopia and Malawi [7]. Health workers (and even lay people) will need to play a role in supporting patients in self-management of their chronic disease, and there is evidence that such strategies have led to improvements in disease outcomes resulting from improved body mass index and blood pressure [21].

A review of chronic disease care in Thailand called for adaptations to human resource strategies to cope with a move beyond prevention-based NCD interventions towards approaches for the treatment and long-term management of NCDs [59]. Thailand has seen success in providing affordable and sustainable long-term care for HIV patients, a model that could be replicated for NCDs: stable patients were distributed from provincial hospitals to local clinics by building AIDS care and management capabilities throughout all levels, particularly relying on nurses. The model is one of decentralized NCD care, necessitating capacity building at community hospitals and local primary care centres [59].

One frequently cited reason as to why the scale-up of cancer control cannot be expanded in low-income countries is the lack of cancer specialists. As mentioned above, an international partnership, including Harvard Medical School, is now providing support and training to physicians in rural Malawi, Rwanda and Haiti [43]. Cancer care including chemotherapy is now delivered by the physicians and nurses in these countries, supported by remote consultants. Although this is a currently a pilot project and funding constraints prevent scale-up, it nevertheless shows the potential for innovative solutions.

6.3.3 Information systems

Health information systems need to be considered at both the clinical individual level and the management level. In general, surveillance of NCDs had not been well integrated into national health information systems in LMICs [6]. The long-term care requirements of chronic conditions are inherently different from the care requirements of acute conditions. Chronic NCDs place a new importance on health information systems, as they need a greater level of organization, often over a patient's lifetime [21]. Clinical monitoring systems can be used to 'identify patients' needs, plan care over time, monitor responses to treatment and assess health outcomes' [21]. Individual patients can be monitored by paper-based records, although these are likely to be superseded by IT systems, including mobile phone technology [21]. In Nigeria, for example, smart phones have been used to monitor patients with tuberculosis, and these lessons could be transferred to support the supervision of patients with chronic NCDs [60]. Kaufman *et al.* (2011) [59] pointed out the need for capacity building in Thailand to focus not only on treatment and management of NCDs but also on reorganizing patient records, drug procurement and storage systems, and on initial reporting [59].

At the management level, the key reason for having effective information systems is to enable monitoring and evaluation of health system performance as measured by selected indicators. South Africa has successfully streamlined its health information system in response to ineffective data collection and poor-quality data [61, 62]. The prior system of uncoordinated but large-scale data collection for numerous programmes (e.g. HIV/AIDS, tuberculosis, and maternal and child health) was producing poor-quality data, was duplicative and was a burden to the health workforce. In response, a system based on essential data was implemented as a major component of the District Health Information System. All programmes were monitored through 75 indicators, and these were continually reviewed over time. Furthermore, each level of the health system was allowed to develop its own data set within the larger framework. Through this mechanism, the system has been effective in providing data at local and national levels [61, 62].

An information-related aspect of NCDs is the implementation and use of guidelines for standardized management and treatment. In reference to chronic respiratory diseases, Aït-Khaled *et al.* [57] stated that, while such guidelines have been proposed for high-income countries, they are rare elsewhere. They recommended that guidelines be adapted to the local context and distributed, in addition to regular, continual monitoring and evaluation of performance indicators.

6.3.4 Medical products, vaccines and technologies

Reducing the burden of NCDs requires a range of technological interventions, which can be used effectively in LMICs. As the technology of interventions to reduce the mortality of those with NCDs is developed, the fixed costs for the health system increase [16]. This is because of an expectation of a lifelong commitment to manage an NCD, which might involve multiple acute episodes. LMICs have to deal with the dual burden of basic/primary healthcare – including essential medicines and technologies – alongside rising demand for goods and services related to NCDs (co-morbidities notwithstanding). Healthcare planners need to identify producers of high-quality generic drugs at affordable prices, add to national lists of essential drugs and consider procurement implications [57]. There is also a need to ensure that health service providers are trained in any new technologies so that they can be delivered effectively.

Production of cheaper, efficacious generic drugs for mental health treatment makes such treatment more accessible in LMICs [28]. However, such developments need to be accompanied by commodity chain improvements in logistics and procurement to eliminate stock-outs. Recombinant therapeutic proteins have been identified as a promising technology for LMICs in tackling NCDs [63], by inserting a gene(s) for a therapeutic protein into a suitable organism (e.g. yeast). Such technology is increasingly being developed by LMIC-based entrepreneurs [63].

Access to medicines in general in LMICs is a complex public health issue, reflecting in part the ability of countries to pay for new medical products that demand high prices in order to recover their high research and development costs. Recent evidence suggests that pharmaceutical manufacturers do not set their prices (including those for NCD treatment) on the basis of a country's income (ability to pay), meaning that LMICs are subject to significant market access restrictions to pharmaceuticals [64]. Mendis *et al.* (2007) [65] assessed the affordability and availability of 32 medicines for the treatment of five NCDs in six LMICs (Bangladesh, Brazil, Malawi, Nepal, Pakistan and Sri Lanka) and found generally low availability of these drugs in the public sector. They concluded that education – of both consumers and healthcare professionals – was essential in order to improve the use of generic medicines in order to improve drug affordability and availability [65].

The interplay between finance and research and development must be considered. It has been suggested that investment in vaccines for infectious diseases in LMICs was in large part reliant on donor funding, without which there would be no market for these vaccines against infectious diseases, which now occur primarily in LMICs [66]. It remains a paradox that many NCDs such as cancer have substantial global research and development investment – much higher than that for neglected tropical diseases [67] – but that this is not translated into affordable and accessible NCD pharma in LMICs, because in such settings the market is not (yet) profitable, although this will change as LMIC populations age and become relatively wealthier. Relatively few efficacy trials for the treatment of NCDs have been performed in LMICs, especially in sub-Saharan Africa [11].

Aït-Khaled *et al.* (2001) [57] discussed chronic respiratory diseases, suggesting that international agencies take the lead in defining essential drugs and equipment and promoting the use of generic drugs, especially for high doses of inhaled corticosteroids, thus making high-quality drugs available at low cost. This would involve the identification of high-quality generic drugs, and national governments adding these to lists of essential drugs and procurement systems. The authors also identified the upgrading of equipment at the district level as another priority area for tackling chronic respiratory disease [57]. New technologies – such as mobile phones – are beginning to be harnessed to deliver individual behavioural change interventions (risk reduction and/or treatment adherence) [68, 69]. NCD programmes can learn from successful interventions in other health conditions such as anti-malaria medicines in Tanzania [7].

6.3.5 Financing

Fiscal resource constraints are a major impediment to the establishment and sustainability of effective health systems management and prevention of NCDs. Healthcare planners and policy makers are faced with changes in behaviour, such as increases in tobacco use, in LMICs against a backdrop of limited fiscal resources [57]. The chronic nature of NCDs has very specific implications for individuals and their families, as expensive and long-term treatment might consume savings or lead to catastrophic costs. In most low-income countries, people pay for the majority of health services that they use – meaning that poorer people with chronic conditions are significantly disadvantaged in accessing healthcare. Even where user fees generate revenue and/or reduce inappropriate service use for health systems, they continue to be a major barrier to use for the poorest.

The majority (60%) of healthcare in LMICs is financed by out-of-pocket expenses, which patients pay for at the point of delivery, compared with 20% in high-income countries [6]. This is unsustainable, particularly so as the level of chronic NCDs rises. High-income countries are almost four times more likely to have NCD services covered by health insurance than low-income countries, meaning that populations in settings with inadequate coverage by health insurance schemes are unlikely to be able to access essential NCD interventions [26].

There are increasing examples of low-cost and cost-effective interventions for NCDs. Financing for universal coverage has been seen in Rwanda where funding from HIV programmes has been used to expand health insurance coverage for poorer people to improve access to health services, including those for NCDs [7]. Social insurance schemes that include NCDs have been demonstrated in Kyrgyzstan, Mexico and Thailand [7], and there are even examples of LMICs with inclusion of cancer treatment in national health insurance programmes: Mexico and Colombia [43]. Healthcare financing and access to treatment for NCDs are being promoted in Pakistan using mobile phones [7].

The ability of health systems to convert public spending on NCDs into improved health outcomes cannot be assumed [9]. There remains a need for all of the functioning components of the health system, from monitoring and surveillance to health information systems, to work together.

Clinical social franchising is a private sector effort to achieve social goals and improve healthcare using a commercial franchise model. A social franchise is a network of private providers operating under contracts with a common agency that provides a common brand of products and services [53]. The model is increasingly being used in LMICs, one of the largest being the USAID-funded NGO Health Service Delivery Program in Bangladesh, which provides primarily family planning and maternal and child health services but also referral for tuberculosis and limited services for other chronic diseases to a catchment population of roughly 20 million in the country [70]. A systematic review of 23 franchises across the globe suggested that franchises in certain contexts can significantly outperform other models of healthcare, particularly in areas of increased client volume and client satisfaction [53].

6.3.6 Leadership/governance

Governance is central and overarches the other building blocks as it lays out the guiding principles, policies and framework of a health system. Leadership or stewardship involves effective implementation of the strategic policy framework through proper oversight, forging strategic partnerships, continuous monitoring and accountability. Accountability has been an increasingly important component of governance with the advent of increased funding through sources such as the Global Alliance for Vaccines and Immunization (GAVI) and Global Fund, and a growing demand to demonstrate results and aid effectiveness.

In 2000, the World Health Assembly endorsed the global strategy for NCD prevention and control, urging member states to develop a national policy to address the growing burden of these diseases. An action plan for implementing the global strategy for NCD prevention and control was drawn up in 2008. Most LMICs still do not have a national NCD policy, which at least partly reflects weak national capacity for policy formation and implementation [5]. Poor stewardship in harnessing an effective health system has been cited as reflecting the wider failure of governance in the country as a whole [18].

A strong case has been made for the adoption of a single NCD policy to address the four major chronic diseases that share common behavioural risk factors [5]. The determinants of the NCDs are outside the health sector and, as such, a national multi-sectoral approach is needed to provide a common platform to combine approaches that involve interventions at the population level and with target groups, combined with legislative change and regulation. Co-morbidities are common, in particular, diabetes with CVDs. Chronic renal disease is related to the four main NCDs, as it is often the result of a failure to address hypertension and diabetes [5]. Thus, some of the neglected NCDs can also be brought under the jurisdiction of the health system with the effective adoption of a single NCD policy. Integration will undoubtedly ensure more efficient use of scarce resources in LMICs. Continuous monitoring and evaluation of interventions are key to assessing their effectiveness [71].

A recent review of Bangladesh, Ethiopia, Kyrgyzstan, Thailand and the Indian state of Tamil Nadu have identified good governance and political commitment as the driving forces facilitating the favourable health outcomes in these regions relative to similar LMICs [18]. Bangladesh has continued to pursue four innovative health policies, despite major political regime changes. These include a population and family planning policy in close partnership with donors and NGO partners, a drug policy to make essential drugs affordable, an initiative to provide door step family planning and maternal and child health services through an extensive network of fieldworkers, and a broad-based policy outside the health sector that focused on increasing levels of education, female empowerment, communication infrastructure and access to mobile technology. Ethiopia, like Bangladesh, has had a turbulent past sharing a common history of civil war, a series of famines, natural calamities and political unrest. Unlike most other LMICs, these two countries have successfully utilized the development assistance they received to expand the health workforce and infrastructure and to ensure a steady supply of drugs. The health success in Kyrgyzstan has been attributed to able leadership who brought about legislative changes for health reform. The health sector in Thailand received patronage from health ministers and senior staff, as well as from the Thai royal family.

6.4 Health System Strengthening and NCDs in LMICs

There is no consensus about what health system strengthening is [2], and there are multiple approaches to health system strengthening [72, 73] and a lack of clarity about the direction that future health system strengthening should take

[74]. The WHO definition serves as a departure point: 'Health system strengthening [i]s defined as improving these six health system building blocks and managing their interactions in ways that achieve more equitable and sustained improvements across health services and health outcomes. It requires both technical and political knowledge and action' [4]. This WHO model is supported by some authors but not universally [73], and there are suggestions that improving health system responsiveness might be a more effective way forward [7].

The 2008 G8 Summit in Tokyo, Japan, focused on three aspects of health system performance – financing, information and the health workforce – and led to a strong G8 commitment for collective action in health system strengthening in low-income countries. Issues of country capacity and ownership in health policy making and implementation remain underdeveloped [72]. The WHO 2008–2013 Action Plan for addressing NDCs in LMICs outlined three main activities: (i) mapping the emergence and consequences of an evolving epidemic; (ii) reducing exposure to common factors; and (iii) strengthening healthcare resources [37]. However, individualized interventions to prevent and reduce NCDs need a well-functioning health system, and it has been argued that NCDs are a 'litmus test' for health systems in LMICs [6].

Many global health initiatives (often condition-specific) incorporate health system strengthening – both directly and indirectly [74]. However, such global health initiatives can lead to a mismatch between activities and resources, and a 2009 review underscored the limited evidence base to show that global health initiatives (e.g. The Global Fund to fight AIDS, Tuberculosis and Malaria (GFATM) and GAVI) had been effective in improving country health systems [75]. Balabanova *et al.* (2010) [18], following a review of GAVI and GFATM, concluded that there was a risk that health system strengthening efforts might 'simply aggravate the current crowded scene of diverse global initiatives'.

While there is increasing agreement that strengthened health systems are essential for improving health outcomes, especially in LMICs, there is less consensus about how to make health systems stronger [74, 75]. There are concerns that a focus on Millennium Development Goal health targets (which do not include an explicit mention of NCDs) has led to too narrow a concentration on Millennium Development Goal-central issues, such as maternal, neonatal and child health, and HIV, without a broader development of the health systems that underpin health improvements [76]. It has also been said that health systems themselves 'have an image problem' [76] – issues such as accountability or planning are less visible or emotive (relative to, for example, child deaths) and thus do not engender the same financial and political support.

The Innovative Care for Chronic Conditions Framework – adapted from the Chronic Care Model (2002) – identifies core building blocks to design health systems in LMICs in order to cope with long-term health conditions. Substantial evidence from high-income countries with strong health systems suggests that this approach is effective; it focuses on partnerships that support patient and family interactions, healthcare organization and community, and a well-coordinated policy and health systems environment. The evidence base for whether this approach works in LMICs is poorly developed and restricted to pilot and small-scale projects, not least because the resource and capacity implications of delivering such a framework is likely to be beyond the scope of many LMICs. Instead, some authors ask how health systems for NCDs in LMICs can build on the achievements of health system strengthening for other outcomes, such as maternal and newborn health [6]. How can NCDs build on the synergies identified by approaches to tackle HIV and tuberculosis, for example? Atun *et al.* (2013) [7] suggested that there are 'unexploited opportunities' for the integration of NCD activities with other health initiatives – for example, through repeated contact with sexual and reproductive health and antenatal care services, which many people – particularly women – use repeatedly over their life course.

6.5 Looking Ahead

Dealing with NCDs equitably represents one strategy for reducing poverty and fostering development in LMICs. Country and global leadership is needed to support health system investment for synergy between vertical and horizontal programmes in LMICs. To date, there have been sporadic and haphazard efforts for partial strengthening of health systems by several agencies with direct support for their own activities, producing an international health architecture that is already complex and fragmented. Different donor funds and agencies fund different elements of health systems with poor coordination, communication and high transaction costs. Integration of health service delivery will create links between prevention and treatment. This synergy is needed for the long-term management of chronic disorders such as HIV/AIDS, diabetes, CVDs and mental illnesses, which require a similar input [18]. An integrated management of a range of chronic diseases in primary care settings is the way forward for LMICs that are faced with a rising burden of NCDs [21]. A single national NCD policy is being advocated by some as a route to ensure the most efficient use of scarce human and financial resources in LMICs [5], although the problem of how to make health systems accountable while avoiding the unintended consequences or pitfalls of targets that distort health system behaviour remains [18].

Our review has shown a large (and growing) number of small-scale and pilot interventions with potentially successful models; we need to understand how effective they might be in health systems with multiple actors (state, private or third sector), and the challenges in taking these pilot interventions to scale. The majority of evidence about what works (effective and cost-effective) in scaling-up NCD interventions is still rooted overwhelmingly in high-income countries – meaning that the limited evidence base of successful NCD interventions in LMICs undermines the potential for evidence-based decision making. A part of this strategy must include how to build research capacity so that the high-quality research that is context-specifically relevant is both produced and consumed by LMICs. The failure to tackle NCDs, to reflect the burden of disease they represent, is argued to be a political failure, rather than a technical problem [77]. The authors argue that, against this backdrop of increasing evidence about what works, there is a need for three strategies to reframe approaches to NCDs: (i) emphasize the interrelationships between NCD, poverty and development; (ii) focus on avoidable mortality as the basis for equitable resource mobilization; and (iii) keep up the pressure established by the United Nations High Level Meeting on NCDs [13, 14, 51].

How will individual health systems cope with the scale of the issue of NCDs as their populations pass through the epidemiological transition and age [78]? Currently, more than 90% of premature mortality attributable to NCDs occurs in LMICs. Nation states need to consider how (and whether) to shift health from a sectoral activity to a 'broad-based multisectoral coalition' in order to tackle issues such as alcohol-related illnesses and obesity [79]. Linked to this are broad questions about whether, and how, there should be a different vision, one that moves away from a narrow focus on health system strengthening towards a broader agenda with coherent policies across a range of sectors (e.g. trade policy, food standards, intellectual property and inequality). For example, enriched genetically modified crops might play a future role in preventing NCDs.

Daar *et al.* [80] used the Delphi method to identify the 'grand challenges' in chronic NCDs and identified six major issues: (i) raising public awareness; (ii) an improved policy environment; (iii) reduced risk factors; (iv) involvement of businesses and communities; (v) addressing the inter-relationships between poverty and urbanization; and (vi) health system reorientation. For example, NCDs were absent from the Millennium Development Goals (agenda and indicators), and the post-2015 agenda should include a global chronic disease goal in order to deal with this lacuna (see Mendis and Chestnov, Chapter 12, this volume). To date, the international donor community has not been particularly forthcoming in making NCD funding, prevention and control a priority, and there is no equivalent to GAVI and GFATM for addressing NCDs.

Health systems in LMICs include a wide range of actors, including: civil society, bi/multi-lateral aid agencies, fixed-base operators and the traditional health sector. These actors are rarely considered in strategies to tackle NCD prevention and care. Traditions of community-based care are rarely considered in strategies to deal with the treatment and management of NCDs. In order to harness these potential resources, there is a need to consider how to develop sustained civil society engagement and advocacy (e.g. patient groups) around NCDs (see also de-Graft Aikins *et al.*, Chapter 9, this volume). Strengthening primary healthcare is just one way to improve NCD prevention and identification, requiring strategies to bring more people into contact with health service points, especially those who are rural and poor. The issue then becomes how to include NCDs in the basic package of essential health services, with an emphasis on those delivered by primary care. We have a relatively poor understanding of the beliefs and attitudes of LMIC healthcare providers towards NCDs, which are likely to influence people's ability to access high-quality NCD care [11].

Broader social mobilization (e.g. the use of traditional and mass media for tobacco control) is one component of this. How can health systems (including traditional- and community-based care) change to provide person-centred care and self-management in order to effectively manage risk factors, episodes of illness and multi-morbidity, in addition to the more traditional patient care? What are the opportunities to focus on modifiable known risk factors (e.g. physical inactivity, an unhealthy diet, and alcohol and tobacco consumption) to encourage individualized risk profiling and management, building on success from elsewhere [81–85]?

Strategies to deal with NCDs need to be context-specific and take account of the demographic change in LMICs. For example, how can continuity of care be provided for NCDs against a backdrop of high levels of population mobility, especially in urban areas in LMICs [11]? Urban–rural differentials in many LMICs mean that this dimension needs to be taken into account. We know that the prevalence of many NCDs is higher in urban areas, and coverage of and access to health services is better in urban areas [86]. Future interventions need to consider how to be effective in the prevention and care of NCDs in rural settings [36], including the need to improve surveillance of NCDs in LMICs, taking into account urban–rural differentials [11].

References

1. Rechel, B., Thomson, S. and van Ginneken, E. (2010) *Health Systems in Transition Template for Authors*. World Health Organization, Denmark, on behalf of the European Observatory on Health Systems and Policies 2010.
2. Smith, R.D. and Hanson, K. (2011) *What is a Health System? Health Systems in Low- and Middle-Income Countries: an Economic and Policy Perspective*. Oxford University Press, Oxford, UK.
3. Bloom, G. and Standing, H. (2008) Future health systems: why future? Why now? *Social Science and Medicine* 66, 2067–2075.
4. WHO (2007) *Everybody's Business: Strengthening Health Systems to Improve Health Outcomes: WHO's framework for action*. World Health Organization, Geneva, Switzerland.
5. Mendis, S. and Fuster, V. (2009) National policies and strategies for noncommunicable diseases. *Nature Reviews Cardiology* 6, 723–727.
6. Samb, B., Desai, N., Nishtar, S., Mendis, S., Bekedam, H., Wright, A., Hsu, J., Martiniuk, A., Celletti, F., Patel, K., Adshead, F., McKee, M., Evans, T., Alwan, A. and Etienne, C. (2010) Prevention and management of chronic disease: a litmus test for health-systems strengthening in low-income and middle-income countries. *Lancet* 376, 1785–1797.
7. Atun, R., Jaffar, S., Nishtar, S., Knaul, F.M., Barreto, M.L., Nyirenda, M., Banatvala, N. and Piot, P. *(*2013) Improving responsiveness of health systems to non-communicable diseases. *Lancet* 381, 690–697.
8. Abegunde, D.O., Mathers, C.D., Adam, T., Ortegon, M. and Strong, K. (2007) The burden and costs of chronic diseases in low-income and middle-income countries. *Lancet* 370, 1929–1938.
9. Adeyi, O., Smith, O. and Robles, S. (2007) Public policy and the challenge of chronic noncommunicable diseases. The World Bank, Washington, DC. <http://siteresources.worldbank.org/INTPH/Resources/PublicPolicyandNCDsWorldBank2007FullReport.pdf>.
10. WHO (2011) *Global Status Report on Noncommunicable Diseases 2010*. World Health Organization, Geneva, Switzerland.
11. Unwin, N., Setel, P., Rashid, S., Mugusi, F., Mbanya, J.C., Kitange, H., Hayes, L., Edwards, R., Aspray, T. and Alberti, K.G. (2002) Noncommunicable diseases in sub-Saharan Africa: where do they feature in the health research agenda? *Bulletin of the World Health Organization* 79, 947–953.
12. Atun, R.A., Gurol-Urganci, I. and McKee, M. (2009) Health systems and increased longevity in people with HIV and AIDS. *British Medical Journal* 338, b2165.
13. Beaglehole, R., Bonita, R., Horton, R., Adams, C., Alleyne, G., Asaria, P., Baugh, V., Bekedam, H., Billo, N., Casswell, S. *et al.* (2011) Priority actions for the non-communicable disease crisis. *Lancet* 377, 1438–1447.
14. Stuckler, D., Basu, S. and McKee, M. (2011) Commentary: UN high level meeting on non-communicable diseases: an opportunity for whom? *British Medical Journal* 343, d5336.

15. WHO (2008) *2008–2013 Action Plan for the Global Strategy for the Prevention and Control of Noncommunicable Diseases*. World Health Organization, Geneva, Switzerland.
16. Allotey, P., Reidpath, D.D., Yasin, S., Chan, C.K. and de-Graft Aikins, A. (2011) Rethinking health-care systems: a focus on chronicity. *Lancet* 377, 450–451.
17. Sanders, D. and Haines, A. (2006) Implementation research is needed to achieve international health goals. *PLoS Medicine* 3, e186.
18. Balabanova, D., McKee, M., Mills, A., Walt, G. and Haines, A. (2010) What can global health institutions do to help strengthen health systems in low income countries? *Health Research Policy and Systems* 8, 22.
19. Woodward, D., Drager, N., Beaglehole, R. and Lipson, D. (2001) Globalization and health: a framework for analysis and action. *Bulletin of the World Health Organization* 79, 875–881.
20. Asaria, P., Chisholm, D., Mathers, C., Ezzati, M. and Beaglehole, R. (2007) Chronic disease prevention: health effects and financial costs of strategies to reduce salt intake and control tobacco use. *Lancet* 370, 2044–2053.
21. Beaglehole, R., Epping-Jordan, J., Patel, V., Chopra, M., Ebrahim, S., Kidd, M. and Haines, A. (2008) Improving the prevention and management of chronic disease in low-income and middle-income countries: a priority for primary health care. *Lancet* 372, 940–949.
22. Ngo, V.K., Rubinstein, A., Ganju, V., Kanellis, P., Loza, N., Rabadan-Diehl, C. and Daar, A.S. (2013) Grand challenges: integrating mental health care into the non-communicable disease agenda. *PLoS Medicine* 10, e1001443.
23. WHO (2000) *The World Health Report 2000: Health Systems: Improving Performance*. World Health Organization, Geneva, Switzerland.
24. WHO (2002) *Innovative Care for Chronic Conditions: Building Blocks for Action: Global Report*. World Health Organization, Geneva, Switzerland.
25. WHO (2012) *65th World Health Assembly. Prevention and Control of Noncommunicable Disease*. World Health Organization, Geneva, Switzerland.
26. WHO (2013) Noncommunicable diseases: Fact sheet. World Health Organization, Geneva, Switzerland <http://www.who.int/mediacentre/factsheets/fs355/en/>.
27. Mazumder, D.N.G., Haque, R., Ghosh, N., De, B.K., Santra, A., Chakraborti, D. and Smith, A.H. (2000) Arsenic in drinking water and the prevalence of respiratory effects in West Bengal, India. *International Journal of Epidemiology* 29, 1047–1052.
28. Jenkins, R., Baingana, F., Ahmad, R., McDaid, D. and Atun, R. (2011) Health system challenges and solutions to improving mental health outcomes. *Mental Health in Family Medicine* 8, 119.
29. Sikder, S., Labrique, A., Ullah, B., Mehra, S., Rashid, M., Ali, H., Jahan, N., Shamim, A.A., West, K.P. Jr and Christian, P. (2012) Care-seeking patterns for fatal non-communicable diseases among women of reproductive age in rural northwest Bangladesh. *BMC Women's Health* 12, 23.
30. Hansen, M.A., Gluckman, P.D., Ma, R.C., Matzen, P. and Biesma, R.G. (2012) Early life opportunities for prevention of diabetes in low and middle income countries. *BMC Public Health* 12, 1025.
31. Wild, S., Roglic, G., Green, A., Sicree R and King, H. (2004) Global prevalence of diabetes: estimates for the year 2000 and projections for 2030. *Diabetes Care* 27, 1047–1053.
32. King, H., Keuky, L., Seng, S., Khun, T., Roglic, G. and Pinget, M. (2005) Diabetes and associated disorders in Cambodia: two epidemiological surveys. *Lancet* 366, 1633–1639.
33. Saquib, N., Khanam, M.A., Saquib, J., Anand, S., Chertow, G.M., Barry, M., Ahmed, T. and Cullen, M.R. (2013) High prevalence of type 2 diabetes among the urban middle class in Bangladesh. *BMC Public Health* 13, 1032.
34. Hwang, C.K., Han, P.V., Zabetian, A., Ali, M.K. and Narayan, K.M. (2012) Rural diabetes prevalence quintuples over twenty-five years in low- and middle-income countries: a systematic review and meta-analysis. *Diabetes Research and Clinical Practice* 96, 271–285.

35. Weber, M.B., Ranjani, H., Meyers, G.C., Mohan, V. and Narayan, K.M. (2011) A model of translational research for diabetes prevention in low and middle-income countries: The Diabetes Community Lifestyle Improvement Program (D-CLIP) trial. *Primary Care Diabetes* 6, 3–9.
36. Farzadfar, F., Murray, C.J., Gakidou, E., Bossert, T., Namdaritabar, H., Alikhani, S., Moradi, G., Delavari, A., Jamshidi, H. and Ezzati, M. (2012) Effectiveness of diabetes and hypertension management by rural primary health-care workers (Behvarz workers) in Iran: a nationally representative observational study. *Lancet* 379, 47–54.
37. Stewart, S. and Sliwa, K. (2009) Preventing CVD in resource-poor areas: perspectives from the 'real-world'. *Nature Reviews Cardiology* 6, 489–492.
38. Gaziano, T.A. (2007) Reducing the growing burden of cardiovascular disease in the developing world. *Health Affairs (Millwood)* 26, 13–24.
39. Paradis, G. and Chiolero, A. (2011) The cardiovascular and chronic diseases epidemic in low- and middle-income countries: a global health challenge. *Journal of the American College of Cardiology* 57, 1775–1777.
40. van de Vijver, S., Oti, S., Addo, J., de Graft-Aikins, A. and Agyemang, C. (2012) Review of community-based interventions for prevention of cardiovascular diseases in low- and middle-income countries. *Ethnicity and Health* 17, 651–676.
41. Lim, S.S., Gaziano, T.A., Gakidou, E., Reddy, K.S., Farzadfar, F., Lozano, R. and Rodgers, A. (2007) Prevention of cardiovascular disease in high-risk individuals in low-income and middle-income countries: health effects and costs. *Lancet* 370, 2054–2062.
42. Kanavos, P. (2006) The rising burden of cancer in the developing world. *Annals of Oncology* 17 (Suppl. 8), viii15–viii23.
43. Farmer, P., Frenk, J., Knaul, F.M., Shulman, L.N., Alleyne, G., Armstrong, L., Atun, R., Blayney, D., Chen, L., Feachem, R., Gospodarowicz, M., Gralow, J., Gupta, S., Langer, A., Lob-Levyt, J., Neal, C., Mbewu, A., Mired, D., Piot, P., Reddy, K.S., Sachs, J.D., Sarhan, M. and Seffrin, J.R. (2010) Expansion of cancer care and control in countries of low and middle income: a call to action. *Lancet* 376, 1186–1193.
44. Boyle, P. and Levin, B. (2008) *World Cancer Report 2008*. International Agency for Research on Cancer, Lyon, France.
45. Boyle, P. and Howell, A. (2010) The globalisation of breast cancer. *Breast Cancer Research* 12, S7.
46. Boyle, P. (2006) The globalisation of cancer. *Lancet* 368, 629–630.
47. Dixon, A., McDaid, D., Knapp, M. and Curran, C. (2006) Financing mental health services in low- and middle-income countries. *Health Policy and Planning* 21, 171–182.
48. Sabir, A.B. and Iftikhar, R. (2006) Promotion of mental health in developing countries: a conceptual system. *Primary Care Mental Health* 4, 29–36.
49. Abel, W., Kestel, D., Eldemire-Shearer, D., Sewell, C. and Whitehorne-Smith, P. (2012) Mental health policy and service system development in the English-speaking Caribbean. *West Indian Medical Journal* 61, 475–482.
50. Alem, A., Jacobsson, L. and Hanlon, C. (2008) Community-based mental health care in Africa: mental health workers' views. *World Psychiatry* 7, 54–57.
51. Beaglehole, R. and Horton, R. (2010) Chronic diseases: global action must match global evidence. *Lancet* 376, 1619–1621.
52. Chowdhury, A.M., Bhuiya, A., Chowdhury, M.E., Rasheed, S., Hussain, Z. and Chen, L.C. (2013) The Bangladesh paradox: exceptional health achievement despite economic poverty. *Lancet* 382, 1734–1745.
53. Beyeler, N., York De La Cruz, A. and Montagu, D. (2013) The impact of clinical social franchising on health services in low-and middle-income countries: a systematic review. *PLoS One* 8, e60669.
54. Gill, G., Yudkin, J., Keen, H. and Beran, D. (2011) The insulin dilemma in resource-limited countries. A way forward? *Diabetologia* 54, 19–24.

55. Balabanova, D., Mills, A., Conteh, L., Akkazieva, B., Banteyerga, H., Dash, U., Gilson, L., Harmer, A., Ibraimova, A., Islam, Z., Kidanu, A., Koehlmoos, T.P., Limwattananon, S., Muraleedharan, V.R., Murzalieva, G., Palafox, B., Panichkriangkrai, W., Patcharanarumol, W., Penn-Kekana, L., Powell-Jackson, T., Tangcharoensathien, V. and McKee, M. (2013) Good health at low cost 25 years on: lessons for the future of health systems strengthening. *Lancet* 381, 2118–2133.
56. Bousquet, J., Dahl, R. and Khaltaev, N. (2007) Global alliance against chronic respiratory diseases. *Allergy* 62, 216–223.
57. Aït-Khaled, N., Enarson, D. and Bousquet, J. (2001) Chronic respiratory diseases in developing countries: the burden and strategies for prevention and management. *Bulletin of the World Health Organization* 79, 971–979.
58. Sepulveda, J. (2006) Foreword. In: Jamison, D.T., Breman, J.G., Measham, A.R., Alleyne, G., Claeson, M., Evans, D.B., Jha, P., Mills, A. and Musgrove, P. (eds) *Disease Control Priorities in Developing Countries.* Oxford University Press, New York, and The World Bank Washington, DC, pp. xiii–xvi.
59. Kaufman, N.D., Chasombat, S., Tanomsingh, S., Rajataramya, B. and Potempa, K. (2011) Public health in Thailand: emerging focus on non-communicable diseases. *International Journal of Health Planning and Management* 26, e197–e212.
60. Dieng, A. and Ekbladh, L. (2012) *Smartphones Improve Supportive Supervision for Tuberculosis in Nigeria.* Health Systems 20/20, Bethesda, Maryland.
61. Shaw, V. (2005) Health information system reform in South Africa: developing an essential data set. *Bulletin of the World Health Organization* 83, 632–636.
62. Prata, N. (2008) Sub-Saharan Africa, health systems of. In: Heggenhougen, K. (ed.) *International Encyclopedia of Public Health.* Academic Press, Oxford, UK, pp. 250–257.
63. Acharya, T., Kennedy, R., Daar, A.S. and Singer, P.A. (2004) Biotechnology to improve health in developing countries: a review. *Memórias do Instituto Oswaldo Cruz* 99, 341–350.
64. Srivastava, D. and McGuire, A. (2013) *Analysis of Prices Paid by Low-income Countries – How Price Sensitive is Government Demand for Medicines?* Working Paper No: 35/2013. London School of Economics. London, UK.
65. Mendis, S., Fukino, K., Cameron, A., Laing, R., Filipe, A. Jr, Khatib, O., Leowski, J. and Ewen, M. (2007) The availability and affordability of selected essential medicines for chronic diseases in six low-and middle-income countries. *Bulletin of the World Health Organization* 85, 279–288.
66. Anderson, G.F. and Chu, E. (2007) Expanding priorities – confronting chronic disease in countries with low income. *New England Journal of Medicine* 356, 209–211.
67. Trouiller, P., Olliaro, P., Torreele, E., Orbinski, J., Laing, R. and Ford, N. (2002) Drug development for neglected diseases: a deficient market and a public-health policy failure. *Lancet* 359, 2188–2194.
68. Nishtar, S., Khalid, F., Ikram, A., Kazi, A., Mirza, Y.A., Khattak, I.U.H., Javad, A., Jaffer, H., Brown K and Badsha, T. (2010) *Protecting the Poor Against Health Impoverishment in Pakistan: Proof of Concept of the Potential Within Innovative Web and Mobile Phone Technologies.* World Health Report 2010, Background Paper 55. World Health Organization, Geneva, Switzerland.
69. Howitt, P., Darzi, A., Yang, G.Z., Ashrafian, H., Atun, R., Barlow, J., Blakemore, A., Bull, A.M., Car, J., Conteh, L., Cooke, G.S., Ford, N., Gregson, S.A., Kerr, K., King, D., Kulendran, M., Malkin, R.A., Majeed, A., Matlin, S., Merrifield, R., Penfold, H.A., Reid, S.D., Smith, P.C., Stevens, M.M., Templeton, M.R., Vincent, C. and Wilson, E. (2012) Technologies for global health. *Lancet* 380, 507–535.
70. Lance, P., Angeles, G. and Kamal, N. (2012) *Smiling Sun Franchise Program (BSSFP) Impact Evaluation Report.* MEASURE Evaluation, Chapel Hill, North Carolina.
71. Bleich, S., Koehlmoos, N.T.L., Rashid, M., Peters, D.H. and Anderson, G. (2011) Non-communicable chronic disease in Bangladesh: overview of existing programs and priorities going forward. *Health Policy* 100, 282–289.

72. Reich, M. and Takemi, K. (2009) G8 and strengthening of health systems: follow-up to the Toyako summit. *Lancet* 373, 508–515.
73. Shakarishvili, G., Atun, R., Berman, P., Hsiao, W., Burgess, C. and Lansang, M.A. (2010) Converging health systems frameworks: towards a concepts-to-actions roadmap for health systems strengthening in low and middle income countries. *Global Health Governance* 3, 1–6.
74. Sundewall, J., Swanson, R.C., Betigeri, A., Sanders, D., Collins, T.E., Shakarishvili, G. and Brugha, R. (2011) Health-systems strengthening: current and future activities. *Lancet* 377, 1222–1223.
75. World Health Organization Maximizing Positive Synergies Collaborative Group (2009) An assessment of interactions between global health initiatives and country health systems. *Lancet* 373, 2137–2169.
76. Travis, P., Bennett, S., Haines, A., Pang, T., Bhutta, Z., Hyder, A.A., Pielemeier, N.R., Mills, A. and Evans, T. (2004) Overcoming health-systems constraints to achieve the Millennium Development Goals. *Lancet* 364, 900–906.
77. Geneau, R., Stuckler, D., Stachenko, S., McKee, M., Ebrahim, S., Basu, S., Chockalingham, A., Mwatsama, M., Jamal, R., Alwan, A. and Beaglehole, R. (2010) Raising the priority of preventing chronic diseases: a political process. *Lancet* 376, 1689–1698.
78. Yang, G., Kong, L., Zhao, W., Wan, X., Zhai, Y., Chen, L.C. and Koplan, J.P. (2008) Emergence of chronic non-communicable diseases in China. *Lancet* 372, 1697–1705.
79. Banatvala, N. and Donaldson, L. (2007) Chronic diseases in developing countries. *Lancet* 370, 2076–2078.
80. Daar, A.S., Singer, P.A., Persad, D.L., Pramming, S.K., Matthews, D.R., Beaglehole, R., Bernstein, A., Borysiewicz, L.K., Colagiuri, S., Ganguly, N., Glass, R.I., Finegood, D.T., Koplan, J., Nabel, E.G., Sarna, G., Sarrafzadegan, N., Smith, R., Yach, D. and Bell, J. (2007) Grand challenges in chronic non-communicable diseases. *Nature* 450, 494–496.
81. Menezes, A.M.B., Perez-Padilla, R., Jardim, J.R., Muiño, A., Lopez, M.V., Valdivia, G., Montes de Oca, M., Talamo, C., Hallal, P.C., Victora, C.G. and the PLATINO Team (2005) Chronic obstructive pulmonary disease in five Latin American cities (the PLATINO study): a prevalence study. *Lancet* 366, 1875–1881.
82. Stevens, G., Dias, R.H., Thomas, K.J., Rivera, J.A., Carvalho, N., Barquera, S., Hill, K. and Ezzati, M. (2008) Characterizing the epidemiological transition in Mexico: national and subnational burden of diseases, injuries, and risk factors. *PLoS Medicine* 5, e125.
83. Krishnan, A., Nongkynrih, B., Kapoor, S.K. and Pandav, C. (2009) A role for INDEPTH Asian sites in translating research to action for non-communicable disease prevention and control: a case study from Ballabgarh, India. *Global Health Action* 2009, 2.
84. Yap, I.K., Brown, I.J., Chan, Q., Wijeyesekera, A., Garcia-Perez, I., Bictash, M., Loo, R.L., Chadeau-Hyam, M., Ebbels, T., De Iorio, M., Maibaum, E., Zhao, L., Kesteloot, H., Daviglus, M.L., Stamler, J., Nicholson, J.K., Elliott, P. and Holmes, E. (2010) Metabolome-wide association study identifies multiple biomarkers that discriminate north and south Chinese populations at differing risks of cardiovascular disease: INTERMAP study. *Journal of Proteome Research* 9, 6647–6654.
85. Miranda, J.J., Gilman, R.H. and Smeeth, L. (2011) Differences in cardiovascular risk factors in rural, urban and rural-to-urban migrants in Peru. *Heart* 97, 787–796.
86. Aspray, T.J., Mugusi, F., Rashid, S., Whiting, D., Edwards, R., Alberti, K.G. and Unwin, N.C. (2000) Essential Non-Communicable Disease Health Intervention Project. Rural and urban differences in diabetes prevalence in Tanzania: the role of obesity, physical inactivity and urban living. *Transactions of the Royal Society of Tropical Medicine and Hygiene* 94, 637–644.

7 Population Surveillance and Chronic Non-communicable Diseases

ANDRE PASCAL KENGNE[1*], JUSTIN BASILE ECHOUFFO-TCHEUGUI[2], SANNI YAYA[3] AND ROHINA JOSHI[4]

[1]*Non-communicable Diseases Research Unit, South African Medical Research Council and University of Cape Town, Cape Town, South Africa;* [2]*Hubert Department of Global Health, Rollins School of Public Health, Emory University, Atlanta, Georgia, USA;* [3]*Faculty of Health Sciences, University of Ottawa, Ottawa, Canada;* [4]*The George Institute for Global Health, The University of Sydney, Sydney, Australia*

7.1 Introduction

Health surveillance is the systematic and on-going tracking and forecasting of population-level health status, events, outcomes, risk/protective factors and other determinants through the collection, integration, analysis and interpretation of data and the timely dissemination of the information to those who need to know, to inform action [1]. The term 'surveillance', in its ancient conception, has its roots in the Latin word '*vigilare*' from which the term 'vigilant' is derived. In its more recent understanding, in the 19th century in particular, it originated from the French root '*sur*' meaning 'over' and '*veiller*' meaning 'to watch' [2]. Therefore, surveillance literally means 'to watch over'; when applied to public health, it means close monitoring of the occurrence of health-related events in the population. Surveillance has a pivotal role in public health by making available the information required by healthcare providers and decision makers, who undertake activities relating to population health assessment, health promotion and protection, as well as disease or injury prevention. Information generated through surveillance is useful for policy and decision making regarding population-level preventative, curative or palliative interventions, but also individual-level interventions, and is relevant for healthcare providers and consumers. While the methods for surveillance were originally developed as part of the efforts to control infectious diseases, the basic concepts of surveillance have been applied to virtually all areas of public health, although the application of surveillance to chronic disease is very recent.

*E-mail: andre.kengne@mrc.ac.za

Indeed, chronic disease surveillance is a developing field worldwide, and systems to achieve this remain less well developed than those for infectious diseases [3].

This chapter elaborates on the lessons learned from specific and potential population-based surveillance initiatives on chronic diseases in low- and middle-income countries (LMICs). It includes a historical perspective on public health surveillance in general and chronic diseases in particular, followed by a description of the scope and data requirement for chronic disease surveillance, and an overview of major initiatives with relevance for chronic disease surveillance in LMICs. The chapter ends with a discussion on the future challenges on the long journey of LMICs towards implementing comprehensive chronic disease surveillance systems.

7.2 Public Health Surveillance: a Historical Perspective

Public health surveillance has been traced back to as early as the time of Pharaoh Menes in the First Dynasty, when it is believed that an epidemic was recorded for the first time in the history of mankind [4]. Mempses probably reigned at the time of the 'great pestilence', which dates back to 3180 years BC. Other major epidemics have been recorded through the history of humanity including devastating ones such as the Plague of Justinian (AD 541–549), which lasted 50 years [5], the Black Death (1348–1351), which lasted for 4 years [4], and the Spanish Influenza (1918), which lasted for 5 months [6]. The earliest records of epidemic events focused on gathering information on health outcomes, risk factors and interventions [7]. By their restriction to simple recording of epidemics, the earliest initiatives did not strictly meet the definition of surveillance. The idea of analysing the data collected to inform health actions has been traced back to Hippocrates (430–370 BC) [8].With regard to disease occurrence, Hippocrates made a distinction between acute conditions with a short duration, and chronic or long-lasting conditions. In his view, endemic diseases were determined by the nature of a certain place, with climatic, hydrological and behavioural determinants being the main drivers [9].

The origins of mortality registration date back to 443 BC and the Roman Empire when a census asked participants to report births and deaths that had occurred in their family over the past 5 years. It is also known that births, deaths, marriages and divorces were recorded routinely by Roman families from as early as the 1st century. In Europe, systematic registration of births and deaths was commenced by the church. 'Ecclesiastical Registers' were the precursor of modern civil registers in which births, deaths, baptisms, marriages and other church-related statistics were recorded. The first Bill of Mortality was issued in 1532, comprising burial lists with causes of death recorded for all those registered in the parish.

The first public action attributable to health surveillance is believed to have occurred during the 1348 epidemic of bubonic plague in Europe, when the Venetian Republic appointed guardians of public health to detect infected passengers aboard the ships and prevent them from coming ashore [10]. This approach, otherwise known as quarantine, was also used in Marseille as a means for controlling the spread of infection [7]. Historically, systematic and on-going disease surveillance through data collection did not start until the year 1532, when the first Bill of Mortality was issued [11]. In 1538, the first mortality registration statistics were used to track the number of people who died from the plague, although data collection was restricted to simply documenting the occurrence of death with no cause recorded. It is only during the subsequent century that comprehensive analysis and reporting of collected data was introduced, with John Graunt being credited for publishing one of the first documents on the use of numerical methods to monitor health events through his book *Natural and Political Observations Made Upon the Bills of Mortality*, which was published in 1662 [11]. The 17th century also witnessed more attempts to record causes of death being initiated, mostly for the purpose of monitoring epidemics. These attempts were essentially based on lay reporting systems also known as 'death searches', which typically involved using women to interview families about the cause of death of their recently deceased member. The Registration Act passed in England in 1837 formalized the 'death search' process by requiring information relating to the cause of death to be recorded.

An early attempt to legislate on surveillance came from Rhodes Island where laws were passed around the 1740s to instruct the report of infectious diseases such as smallpox, yellow fever or cholera [12]. A link of surveillance to policy formulation was achieved in 1776 when Johann Peter Frank recommended a more extensive health surveillance in Germany, to support public health efforts in the areas of school health, injury prevention, maternal and child health, public water and sewage disposal [12]. Other instances of the use of surveillance data to influence legislation around the same period came from France and Great Britain [7].

The modern concept of surveillance is believed to have started with William Farr, who was the Superintendent of the Statistical Department in the General Registrar's Office of Great Britain between 1839 and 1879. During this period, Farr compiled, analysed and interpreted vital statistics data, as well as regularly reporting these to the authorities and general public [13]. In doing so, Farr laid the foundations for the modern concepts of mortality surveillance and classification of diseases. Other major contributions to the development and application of health surveillance across the 19th century include those of Edwin Chadwick and John Snow in Great Britain, Lemuel Shattuck in the USA and Louis-René Villermé in France [4, 13].

The first international list of causes of death was established in the early 1890s, but the full internationalization of health surveillance mostly occurred during the 20th century, a period during which health surveillance concepts were expanded and diversified. The Epidemiological Surveillance Unit was established within the Division of Communicable Diseases at the World Health Organization (WHO) headquarters in 1965 [14], followed by publication of the WHO's first report on communicable disease surveillance [15]; then in 1968, the 21st World Health Assembly established surveillance as an essential function of public health practice [10]. The advent of microcomputers in the 1980s was instrumental in shaping the ways surveillance data are increasingly being assembled, analysed and disseminated through global network systems. In recent decades, the concept of health surveillance has been further refined and its scope broadened to include chronic diseases and other aspects of health.

7.3 Development of Chronic Disease Surveillance

Although health surveillance has been conducted for centuries as described above, its application to chronic disease is very recent [16]. In the USA, for instance, it is only about a century ago that cancer reporting was commenced in New York State in 1911, followed by the establishment of the first population-based cancer registry in Connecticut in 1935 and later by major community-based cohort studies such as the landmark Framingham Heart Study [17]. In the early 1980s, the USA established the Behavioural Risk Factor Surveillance System to continuously collect data on key behavioural determinants of health nationwide [18]. The potential utility of health surveillance in addressing chronic diseases at the global level was recognized at the 21st World Health Assembly, when it was recommended that surveillance principles should be applied to non-infectious health problems like cancers and atherosclerosis and to social problems such as drug addiction [19]. However, interest in chronic disease surveillance mostly remained the concern of developed countries until the 1990s, when it became obvious that the greatest impact of non-communicable diseases (NCDs) was increasingly in LMICs. At the 53rd World Health Assembly in 2000, a resolution was passed on a 'Global strategy for prevention and control of noncommunicable diseases' [20]. The resolution positioned surveillance as a key objective of the global strategy, by stressing the need to map the emerging epidemics of NCDs and to analyse their social, economic, behavioural and political determinants with particular reference to poor and disadvantaged populations, in order to provide guidance for policy, legislative and financial measures related to the development of an environment supportive of control [20].

In September 1999, the first global conference on risk factor surveillance was held in Atlanta (Georgia), co-organized by the US Centers for Disease Control and Prevention (CDC) and the Finnish National Public Health Institute (KTL), with additional support from the NCD surveillance department of the WHO. This conference is credited as being a landmark event for the development of an international collaboration towards global NCD surveillance [21]. Subsequent conferences were held in Finland (2001), Australia (2003), Uruguay (2005), Italy (2007) [22], Canada (2011) and China (2013). The conference in Italy was followed by the creation in 2008 of a Global Working Group termed the World Alliance for Risk Factor Surveillance (WARFS) by the International Union for Health Promotion and Education (IUHPE) [22]. The mission of WARFS is to support the development of behavioural risk factor surveillance as a tool for evidence-based public health, thus acknowledging its importance in informing, monitoring and evaluating disease prevention and health promotion policies, services and interventions [22]. WARFS has so far produced and updated a draft white paper on surveillance [2], and co-organized global behavioural risk factor surveillance conferences.

In general, the development of chronic disease surveillance in developing countries is a work in progress [23], largely driven by international efforts led by the WHO [24], or bilateral collaborations between developed and developing countries. For instance, since 2006, the CDC has embarked on a collaboration with Brazil for NCD surveillance, whereby CDC is providing an extensive and ongoing technical support resulting in the development of a behavioural risk factor surveillance system across Brazil's state capitals. Furthermore, the CDC has provided guidance on policy development, programme planning and evaluation of physical activity in about 300 municipalities in Brazil. The efforts of the CDC are being supported by the Brazilian Health and Disease Surveillance System funds provided to the CDC Foundation [25]. A similar collaboration for behavioural risk factor surveillance also exists between the CDC and China [26].

7.4 Scope of Chronic Disease Surveillance

Chronic disease surveillance refers to surveillance of the whole spectrum of chronic diseases including determinants, events, health service utilization and outcomes of care. Selection of conditions for inclusion in the surveillance system varies across countries and settings, with the preference often given to important chronic diseases and risk factors that are amenable to prevention and control (Table 7.1). Surveillance systems and requirements for chronic diseases have evolved over time, largely paralleling the progress in our understanding of the complexity of the causes of chronic diseases, to include monitoring of trends in behavioural, occupational and environmental risk factors, as well as health conditions such as disabilities. Furthermore, there has been a growing awareness of the impact of the built environment on the physical and mental health of populations [27]. Therefore, several new surveillance methodologies have been developed to

Table 7.1. Clusters of preventable chronic diseases, risk factors and determinants.

Risk and protective factors	Biological risk factors/ markers	Preventable chronic disease and conditions
Behavioural factors	Obesity	Ischaemic heart disease
Diet	Hypertension	Stroke
Physical activity	Dyslipidaemia	Type 2 diabetes
Smoking	Impaired glucose regulation	Renal disease
Alcohol misuse	Proteinuria	Chronic obstructive pulmonary disease (COPD) and asthma
Psychosocial factors		Certain cancers
'Sense of control'		Mental health problem/depression
Social support/social exclusion		Oral health
Resilience and emotional well-being		Musculoskeletal conditions
Early life factors		
Maternal health		
Low birthweight		
Childhood infections		
Abuse and neglect		
Non-modifiable factors: Age, sex, ethnicity, genetic make-up, family history		
Socio-environmental determinants (may or may not be modifiable): socio-economic status, community characteristics (e.g. presence/absence of social capital), work conditions, environmental health, etc.		

monitor the health of populations in the context of their residential communities, involving a complex interaction of health determinants, health outcomes, physical measurements, biological samples, policies and the built environment [28].

Population-based data are essential for chronic disease surveillance, and provide valuable information for the planning and evaluation of disease prevention, treatment and control strategies [3]. However, the sources of data for chronic disease surveillance vary substantially; they can include a notifiable diseases system, vital statistics, sentinel surveillance, registries, health surveys, administrative data collection systems and a census (Table 7.2). The nature of chronic diseases, however, renders some data-gathering systems less attractive. Indeed, the factors for chronic diseases most amenable to public health interventions are disease precursors, which are present years before the disease becomes evident. Furthermore, some risk factors for diseases and related complications are simply not known on an individual level, and there are future issues for planning related to

Table 7.2. Scope and potential sources of data required for chronic disease surveillance (From [1]).

Determinants	← Pre-clinical	← Clinical	← Outcomes
Data examples			
Genetics	*Screening*	*Diagnosis*	*Mortality*
Prevalence of breast cancer gene; familial disease	PAP testing; blood pressure; blood glucose; blood lipids	Modes of diagnosis; time to diagnosis	Cause specific deaths; survival rates
Risk behaviour	*Risk reduction*	*Treatment and procedures*	*Morbidity*
Smoking; dietary fat intake	Smoking cessation; programme uptake; physical activity rates	Surgery; systemic therapy; radiation; palliation	Complications; degree of disability; quality of life
Environment			
Occupational exposure			
Socio-economic		*Service use*	
Housing; income level; education		Hospitalization; physician visits; home care; ambulatory care; palliative care	
		Pharmaceutical	
		Drug use; Complications and interactions	
Data sources			
Surveys; census; workplace monitoring	Screening databases; surveys; public health programme databases; primary care physicians	Hospital databases; discharge abstract databases; registry data	Vital statistics; coroner's database

co-morbidity [1]. The pros and cons of each data source are described in detail elsewhere [1, 10, 16].

7.5 Opportunities/Experiences of Chronic Disease Surveillance in Developing Countries

7.5.1 Notifiable diseases systems and chronic disease surveillance in developing countries

Diseases/health threat notification systems exist in many countries worldwide, including LMICs. Such systems, mostly put into place by countries to fulfil their international obligations, have been geared towards the notification of a few infectious diseases [29]. In some countries, however, NCDs such as lead poisoning have been historically part of the list of notifiable diseases [30]. Disease notification is a case-based system whereby health workers coming into contact with patients (or test results) with a suspected notifiable medical condition are required to report the case to the health authorities for follow-up and action. In South Africa (a major global lead producer), where reporting lead poisoning is a legal requirement, it has been suggested that under-reporting of cases makes the disease notification pathway a less reliable source of data for monitoring the harmful effect of lead poisoning on the health of populations [31].

There have also been initiatives within countries to legislate on the notification for some major NCDs, but not necessarily for the purpose of immediate action as expected in the traditional disease notification system. In 2011 for instance, South Africa promulgated a new legislation on cancers, which makes it compulsory for every healthcare worker who has diagnosed a new case of cancer to notify it on an indicated form [32]. However, the completed form is instead submitted to the National Cancer Register to improve cancer reporting and monitoring [32]. The Integrated Disease Surveillance Project in India run by the Ministry of Health and Family Welfare, Government of India, is another example of disease surveillance where a number of communicable diseases and NCDs including risk factors for NCDs and road traffic crashes are recorded and reported regularly.

7.5.2 Population-based disease registries

Cancer is perhaps the chronic condition for which the culture of disease registry is most well-grounded, especially in developed countries and increasingly more so in developing nations (see Adeloye and Grant, Chapter 2, this volume). As of 2012, 25 cancers registries based in 19 sub-Saharan African countries were affiliated with the African Cancer Registry Network, a member of the Global Initiative for Cancer Registries Development (GICR) [33]. The Indian National Cancer Registry was launched in 1981 and as of 2013, there are 23 population-based cancer registries in the country [34]. The GLOBOCAN project, an initiative of the International Agency for Research on Cancer (IARC), uses data from cancer registries to provide contemporary estimates of the incidence of, mortality, prevalence and disability-adjusted life years from major types of cancers, at a national level, for 184 countries around the world [33]. IARC is a specialized cancer agency of the WHO, with particular interest in conducting research in LMICs.

Population-based stroke registries are also becoming commonplace in developing countries [35, 36], probably popularized by the WHO STEPwise approach to Surveillance (STEPS), which is described in greater detail in the next section. Examples include the following stroke registries: Trivandrum [37] and Mumbai [38] in India, North Beijing in China [39], Matao in Brazil [40] and Surulere in Nigeria [41]. Community-based registries have also been implemented in some countries for diabetes, mostly to quantify the incidence of type 1 diabetes. Some examples include the following diabetes registries: Avellaneda in Argentina [42], Passo Fundo in Brazil [43], Benghazi in Libya [44], Beja-Monastir-Gafsa in Tunisia [45], Dhaka in Bangladesh [46] and Karnataka in India [47].

7.5.3 Vital statistics and causes of death

The critical importance of reliable, valid and comparable information about mortality and causes of death in monitoring health and planning health services for populations has been widely acknowledged [48, 49]. Data collection on vital statistics and causes of death started in western countries in the 17th century with northern European countries including Denmark, Finland, Norway and Sweden setting up civil registration systems following the initiation of such a system in England. However, some high-income countries including Australia, Canada and New Zealand only started civil registration in the 20th century, while vital statistic data collection in the USA became systematic, compulsory and complete for the whole country only in 1930. Vital statistic data collection in LMICs probably only started in the 19th century, with some attempts reported in the Middle East and Asia in particular. For instance, civil registration was started in Egypt in 1839 and become compulsory after 1912, while in India it was commenced in 1850 and modernized throughout the 20th century. In Africa, Mauritius was the first country to pass a law on civil registration with Cape Verde, Central African Republic, Congo and Mauritius commencing civil registration in the 19th century, while it was established in other countries in the region only in the 20th century. While robust systems for documenting death and the causes are currently in place in most developed countries, few developing countries have such data [48], and even fewer have assessed the quality of their mortality data [50]. During the 1965–2004 period, 25–28% of the global population was living in countries with complete (i.e. at least 90% of events recorded) death registration. This proportion was 2–7% in Africa, 1% in South-east Asia and 10–13% in the Western Pacific [50]. The few developing countries that conducted periodic assessment of mortality statistics are South Africa [51], China [52], India [53] and Brazil [54].

Where available, vital statistics data may not be suitable for chronic disease surveillance when information on the causes of death and/or risk factors for chronic diseases is missing, under-reported or inaccurate. For instance, numerous studies including in developed countries have shown that a condition like diabetes mellitus is often and by a large proportion under-reported on death certificates [16, 55, 56]. Nevertheless, in a developing country like South Africa, improvement in the completeness and quality of vital statistics data reporting has significantly contributed to a better quantification of the contribution of chronic diseases and risk factors to the burden of diseases at the national level [57–66]. Another illustration of the use of vital statistics data for the purpose of chronic disease surveillance comes from the Seychelles, where Stringhini *et al.* [67] used death certificate reports for the 1989–2010 period to describe the changing patterns of mortality due to stroke and myocardial infarction. They showed that, over a 22-year period, age-standardized mortality rate (men/women) declined by 44/39% for stroke and by 50/53% for myocardial infarction [67]. This pattern is in sharp contrast to suggested increasing trends in other countries of the region, probably reflecting differing stages of the epidemiological transition and differences across countries in the response to emerging chronic diseases. However, the findings from the Global Burden of Disease 2010 study [29] suggested a declining age-standardized mortality due to cardiovascular disease in Africa, although the confidence interval around these estimates was very broad, reflecting the limitations of the data [68].

7.5.4 Health surveys

The WHO's STEPwise approach to Surveillance (STEPS)

STEPS is a standardized method for collecting, analysing and disseminating data in WHO member countries, with a specific focus on LMICs. The STEPS approach focuses on collecting core data on established risk factors/determinants of disease burden. The STEPS approach is flexible enough to allow each country to expand on the core variables and risk factors, and to incorporate optional modules related to local or regional interests. The WHO expects that by using the same standardized questions and protocols, information collected can be used not only for monitoring within-country trends but also for making comparisons across countries. STEPS encourages the collection of small amounts of useful information on a regular and continuous basis. There are currently two primary STEPS surveillance systems: the STEPwise approach to risk factor surveillance and the STEPwise approach to stroke surveillance (STEPS Stroke) [69].

The STEPwise approach to risk factor surveillance is implemented through STEPS instruments, which cover three different levels of 'steps' of risk factor assessment comprising: (i) a questionnaire; (ii) physical assessments; and (iii) biochemical measurements. For each of the steps, WHO further distinguishes core items, expanded items and optional items (Box 7.1).

STEPS Stroke was developed as a collaborative effort between the WHO and the International Stroke Society [69], which subsequently merged with World Stroke Federation to form the World Stroke Organization. The STEPS Stroke instruments also cover three different 'steps' of stroke case findings for a defined population, and target data collection with different levels of complexity (Box 7.2).

Both the STEPS for risk factors and STEPS Stroke instruments are conceived as a comprehensive package to assist countries/investigators in collecting relevant

Box 7.1. STEPS risk factors core, expanded and optional items

	Core items	Expanded items	Optional items
Step 1: Behavioural measures	Basic demographic information, including age, sex, literacy and highest level of education	Expanded demographic information including years at school, ethnicity, marital status, employment status, household income	Mental health, intentional and unintentional injury and violence, oral health and sexual behaviours
	Tobacco use	Smokeless tobacco use	
	Alcohol consumption	Past 7 days drinking	
	Fruit and vegetables consumption	Oil and fat consumption	
	Physical activity		Objective measure of physical activity behaviour
		History of blood pressure, treatment for raised blood pressure	
		History of diabetes, treatment for diabetes	
Step 2: Physical measurements	Weight and height, waist circumference, blood pressure	Hip circumference	Skin fold thickness, assessment of physical fitness
Step 3: Biochemical measurements	Fasting blood sugar, total cholesterol	High-density lipoprotein (HDL)-cholesterol and fasting triglycerides	Oral glucose tolerance test, urine examination, salivary cotinine

data, and also in converting the data into surveillance products to assist action, with assistance from the WHO, where relevant. There is accumulating evidence to suggest a progressive uptake of STEPS for risk factors in developing countries, but little on STEPS Stroke. As of 2013, about 85 countries across the six WHO regions have conducted STEPS surveys and published their results in the form of country reports, data books, fact sheets, journal articles, presentations or posters [70]. Some countries have conducted more than one survey; hence, it is difficult and perhaps premature to ascertain whether the whole cycle of surveillance based on the STEPS approaches is occurring at the level of countries.

The MEASURE Demographic Health Survey (DHS) project

The DHS project is an on-going initiative, funded primarily by the US Agency for International Development, with additional contribution from other donors as well as the beneficiary countries, to support the conduct of population-based survey data collection on a range of areas in LMICs. The DHS was established in 1984

Box 7.2. STEPS Stroke core items [69].

	Core items	Expanded items	Provides data on:
Step 1: Hospitalized events (fatal and non-fatal)	Demographic information Time of onset Vital status day 10	Treatment Disability Type of stroke	Stroke admissions and hospital case fatality
Step 2: Fatal events in the community	Demographic information Death certificates, or verbal autopsy	Autopsy/necropsy reports Type of stroke	Stroke deaths
Step 3: Non-fatal events in the community	Demographic information Time of onset Vital status day 10	Treatment Disability Type of stroke	Stroke incidence and case fatality
Step 3: Biochemical measurements	Fasting blood sugar, total cholesterol	High-density lipoprotein (HDL)-cholesterol and fasting triglycerides	Oral glucose tolerance test, urine examination, salivary cotinine

as an evolution from two major survey programmes for developing countries started in the mid- and late 1970s: the World Fertility Survey (WFS) and the Contraceptive Prevalence Surveys (CPSs) [71]. The WFS programme aimed to provide countries with accurate data on fertility and its determinants, as well as on other demographic variables. The primary aim of the CPSs was to produce information for managing and evaluating family-planning programmes [71]. The WFS took place from 1973 to 1984, and the CPSs from 1977 to 1985. The WFS programme conducted surveys in 41 developing countries and collaborated on surveys in 20 developed countries, while the CPS programme carried out 43 surveys in 33 countries [72]. In line with its two ancestors, the DHS originally aimed to collect comparable population-based data on fertility, contraception, maternal and child health, and nutrition in developing countries [73]. The first DHS was conducted in 1985, and since then over 230 such surveys have been conducted in 90 countries [73]. Over time, the amount and scope of data collected by the DHS have expanded considerably, with new questions, modules on behaviour (e.g. alcohol consumption, tobacco use) and biomarkers being introduced at regular intervals over the course of the programme (Fig. 7.1) [74]. The DHS typically takes place once every 5 years, although a few countries have surveys at lesser intervals [72].

It follows from the above description of the initial concept and subsequent updates of the DHS, that it has not yet embraced the full spectrum of NCDs. However, the DHS has great potential for informing NCD surveillance in developing countries. Many such countries including the poorest have already conducted at least one DHS survey [75]. For instance, of the 236 DHSs conducted between 1985 and 2010, 49% were conducted in sub-Saharan Africa, 20% in Asia and 18% in Latin America and the Caribbean [73]. During that same time interval, countries had conducted a median of two surveys (range 1–10) [73]. There is

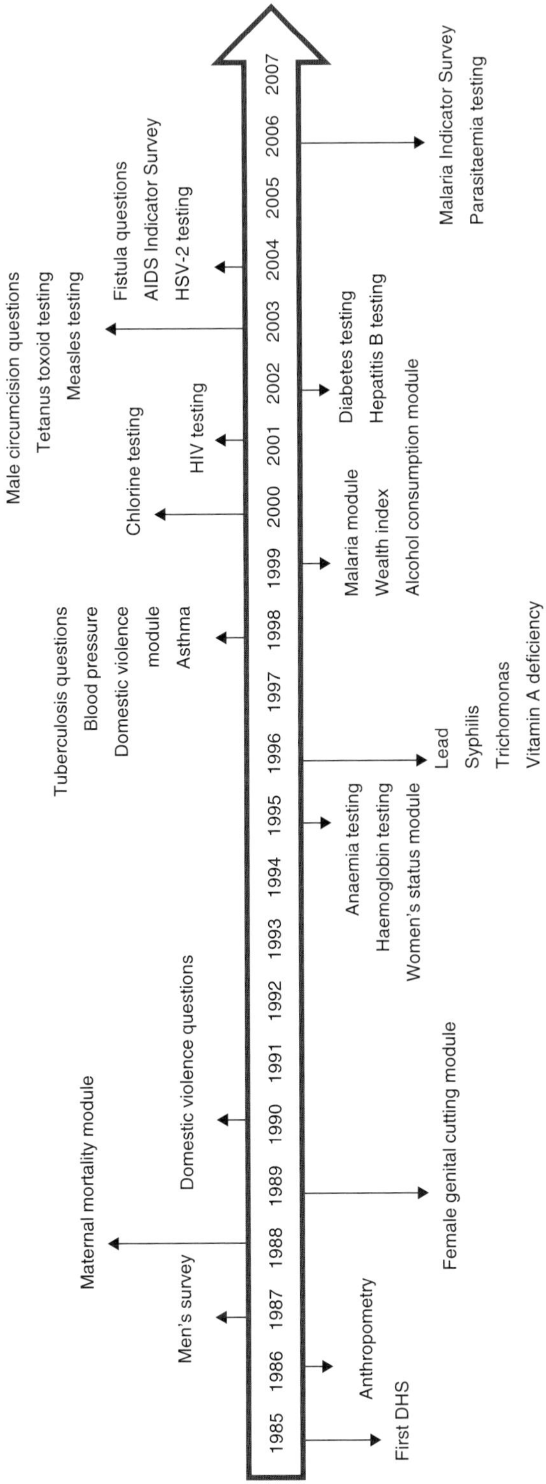

Fig. 7.1. Demographic and Health Survey (DHS) timeline: key survey questions, modules and biomarker milestones, 1985–2006. (Adapted with permission from [74]).

therefore an opportunity to use the DHS platform for acquiring data for NCD surveillance (as a by-product), an approach that has already been used in some developing countries. The 2002 DHS survey in Uzbekistan measured blood pressure and levels of other common cardiovascular risk factors including biological markers, and was subsequently used to describe their epidemiology in the country [75, 76]. However, the traditional focus of the DHS on children and women only is a major limitation of its use for NCD surveillance [77].

So far, a major contribution of the DHS has been to provide information about the patterns of excess weight, a risk factor for many NCDs, building on anthropometric data that are collected routinely across most surveys [74, 78–81]. For instance, Martorell *et al.* [79], used data for 39 DHSs from 38 countries and comprising 147,938 non-pregnant women aged 15–49 years to provide comparative prevalence figures for obesity in women across several developing regions. Using 71 DHSs conducted in 50 countries and totalling 150,482 children aged 12–60 months, Martorell *et al.* derived equivalent figures for children [78]. More recently, Lopez-Arana *et al.* [80, 82] used DHS data to describe the varying trends of overweight and risk factors in women from 33 LMICs between 1992 and 2009. Other investigators around the world have also reported comparative figures for overweight/obesity, body mass index and risk factors based on DHS data [74, 81, 83–92].

The Global Tobacco Surveillance System (GTSS)

The GTSS is credited as being the largest public health surveillance system ever developed and maintained [93]. The GTSS aims to enhance country capacity to design, implement and evaluate tobacco control interventions, and to monitor key initiatives of the WHO's Framework Convention on Tobacco Control (FCTC) and components of the WHO MPOWER technical package [94]. The WHO, CDC and the Canadian Public Health Association (CPHA) began development of the GTSS in 1998 [95]. The GTSS includes the collection of data through four surveys: the Global Youth Tobacco Survey (GYTS); the Global School Personnel Survey (GSPS); the Global Health Professions Student Survey (GHPSS) and the Global Adult Tobacco Survey (GATS). The GYTS focuses on youths aged 13–15 and collects information in schools. The GSPS surveys teachers and administrators from the same schools that participate in the GYTS. The GHPSS focuses on third-year students pursuing degrees in dentistry, medicine, nursing and pharmacy. The GATS is a nationally representative household survey that monitors tobacco use among adults aged 15 years and older.

The different components of GTSS were developed and introduced over time, with GYTS being the first (introduced in 1999) and GATS the last (introduced in 2007). Accordingly, the number of countries that have already adopted each of the components and the number of such surveys already conducted vary widely. As of 2008, the GYTS had been conducted in at least 154 countries around the world, and more than once in 107 countries. Over 800 samples had been drawn, covering over 2 million students in 11,000 schools [96]. By 2008, unlike GYTS, GSPS, which was introduced in 2000, had a rather limited global coverage, with most surveys conducted in African countries. By this time, 74 WHO member countries had conducted at least one such survey, with 19 of them having conducted more than one survey [96]. By comparison, the GHPSS, which only started in 2005, had already been conducted in 50 countries by 2008 [96].

One of the earliest scientific comparative reports from GTSS dates back to 2000 and was based on data from 12 of the 13 developing countries in which the first GYTSs were conducted in 1999 [97]. Since then, many other comparative reports, based on data from an increasing number of countries, have been made available [93–95, 97–102]. Numerous other scientific papers and reports have been published from the GTSS data [96], including the GTSS Atlas, which aims to map the coverage of the surveys and provides data on the various elements of a comprehensive tobacco control strategy as outlined in the WHO FCTC and MPOWER Technical Package [25].

The International Network for the Demographic Evaluation of Populations and Their Health (INDEPTH) Network

The INDEPTH network is a global network of members who conduct longitudinal health and demographic evaluation of populations in LMICs [102]. INDEPTH aims to strengthen the global capacity for health and demographic surveillance systems (HDSSs), and to mount multi-site research to guide health priorities and policies in LMICs, based on up-to-date scientific evidence. The INDEPTH network was established in 1998 by a consortium of 17 demographic surveillance sites from 13 countries across Africa and Asia, as a mid-term response to the lack of reliable population-based data on health across LMICs in Africa, Asia and Oceania [103]. The headquarters of the INDEPTH Network is in Accra, Ghana. As of 2013, the network comprised 48 HDSS sites operated by 40 centres in 20 countries across participating continents, through which a total population of about 3.2 million people has been followed [102, 103].

The initial focus of INDEPTH included: data analysis and capacity strengthening, technical support to field sites, comparative assessments of mortality, reproductive health, malaria, and applications to policy and practice [104]. INDEPTH sites aim to collect epidemiological data on exposures and outcomes on all individuals within a defined population on a longitudinal basis. While issues covered by participating centres may expand with time, at the inception most centres would focus on areas considered to be of major interest locally or nationally. This has an implication in the sense that INDEPTH data at some time points may not be appropriate to inform emerging health issues for instance. Population size across centres ranged from tens of thousands up to around a quarter of a million. At the start of each INDEPTH centre, a baseline census is conducted to collect data on all individuals within the community and the social units in which they live. The dynamic cohort model (Fig. 7.2) is then used to update the database at a frequency that is a function of a combination of several factors relating to the context, resources availability, age range of the population and outcomes of interest. At each update cycle, data are collected on a series of core parameters comprising: (i) the social unit, which in some centres includes information on socio-economic status; (ii) births; (iii) migrations; (iv) deaths; and (v) causes of death, essentially using verbal autopsy interviews.

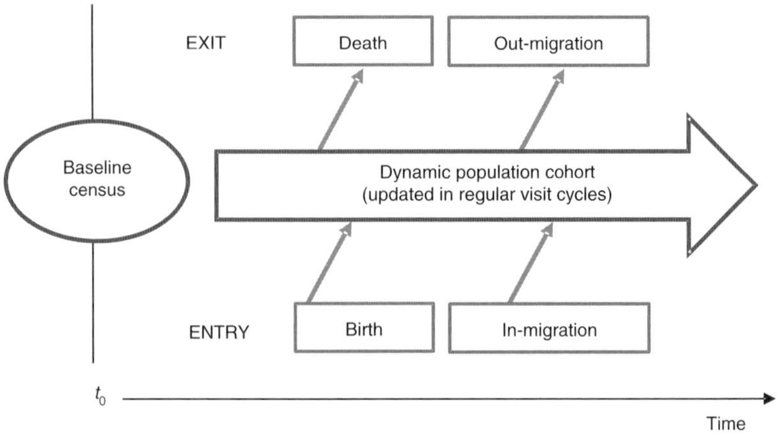

Fig. 7.2. Conceptual structure of the dynamic cohort model used by INDEPTH sites. (Adapted with permission from [102]).

There may be only a limited potential to monitor non-fatal NCD-related health outcomes across the INDEPTH sites, but the focus of INDEPTH on mortality is a huge asset for monitoring the contribution of NCDs to mortality occurrence. The extent of data collection on determinants of NCDs also varies significantly across INDEPTH sites, being non-existent in some centres [105, 106], while a few others have evolved with time into community-based laboratories for the study and monitoring of chronic diseases [107]. For instance, through a series of nested cohorts, the Agincourt HDSS has made significant contributions to the study and monitoring of key NCDs at the population level in recent years in South Africa [107]. Data from INDEPTH centres have also been used to inform aspects of NCD surveillance in other countries. This contribution is not covered in further detail here. A major step in using cross-site INDEPTH data to investigate NCDs was achieved during 2009–2010 through a series of publications from Asian sites on a number of risk factors for NCDs including alcohol consumption [108], blood pressure [109], physical activity [110], diets [111], smoking [112] and excess weight [113].

The Living Standards Measurement Study (LSMS)

The LSMS is a survey series that has been conducted by the World Bank since the 1980s. It was established as a means for exploring avenues for improving the type and quality of household data collected by statistical offices in developing countries, with a goal of fostering the use of household data as a basis for policy decision making [114]. The main objective of LSMS surveys is to collect household data that can be used to assess household welfare, to understand household behaviour and to evaluate the effect of various government policies on the living conditions of the population. Accordingly, LSMS surveys collect data on various dimensions of household well-being, including consumption, income, savings, employment, health, education, fertility, nutrition, housing and migration [114].

The first two LSMS surveys were conducted in the Cote d'Ivoire and Peru in 1985–1986. Thereafter, the surveys were extended to other developing countries. However, it is challenging to know the exact number of such surveys conducted so far. While a number of surveys have been conducted under the LSMS appellation, it is not always obvious to assess the degree of the World Bank's contribution from the study documentation [115]. As of 2005, about 60 LSMS surveys had been conducted in 40 countries [116]. There is a high level of LSMS questionnaire customization for each country, which has led to variations in the overall content of the survey instruments as well as the inclusion of new modules and topics over the years. In Bosnia and Herzegovina, for instance, in 2001 the health module was expanded to incorporate questions on depression in an effort to measure the incidence of this mental health ailment and identify the linkages between it and other aspects of welfare and labour market participation [116]. A potential utility of LSMS survey in informing chronic disease research and surveillance is supported by the LSMS working paper number 131 on chronic illness and retirement in Jamaica [117].

Survey of Ageing and Health

The WHO Study on global AGEing and adult Health (SAGE) is part of an on-going initiative by the WHO to compile comprehensive longitudinal information on the health and well-being of adult populations and the ageing process [118]. The core SAGE collects data on adults aged 50 years and older, including a smaller comparison sample of younger adults aged 18–49 years, from nationally representative samples in six countries comprising China, Ghana, India, Mexico, Russian Federation and South Africa. Additionally, eight health and demographic surveillance sites in Bangladesh, Ghana, India, Indonesia, Kenya, South Africa, Tanzania and Vietnam with an additional combined sample size of over 45,000 people form a part of SAGE [118, 119]. SAGE is supported by the US National Institute on Aging, Division of Behavioural and Social Research. SAGE was designed to provide results that are comparable with ageing studies in developed countries.

Baseline SAGE data collection (wave 0) occurred in 2002–2004 as part of the World Health Survey. The second round of data collection (wave 1) was completed during 2007–2010 and a third round (wave 2) was scheduled to start in the second half of 2013 [118]. Given the spectrum of diseases susceptible to affect elderly people, SAGE has a major focus on chronic diseases and risk factors. Health outcomes data within SAGE will accumulate over time, however the baseline data have already been a source of valuable information on the distribution of risk factors [120–122] and health inequalities [123] across participating countries.

National Health and Nutrition Examination Survey (NHNES)

The NHNES is a USA survey programme of research, conceived to assess the health and nutrition status of adults and children in the country, and to track changes over time. It comprises interviews and physical examinations on a nationally representative sample. Interviews usually include questions on demographics, socio-economic, and dietary and health status. Examinations consist of medicals, physiological measurements and laboratory tests. The first such survey was conducted in the USA in 1971. Over time and mostly inspired by the USA models, some LMICs have implemented similar surveys, one prominent example being the China Health and Nutrition Survey (CHNS). The CHNS is a collaborative effort between the University of North Carolina and the Chinese Center for Disease Control and Prevention [124]. The first CHNS was conducted in 1989, and by 2011, eight such surveys had been conducted [124]. Just like the sister programme in the USA, the CHNS has been a powerful source of information on the distribution and time trends in population levels of risk factors for chronic diseases such as obesity [125–128]. Recent extension of the CHNS measurements to blood analytes will further broaden the scope of its applicability to chronic disease surveillance [128]. Other LMICs that have recently conducted health and nutrition surveys with relevance for chronic disease monitoring include the Philippines [129–130], Argentina [131], South Africa [132] and Mexico [133–136].

7.5.5 Other major within-countries initiatives on chronic disease surveillance

Although the focus of this chapter is primarily on global initiatives, it is worth mentioning that a number of major within-countries initiatives of chronic diseases surveillance have been undertaken in some LMICs. Examples of such important undertakings, especially in relation to cardiovascular risk factor monitoring, include the Indian Council of Medical Research – India Diabetes (ICMR-INDIAB) [137–139], which aims to describe trends in diabetes over time, the CARRS (Centre for Cardiometabolic Risk Reduction in South Asia) Surveillance Study, which builds on the WHO STEPS approach to capture prevalence of risk factors and their socio-economic impact in serial representative surveys to understand trends in both India and Pakistan [140]; and the China Chronic Disease and Risk Factor Surveillance (CCDRFS), which aims to monitor risk factors for chronic diseases across mainland China [23, 141–143].

7.5.6 The Global Burden of Disease (GBD) project

The GBD project is not a surveillance system per se but rather uses data from multiple sources and applies sophisticated statistical methods to provide comparable estimates of the contribution of major conditions or risk factors to the global burden of diseases and disability. The GBD study was launched in 1991 as a collaborative effort between the WHO and the World Bank to provide a comprehensive and internally consistent source of information on the global burden of diseases, injuries and risk factors [144]. Before then, available information on mortality and health in populations in all regions around the world was rather fragmentary and sometimes inconsistent. The first GBD study [145] quantified the health effects of over 100 diseases and injuries for eight regions of the world in 1990 [146]. The GBD study of 1990 introduced a new metric known as DALY (disability-adjusted life year), as a single measure to quantify the burden of diseases, injuries and risk factors [145]. DALY is a time-based measure that combines years of life lost due to premature mortality and years lived with a disability. These 1990 estimates were updated for the years 2000–2002 and included a more extensive analysis of the mortality and burden of disease attributable to 26 global risk factors using a consistent analytic framework known as the Comparative Risk Factor Assessment. Subsequent updates were for the year 2004 [29] and more recently for 2010 [147]. The GBD study 2010 is so far the largest of the GBD studies in terms of both diseases/conditions studied and the number of countries covered around the world (187 countries in total) [147]. The significant contribution that the GBD studies have made in raising the profile of chronic diseases in developing countries, directing more international attention to these conditions and shaping countries' responses, is beyond any doubt. The limited or non-existant capacity within most developing countries to accurately and regularly collect and process surveillance data for chronic diseases suggests that many of these countries will continue to rely on sources of processed surveillance data such as the GBD studies.

7.6 Concluding Remarks

Scientific evidence to support the growing importance of chronic diseases in developing countries has mostly accumulated over the last two decades. Consequently, these countries are still challenged with finding and applying the most appropriate locally relevant prevention and control solutions, and accordingly the best strategies and tools for monitoring the effects of the solutions and changing patterns of chronic diseases over time. Lessons learned from monitoring chronic diseases in developed countries suggest that the scope of data needs for chronic disease surveillance is very broad, and that no single data-gathering system is able to provide the mix of data required for a comprehensive surveillance [1, 16, 21]. Therefore, population-based data collection is essential and, coupled with health facility-based data collection, forms the backbone of chronic disease surveillance.

In developed countries with advanced systems for chronic disease surveillance (e.g. the USA), population-based collection of surveillance data has used multiple sources including some initially established for other purposes in addition to the ones specifically developed for the purpose of surveillance. These sources have included: the notifiable disease system, vital statistics, disease registries, health surveys, censuses and sentinel surveillance [148]. This mix of data feeds is lacking in developing countries, which largely have yet to build the basic blocks for an on-going surveillance system for chronic diseases (see also Coast *et al.*, Chapter 6, this volume).

Setting up and maintaining a system for on-going chronic disease surveillance requires substantial investments in terms of human skills and time, as well as financial resources. The level of such investments required to achieve a comprehensive NCD surveillance in LMICs can quickly become prohibitive, particularly when the baseline is the quasi-absence of any data-gathering framework to build upon. It is therefore important for LMICs to make strategic decisions both in terms of the scope of their surveillance data needs and the possible pathways for making such data available, while accounting for the downstream challenges to process and convert the data collected into outputs that will efficiently inform action. Whenever there is already an existing opportunity within countries for regular contact with the population, which can be capitalized upon to gather data for chronic diseases surveillance, building surveillance upon such an opportunity is likely to be more feasible and cost-effective than setting up a completely new system. Where countries are contemplating starting a new data-gathering system, there are potential major advantages in adapting an existing international system as opposed to setting up a country-specific system. Such advantages include cross-country learning, resources and expertise sharing, and performance comparisons.

References

1. Health Canada (2003) *Chronic Disease Surveillance in Canada – A Background Paper*. Health Surveillance Coordination Division, Centre for Surveillance Coordination, Population and Public Health Branch, Health Canada, Canada.
2. Campostrini, S., McQueen, D., Taylor, A. and Daly, A. (2011) *The IUHPE WARFS GWG White Paper on Surveillance and Health Promotion* <http://www.iuhpe.org/uploaded/Activities/Scientific_Affairs/GWG/WARFS_white_paper_draft_may_2011.pdf>.
3. Thacker, S.B., Stroup, D.F. and Rothenberg, R.B. (1995) Public health surveillance for chronic conditions: a scientific basis for decisions. *Statistics in Medicine* 14, 629–641.
4. Choi, B.C. and Pak, A.W. (2001) Lessons for surveillance in the 21st century: a historical perspective from the past five millennia. *Sozial- und Praventivmedizin* 46, 361–368.
5. Tsiamis, C. (2010) Epidemic waves during Justinian's plague in the Byzantine Empire (6th–8th c. AD). *Vesalius* 17, 36–41.
6. Yang, B. (2004) The epic story of the deadliest plague in history. *Discovery Medicine* 4, 482–487.
7. Choi, B.C.K. (2012) The past, present, and future of public health surveillance. *Scientifica* 2012, 875253.
8. Eylenbosh, W.J. and Noah, N.D. (1988) Historical aspects. In: Eylenbosh, W.J. and Noah, N.D. (eds) *Surveillance in Health and Disease*. Oxford University Press, Oxford, UK.
9. Waltner-Toews, D. (2001) An ecosystem approach to health and its applications to tropical and emerging diseases. *Cadernos de Saude Publica* 17, 7–22.
10. Declich, S. and Carter, A.O. (1994) Public health surveillance: historical origins, methods and evaluation. *Bulletin of the World Health Organization* 72, 285–301.
11. Graunt, J. (1939) *Natural and Political Observations Made Upon the Bills of Mortality, London 1662*. Johns Hopkins University Press, Baltimore, Maryland.
12. Thacker, S.B. and Berkelman, R.L. (1988) Public health surveillance in the United States. *Epidemiologic Reviews* 10, 164–190.
13. Langmuir, A.D. (1963) The surveillance of communicable diseases of national importance. *New England Journal of Medicine* 268, 182–192.
14. Raska, K. (1966) National and international surveillance of communicable diseases. *WHO Chronicle* 20, 315–321.
15. Lucas, A.O. (1968) The surveillance of communicable diseases. *WHO Chronicle* 22, 439–444.
16. Wegner, M.V., Rohan, A.M. and Remington, P.L. (2010) Chronic disease surveillance. In: Remington, P.L., Brownson, R.C. and Wegner, M.V. (eds) *Chronic Disease Epidemiology and Control*, 3rd edn. American Public Health Association, Washington, DC.
17. Brownson, R.C. and Bright, F.S. (2004) Chronic disease control in public health practice: looking back and moving forward. *Public Health Reports* 119, 230–238.
18. CDC (2013) *Behavioral Risk Factor Surveillance System*. Centers for Diseases Control and Prevention, Atlanta, Georgia <http://www.cdc.gov/brfss/about/about_brfss.htm>.

19. WHO (1968) *Report of the Technical Discussion at the 21st World Health Assembly on National and Global Surveillance of Communicable Disease*. World Health Organization, Geneva, Switzerland.
20. WHO (2000) Global strategy for the prevention and control of noncommunicable diseases. Report by the Director-General. In: *53rd World Health Assembly*. Provisional agenda item 12.11 A53/14). World Health Organization, Geneva, Switzerland.
21. Puska, P. (2003) Why is global surveillance necessary? Towards global surveillance of non-communicable disease risk factors: developments and challenges. In: McQueen, D.V. and Puska, P. (eds) *Global Behavioral Risk Factors Surveillance*. Kluwer Academic/Plenum Publishers, New York.
22. Campostrini, S., McQueen, D.V. and Evans, L. (2009) Health promotion and surveillance: the establishment of an IUHPE global working group. *Global Health Promotion* 16, 58–60.
23. Li, Y., Wang, L., Jiang, Y., Zhang, M. and Wang, L. (2013) Risk factors for noncommunicable chronic diseases in women in China: surveillance efforts. *Bulletin of the World Health Organization* 91, 650–660.
24. WHO (2009) *2008–2013 Action Plan for the Global Strategy for the Prevention and Control of Non-communicable Diseases*. World Health Organization, Geneva, Switzerland <http://www.who.int/nmh/publications/ncd_action_plan_en.pdf>.
25. CDC (2013) *CDC in Brazil – Fact Sheet*. Centers for Disease Control and Prevention, Atlanta, Georgia <http://www.cdc.gov/globalhealth/countries/brazil/pdf/brazil.pdf>.
26. CDC (2013) *Global Health – China*. Centers for Disease Control and Prevention Atlanta, Georgia <http://www.cdc.gov/globalhealth/countries/china>.
27. Jackson, R.J. (2003) The impact of the built environment on health: an emerging field. *American Journal of Public Health* 93, 1382–1384.
28. University of Wisconsin School of Medicine and Public Health. (2013) *Survey of the Health of Wisconsin* <http://www.med.wisc.edu/show/survey-of-the-health-of-wisconsin/35828>.
29. WHO (2008) *The Global Burden of Disease: 2004 Update*. World Health Organization, Geneva, Switzerland.
30. South African National Department of Health (2013) *Disease Notification System*. World Health Organization, Geneva, Switzerland <http://www.doh.gov.za>.
31. Mathee, A. (2012) Lead poisoning. In: van Niekerk, A., Suffla, S. and Seedat, M. (eds) *Crime, Violence and Injury in South Africa: 21st Century Solution for Child Safety*. South African Medical Research Council, Cape Town, South Africa.
32. South African National Department of Health (2011) *National Health Act, 2003 (Act No. 61 of 2003) – Regulations Relating to Cancer Registration*. South African National Department of Health, Pretoria, South Africa.
33. WHO (2013) *Chronic Diseases and Health Promotion – STEPS Country Reports*. World Health Organization, Geneva, Switzerland <http://www.who.int/chp/steps/reports/en/index.html>.
34. National Cancer Registry Programme (2012) *National Cancer Registry Programme*. Indian Council of Medical Research, India <http://www.ncrpindia.org>.
35. Feigin, V.L., Lawes, C.M., Bennett, D.A. and Anderson, C.S. (2003) Stroke epidemiology: a review of population-based studies of incidence, prevalence, and case-fatality in the late 20th century. *Lancet Neurology* 2, 43–53.
36. Feigin, V.L., Lawes, C.M., Bennett, D.A., Barker-Collo, S.L. and Parag, V. (2009) Worldwide stroke incidence and early case fatality reported in 56 population-based studies: a systematic review. *Lancet Neurology* 8, 355–369.
37. Sridharan, S.E., Unnikrishnan, J.P., Sukumaran, S., Sylaja, P.N., Nayak, S.D., Sarma, P.S. and Radhakrishnan, K. (2009) Incidence, types, risk factors, and outcome of stroke in a developing country: the Trivandrum Stroke Registry. *Stroke* 40, 1212–1218.
38. Dalal, P.M., Malik, S., Bhattacharjee, M., Trivedi, N.D., Vairale, J., Bhat, P., Deshmukh, S., Khandelwal, K. and Mathur, V.D. (2008) Population-based stroke survey in Mumbai, India: incidence and 28-day case fatality. *Neuroepidemiology* 31, 254–261.

39. Fang, X.H., Wang, W.H., Zhang, X.Q., Liu, H.J., Zhang, H.M., Qin, X.M., Wang, Z.C., Ji, X.M. and Li, L.M. (2012) Incidence and survival of symptomatic lacunar infarction in a Beijing population: a 6-year prospective study. *European Journal of Neurology* 19, 1114–1120.
40. Minelli, C., Fen, L.F. and Minelli, D.P. (2007) Stroke incidence, prognosis, 30-day, and 1-year case fatality rates in Matao, Brazil: a population-based prospective study. *Stroke* 38, 2906–2911.
41. Danesi, M.A., Okubadejo, N.U., Ojini, F.I. and Ojo, O.O. (2013) Incidence and 30-day case fatality rate of first-ever stroke in urban Nigeria: the prospective community based Epidemiology of Stroke in Lagos (EPISIL) phase II results. *Journal of the Neurological Sciences* 331, 43–47.
42. Sereday, M.S., Martí, M.L., Damiano, M.M. and Moser, M.E. (1994) Establishment of a registry and incidence of IDDM in Avellaneda, Argentina. *Diabetes Care* 17, 1022–1025.
43. Lisboa, H.R., Graebin, R., Butzke, L. and Rodrigues, C.S. (1998) Incidence of type 1 diabetes mellitus in Passo Fundo, R.S., Brazil. *Brazilian Journal Of Medical and Biological Research* 31, 1553–1556.
44. Kadiki, O.A. and Roaeid, R.B. (2002) Incidence of type 1 diabetes in children (0–14 years) in Benghazi Libya (1991–2000). *Diabetes and Metabolism* 28, 463–467.
45. Ben Khalifa, F., Mekaouar, A., Taktak, S., Hamhoum, M., Jebara, H., Kodia, A., Zouari, B. and Chakroun, M. (1997) A five-year study of the incidence of insulin-dependent diabetes mellitus in young Tunisians (preliminary results). *Diabetes and Metabolism* 23, 395–401.
46. Nizam, S., Khalequzzaman, M., Yatsuya, H., Khanam, P.A., Sayeed, M.A., Naito, H. and Nakajima, T. (2012) Incidence of young onset insulin-requiring diabetes mellitus among 18- to 30-year-olds in Dhaka, Bangladesh (1994–2003). *Nagoya Journal of Medical Science* 74, 149–156.
47. Kumar, P., Krishna, P., Reddy, S.C., Gurappa, M., Aravind, S.R. and Munichoodappa, C. (2008) Incidence of type 1 diabetes mellitus and associated complications among children and young adults: results from Karnataka Diabetes Registry 1995–2008. *Journal of Indian Medical Association* 106, 708–711.
48. Mathers, C.D., Fat, D.M., Inoue, M., Rao, C. and Lopez, A.D. (2005) Counting the dead and what they died from: an assessment of the global status of cause of death data. *Bulletin of the World Health Organization* 83, 171–177.
49. Joshi, R., Kengne, A.P. and Neal, B. (2009) Methodological trends in studies based on verbal autopsies before and after published guidelines. *Bulletin of the World Health Organization* 87, 678–682.
50. Mahapatra, P., Shibuya, K., Lopez, A.D., Coullare, F., Notzon, F.C., Rao, C., Szreter, S. and Monitoring Vital Events (2007) Civil registration systems and vital statistics: successes and missed opportunities. *Lancet* 370, 1653–1663.
51. Joubert, J., Rao, C., Bradshaw, D., Vos, T. and Lopez, A.D. (2013) Evaluating the quality of national mortality statistics from civil registration in South Africa, 1997–2007. *PloS One* 8, e64592.
52. Rao, C., Lopez, A.D., Yang, G., Begg, S. and Ma, J. (2005) Evaluating national cause-of-death statistics: principles and application to the case of China. *Bulletin of the World Health Organization* 83, 618–625.
53. Mahapatra, P. and Chalapati Rao, P.V. (2001) Cause of death reporting systems in India: a performance analysis. *National Medical Journal of India* 14, 154–162.
54. Franca, E., de Abreu, D.X., Rao, C. and Lopez, A.D. (2008) Evaluation of cause-of-death statistics for Brazil, 2002–2004. *International Journal of Epidemiology* 37, 891–901.
55. Evans, J.M., Barnett, K.N., McMurdo, M.E. and Morris, A.D. (2008) of diabetes on death certificates of 1872 people with type 2 diabetes in Tayside, Scotland. *European Journal of Public Health* 18, 201–203.
56. Lu, T.H., Hsu, P.Y., Bjorkenstam, C. and Anderson, R.N. (2006) Certifying diabetes-related cause-of-death: a comparison of inappropriate certification statements in Sweden, Taiwan and the USA. *Diabetologia* 49, 2878–2881.

57. Mayosi, B.M., Flisher, A.J., Lalloo, U.G., Sitas, F., Tollman, S.M. and Bradshaw, D. (2009) The burden of non-communicable diseases in South Africa. *Lancet* 374, 934–947.
58. Bertram, M.Y., Katzenellenbogen, J., Vos, T., Bradshaw, D. and Hofman, K.J. (2013) The disability adjusted life years due to stroke in South Africa in 2008. *International Journal of Stroke* 8, 76–80.
59. Joubert, J., Norman, R., Lambert, E.V., Groenewald, P., Schneider, M., Bull, F., Bradshaw, D. and the South African Comparative Risk Assessment Collaborating Group (2007) Estimating the burden of disease attributable to physical inactivity in South Africa in 2000. *South African Medical Journal* 97, 725–231.
60. Joubert, J., Norman, R., Bradshaw, D., Goedecke, J.H., Steyn, N.P., Puoane, T. and the South African Comparative Risk Assessment Collaborating Group (2007) Estimating the burden of disease attributable to excess body weight in South Africa in 2000. *South African Medical Journal* 97, 683–690.
61. Schneider, M., Norman, R., Steyn, N., Bradshaw, D. and the South African Comparative Risk Assessment Collaborating Group (2007) Estimating the burden of disease attributable to low fruit and vegetable intake in South Africa in 2000. *South African Medical Journal* 97, 717–723.
62. Norman, R., Bradshaw, D., Schneider, M., Joubert, J., Groenewald, P., Lewin, S., Steyn, K., Vos, T., Laubscher, R., Nannan, N., Nojilana, B., Pieterse, D. and the South African Comparative Risk Assessment Collaborating Group (2007) A comparative risk assessment for South Africa in 2000, towards promoting health and preventing disease. *South African Medical Journal* 97, 637–641.
63. Norman, R., Gaziano, T., Laubscher, R., Steyn, K., Bradshaw, D. and the South African Comparative Risk Assessment Collaborating Group (2007) Estimating the burden of disease attributable to high blood pressure in South Africa in 2000. *South African Medical Journal* 97, 692–698.
64. Norman, R., Bradshaw, D., Lewin, S., Cairncross, E., Nannan, N., Vos, T. and South African Comparative Risk Assessment Collaborating Group (2010) Estimating the burden of disease attributable to four selected environmental risk factors in South Africa. *Review on Environmental Health* 25, 87–119.
65. Groenewald, P., Vos, T., Norman, R., Laubscher, R., van Walbeek, C., Saloojee, Y., Sitas, F., Bradshaw, D. and the South African Comparative Risk Assessment Collaborating Group (2007) Estimating the burden of disease attributable to smoking in South Africa in 2000. *South African Medical Journal* 97, 674–81.
66. Bradshaw, D., Norman, R., Pieterse, D., Levitt, N.S. and the South African Comparative Risk Assessment Collaborating Group (2007) Estimating the burden of disease attributable to diabetes in South Africa in 2000. *South African Medical Journal* 97, 700–706.
67. Stringhini, S., Sinon, F., Didon, J., Gedeon, J., Paccaud, F. and Bovet, P. (2012) Declining stroke and myocardial infarction mortality between 1989 and 2010 in a country of the African region. *Stroke* 43, 2283–2288.
68. Roth, G.A. and Murray, C.J. (2013) The Global Burden of Disease Study 2010 does not show a rise in the age-standardized mortality rate for cardiovascular disease in sub-Saharan Africa. *Progress in Cardiovascular Diseases* 56, 278–280.
69. WHO (2006) *WHO STEPS Stroke Manual: the WHO STEPwise Approach to Stroke Surveillance.* World Health Organization, Geneva, Switzerland.
70. WHO (2013) *STEPwise Approach to Surveillance (STEPS).* World Health Organization, Geneva, Switzerland <http://www.who.int/chp/steps/en>.
71. Anderson, J.E. and Cleland, J.G. (1984) The World Fertility Survey and Contraceptive Prevalence Surveys: a comparison of substantive results. *Studies in Family Planning* 15, 1–13.
72. Vaessen, M., Thiam, M. and Le, T. (2005) The Demographic and Health Surveys. In: *Household Sample Surveys in Developing and Transition Countries.* United Nations, New York, pp. 495–522.
73. Short Fabic, M., Choi, Y. and Bird, S. (2012) A systematic review of demographic and health surveys: data availability and utilization for research. *Bulletin of the World Health Organization* 90, 604–612.

74. Corsi, D.J., Neuman, M., Finlay, J.E. and Subramanian, S.V. (2012) Demographic and health surveys: a profile. *International Journal of Epidemiology* 41, 1602–1613.
75. Mishra, V., Arnold, F., Semenov. G., Hong, R. and Mukuria, A. (2005) *Epidemiology of Obesity and Hypertension in Uzbekistan*. DHS Working Papers. USAID, Washington, DC.
76. Mishra, V., Agrawal, P., Arnold, F., Hong, R., and Macro, I.C.F. (2009) *Effects of Obesity on the Markers of Cardiovascular Disease in Tashkent City, Uzbekistan: Evidence from a Population-Based Health Examination Survey*. DHS Working Papers, USAID, Washington, DC.
77. Corsi, D.J., Finlay JE. and Subramanian, S.V. (2012) Weight of communities: a multilevel analysis of body mass index in 32,814 neighborhoods in 57 low- to middle-income countries (LMICs). *Social Science and Medicine* 75, 311–322.
78. Martorell, R., Khan, L.K., Hughes, M.L. and Grummer-Strawn, L.M. (2000) Overweight and obesity in preschool children from developing countries. *International Journal of Obesity and Related Metabolic Disorders* 24, 959–967.
79. Martorell, R., Khan, L.K., Hughes, M.L. and Grummer-Strawn, L.M. (2000) Obesity in women from developing countries. *European Journal of Clinical Nutrition* 54, 247–252.
80. Lopez-Arana, S., Avendano, M., van Lenthe, F.J. and Burdorf, A. (2014) Trends in overweight among women differ by occupational class: results from 33 low- and middle-income countries in the period 1992–2009. *International Journal of Obesity* 38, 97–105.
81. Popkin, B.M. and Slining, M.M. (2013) New dynamics in global obesity facing low- and middle-income countries. *Obesity Reviews* 14, 11–20.
82. Lopez-Arana, S., Burdorf, A. and Avendano, M. (2013) Trends in overweight by educational level in 33 low- and middle-income countries: the role of parity, age at first birth and breastfeeding. *Obesity Reviews* 14, 806–817.
83. Ziraba, A.K., Fotso, J.C. and Ochako, R. (2009) Overweight and obesity in urban Africa: a problem of the rich or the poor? *BMC Public Health* 9, 465.
84. Razak, F., Corsi, D.J. and Subramanian, S.V. (2013) Change in the body mass index distribution for women: analysis of surveys from 37 low- and middle-income countries. *PLoS Medicine* 10, e1001367.
85. Jones-Smith, J.C., Gordon-Larsen, P., Siddiqi, A. and Popkin, B.M. (2012) Is the burden of overweight shifting to the poor across the globe? Time trends among women in 39 low- and middle-income countries (1991–2008). *International Journal of Obesity* 36, 1114–1120.
86. Jones-Smith, J.C., Gordon-Larsen, P., Siddiqi, A. and Popkin, B.M. (2011) Cross-national comparisons of time trends in overweight inequality by socioeconomic status among women using repeated cross-sectional surveys from 37 developing countries, 1989–2007. *American Journal of Epidemiology* 173, 667–675.
87. Kim, S.A., Stein, A.D. and Martorell, R. (2007) Country development and the association between parity and overweight. *International Journal of Obesity* 31, 805–812.
88. Subramanian, S.V., Perkins, J.M., Özaltin, E. and Davey Smith, G. (2011) Weight of nations: a socioeconomic analysis of women in low- to middle-income countries. *American Journal of Clinical Nutrition* 93, 413–421.
89. Balarajan, Y. and Villamor, E. (2009) Nationally representative surveys show recent increases in the prevalence of overweight and obesity among women of reproductive age in Bangladesh, Nepal, and India. *Journal of Nutrition* 139, 2139–2144.
90. Neuman, M., Finlay, J.E., Davey Smith, G. and Subramanian, S.V. (2011) The poor stay thinner: stable socioeconomic gradients in BMI among women in lower- and middle-income countries. *American Journal of Clinical Nutrition* 94, 1348–1357.
91. Kim, S.A., Yount, K.M., Ramakrishnan, U. and Martorell, R. (2007) The relationship between parity and overweight varies with household wealth and national development. *International Journal of Epidemiology* 36, 93–101.
92. de Onis, M. and Blossner, M. (2000) Prevalence and trends of overweight among preschool children in developing countries. *American Journal of Clinical Nutrition* 72, 1032–1039.

93. Global Tobacco Surveillance System Collaborating Group (2005) Global Tobacco Surveillance System (GTSS): purpose, production, and potential. *Journal of School Health* 75, 15–24.
94. Warren, C.W., Lea, V., Lee, J., Jones, N.R., Asma, S. and McKenna, M. (2009) Change in tobacco use among 13–15 year olds between 1999 and 2008, findings from the Global Youth Tobacco Survey. *Global Health Promotion* 16, 38–90.
95. Warren, C.W., Jones, N.R., Eriksen, M.P., Asma, S. and the Global Tobacco Surveillance System (GTSS) Collaborative Group (2006) Patterns of global tobacco use in young people and implications for future chronic disease burden in adults. *Lancet* 367, 749–753.
96. Warren, C.W., Lee, J., Lea, V., Goding, A., O'Hara, B., Carlberg, M., Asma, S. and McKenna, M. (2009) Evolution of the Global Tobacco Surveillance System (GTSS) 1998–2008. *Global Health Promotion* 16, 4–37.
97. Warren, C.W., Riley, L., Asma, S., Eriksen, M.P., Green, L., Blanton, C., Loo, C., Batchelor, S. and Yach, D. (2000) Tobacco use by youth: a surveillance report from the Global Youth Tobacco Survey project. *Bulletin of the World Health Organization* 78, 868–876.
98. Global Youth Tobacco Survey Collaborating Group (2003) Differences in worldwide tobacco use by gender: findings from the Global Youth Tobacco Survey. *Journal of School Health* 73, 207–215.
99. King, B.A., Mirza, S.A., Babb, S.D. and the GATS Collaborating Group (2013) A cross-country comparison of secondhand smoke exposure among adults: findings from the Global Adult Tobacco Survey (GATS). *Tobacco Control* 22, e5.
100. Warren, C.W., Jones, N.R., Peruga, A., Chauvin, J., Baptiste, J.P., Costa de Silva, V., el Awa, F., Tsouros, A., Rahman, K., Fishburn, B., Bettcher, D.W., Asma, S. and the CDC (2008) Global youth tobacco surveillance, 2000–2007. *MMWR Surveillance Summaries* 57, 1–28.
101. Sinha, D.N., Palipudi, K.M., Rolle, I., Asma, S. and Rinchen, S. (2011) Tobacco use among youth and adults in member countries of South-East Asia region: review of findings from surveys under the Global Tobacco Surveillance System. *Indian Journal of Public Health* 55, 169–176.
102. International Network for the Demographic Evaluation of Populations and Their Health (2013) *The INDEPTH Network: Better Health Information for Better Health Policy* <http://www.indepth-network.org>.
103. Sankoh, O. and Byass, P. (2012) The INDEPTH Network: filling vital gaps in global epidemiology. *International Journal of Epidemiology* 41, 579–588.
104. International Network for the Demographic Evaluation of Populations and Their Health (1998) *Founding Document* <http://indepth-network.org/index.php?option=com_content&task=view&id=43>.
105. Scott, J.A., Bauni, E., Moisi, J.C., Ojal, J., Gatakaa, H., Nyundo, C., Molyneux, C.S., Kombe, F., Tsofa, B., Marsh, K., Peshu, N. and Williams, T.N. (2012) Profile: the Kilifi Health and Demographic Surveillance System (KHDSS). *International Journal of Epidemiology* 41, 650–657.
106. Rossier, C., Soura, A., Baya, B., Compaoré, G., Dabiré, B., Dos Santos, S., Duthé, G., Gnoumou, B., Kobiané, J.F., Kouanda, S., Lankoandé, B., Legrand, T., Mbacke, C., Millogo, R., Mondain, N., Montgomery, M., Nikiema, A., Ouili, I., Pison, G., Randall, S., Sangli, G., Schoumaker, B. and Zourkaleini, Y. (2012) Profile: the Ouagadougou Health and Demographic Surveillance System. *International Journal of Epidemiology* 41, 658–666.
107. Kahn, K., Collinson, M.A., Gómez-Olivé, F.X., Mokoena, O., Twine, R., Mee, P., Afolabi, S.A., Clark, B.D., Kabudula, C.W., Khosa, A., Khoza, S., Shabangu, M.G., Silaule, B., Tibane, J.B., Wagner, R.G., Garenne, M.L., Clark, S.J. and Tollman, S.M. (2012) Profile: Agincourt health and socio-demographic surveillance system. *International Journal of Epidemiology* 41, 988–1001.
108. Huu Bich, T., Thi Quynh Nga, P., Ngoc Quang, L., Van Minh, H., Ng, N., Juvekar, S., Razzaque, A., Ashraf, A., Masud Ahmed, S., Soonthornthada, K. and Kanungsukkasem, U. (2009) Patterns of alcohol consumption in diverse rural populations in the Asian region. *Global Health Action* 2, doi: 10.3402/gha.v2i0.2017.

109. Van Minh, H., Soonthornthada, K., Ng, N., Juvekar, S., Razzaque, A., Ashraf, A., Ahmed, S.M., Bich, T.H. and Kanungsukkasem, U. (2009) Blood pressure in adult rural INDEPTH population in Asia. *Global Health Action* 2, doi: 10.3402/gha.v2i0.2010.
110. Ng, N., Hakimi, M., Van Minh, H., Juvekar, S., Razzaque, A., Ashraf, A., Masud Ahmed, S., Kanungsukkasem, U., Soonthornthada, K. and Huu Bich, T. (2009) Prevalence of physical inactivity in nine rural INDEPTH Health and Demographic Surveillance Systems in five Asian countries. *Global Health Action* 2, doi: 10.3402/gha.v2i0.1985.
111. Kanungsukkasem, U., Ng, N., Van Minh, H., Razzaque, A., Ashraf, A., Juvekar, S., Masud Ahmed, S. and Huu Bich, T. (2009) Fruit and vegetable consumption in rural adults population in INDEPTH HDSS sites in Asia. *Global Health Action* 2, doi: 10.3402/gha.v2i0.1988.
112. Ashraf, A., Quaiyum M.A., Ng, N., Van Minh, H., Razzaque, A., Masud Ahmed, S., Hadi, A., Juvekar, S., Kanungsukkasem, U., Soonthornthada, K. and Huu Bich, T. (2009) Self-reported use of tobacco products in nine rural INDEPTH Health and Demographic Surveillance Systems in Asia. *Global Health Action* 2, doi: 10.3402/gha.v2i0.1997.
113. Razzaque, A., Nahar, L., Van Minh, H., Ng, N., Juvekar, S., Ashraf, A., Ahmed, S.M., Soonthornthada, K., Kanungsukkasem, U. and Huu Bich, T. (2009) Social factors and overweight: evidence from nine Asian INDEPTH Network sites. *Global Health Action* 2, doi: 10.3402/gha.v2i0.1991.
114. Grosh, M.E. and Glewwe, P. (1995) *A Guide to Living Standards Measurement Study Surveys and Their Data Sets*. Living Standards Measurement Study Working Paper No. 120. World Bank, Washington, DC.
115. Global Health Data Exchange (2013) *Living Standards Measurement Study (LSMS)*. World Bank, Washington, DC <http://ghdx.healthmetricsandevaluation.org/series/living-standards-measurement-study-lsms>.
116. Scott, K., Steele, D. and Temesgen, T. (2005) Living standards measurement study surveys. In: *Household Sample Surveys in Developing and Transition Countries*. United Nations, New York.
117. Handa, S. and Neitzert, M. (1998) *Chronic Illness and Retirement in Jamaica*. World Bank, Washington, DC.
118. Kowal, P., Chatterji, S., Naidoo, N., Biritwum, R., Fan, W., Lopez Ridaura, R., Maximova, T., Arokiasamy, P., Phaswana-Mafuya, N., Williams, S., Snodgrass, J.J., Minicuci, N., D'Este, C., Peltzer, K., Boerma, J.T. and the SAGE Collaborators (2012) Data resource profile: the World Health Organization Study on global AGEing and adult health (SAGE). *International Journal of Epidemiology* 41, 1639–1649.
119. Kowal, P., Kahn, K., Ng, N., Naidoo, N., Abdullah, S., Bawah, A., Binka, F., Chuc, N.T., Debpuur, C., Ezeh, A., Xavier Gómez-Olivé, F., Hakimi, M., Hirve, S., Hodgson, A., Juvekar, S., Kyobutungi, C., Menken, J., Van Minh, H., Mwanyangala, M.A., Razzaque, A., Sankoh, O., Kim Streatfield, P., Wall, S., Wilopo, S., Byass, P., Chatterji, S. and Tollman, S.M. (2010) Ageing and adult health status in eight lower-income countries: the INDEPTH WHO-SAGE collaboration. *Global Health Action* 3, doi: 10.3402/gha.v3i0.5302.
120. Yawson, A.E., Baddoo, A., Hagan-Seneadza, N.A., Calys-Tagoe, B., Hewlett, S., Dako-Gyeke, P., Mensah, G., Minicuci, N., Naidoo, N., Chatterji, S., Kowal, P. and Biritwum, R. (2013) Tobacco use in older adults in Ghana: sociodemographic characteristics, health risks and subjective wellbeing. *BMC Public Health* 13, 979.
121. Hosseinpoor, A.R., Bergen, N., Kunst, A., Harper, S., Guthold, R., Rekve, D., d'Espaignet, E.T., Naidoo, N. and Chatterji, S. (2012) Socioeconomic inequalities in risk factors for non-communicable diseases in low-income and middle-income countries: results from the World Health Survey. *BMC Public Health* 12, 912.
122. Phaswana-Mafuya, N., Peltzer, K., Chirinda, W., Musekiwa, A., Kose, Z., Hoosain, E., Davids, A. and Ramlagan, S. (2013) Self-reported prevalence of chronic non-communicable diseases and associated factors among older adults in South Africa. *Global Health Action* 6, doi: 10.3402/gha.v6i0.20936.

123. Ng, N., Kowal, P., Kahn, K., Naidoo, N., Abdullah, S., Bawah, A., Binka, F., Chuc, N.T., Debpuur, C., Egondi, T., Xavier Gómez-Olivé, F., Hakimi, M., Hirve, S., Hodgson, A., Juvekar, S., Kyobutungi, C., Van Minh, H., Mwanyangala, M.A., Nathan, R., Razzaque, A., Sankoh, O., Kim Streatfield, P., Thorogood, M., Wall, S., Wilopo, S., Byass, P., Tollman, S.M. and Chatterji, S. (2010) Health inequalities among older men and women in Africa and Asia: evidence from eight Health and Demographic Surveillance System sites in the INDEPTH WHO-SAGE Study. *Global Health Action* 3, doi: 10.3402/gha.v3i0.5420.
124. Popkin, B.M., Du, S., Zhai, F. and Zhang, B. (2010) Cohort profile: the China Health and Nutrition Survey – monitoring and understanding socio-economic and health change in China, 1989–2011. *International Journal of Epidemiology* 39, 1435–1440.
125. Xi, B., Liang, Y., He, T., Reilly, K.H., Hu, Y., Wang, Q., Yan, Y. and Mi, J. (2012) Secular trends in the prevalence of general and abdominal obesity among Chinese adults, 1993–2009. *Obesity Reviews* 13, 287–296.
126. Liang, Y.J., Xi, B., Song, A.Q., Liu, J.X. and Mi, J. (2012) Trends in general and abdominal obesity among Chinese children and adolescents 1993–2009. *Pediatric Obesity* 7, 355–364.
127. Du, T., Sun, X., Yin, P., Huo, R., Ni, C. and Yu, X. (2013) Increasing trends in central obesity among Chinese adults with normal body mass index, 1993–2009. *BMC Public Health* 13, 327.
128. Yan, S., Li, J., Li, S., Zhang, B., Du, S., Gordon-Larsen, P., Adair, L. and Popkin, B. (2012) The expanding burden of cardiometabolic risk in China: the China Health and Nutrition Survey. *Obesity Reviews* 13, 810–821.
129. Morales, D.D., Punzalan, F.E., Paz-Pacheco, E., Sy, R.G., Duante, C.A. and the National Nutrition and Health Survey: 2003 Group (2008) Metabolic syndrome in the Philippine general population: prevalence and risk for atherosclerotic cardiovascular disease and diabetes mellitus. *Diabetes and Vascular Disease Research* 5, 36–43.
130. Department of Science and Technology Research and Development Institute (2008) *National Nutrition Survey Results 2008* <http://www.fnri.dost.gov.ph>.
131. Duran, P., Mangialavori, G., Biglieri, A., Kogan, L. and Abeyá Gilardon, E. (2009) [Nutrition status in Argentinean children 6 to 72 months old: results from the National Nutrition and Health Survey (ENNyS)]. *Archivos Argentinos de Pediatria* 107, 397–404 (in Spanish).
132. Reddy, P., Shisana, O., Labadarios, D., Rehle, T., Simbayi, L., Zuma, K., Dhansay, A., Parker, W., Naidoo, P., Mchiza, Z., Steyn, N.P., Makoae, M., Ramlagan, S., Zungu, N., Evans, M.G., Faber, M., Hoosain, E., Hongoro, C., Dwane, N., Maluleke, T. and Jacobs, L. (2014) *The South African National Health and Nutrition Examination Survey, 2012: SANHANES-1: the Health and Nutritional Status of the Nation*. Human Sciences Research Council, Pretoria, South Africa.
133. Medina, C., Janssen, I., Campos, I. and Barquera, S. (2013) Physical inactivity prevalence and trends among Mexican adults: results from the National Health and Nutrition Survey (ENSANUT) 2006 and 2012. *BMC Public Health* 13, 1063.
134. Ponce, X., Rodríguez-Ramírez, S., Mundo-Rosas, V., Shamah, T., Barquera, S. and González de Cossio, T. (2013) Dietary quality indices vary with sociodemographic variables and anthropometric status among Mexican adults: a cross-sectional study. Results from the 2006 National Health and Nutrition Survey. *Public Health Nutrition* 17, 1717–1728.
135. Ramirez-Silva, I., Rivera, J.A., Ponce, X. and Hernández-Avila, M. (2009) Fruit and vegetable intake in the Mexican population: results from the Mexican National Health and Nutrition Survey 2006. *Salud Pública de México* 51, S574–S585.
136. Rtveladze, K., Marsh, T., Barquera, S., Sanchez Romero, L.M., Levy, D., Melendez, G., Webber, L., Kilpi, F. and McPherson, K. (2013) Obesity prevalence in Mexico: impact on health and economic burden. *Public Health Nutrition*, 17, 233–239.
137. Anjana, R.M., Pradeepa, R., Deepa, M., Datta, M., Sudha, V., Unnikrishnan, R., Nath, L.M., Das, A.K., Madhu, S.V., Rao, P.V., Shukla, D.K., Kaur, T., Ali, M.K. and Mohan, V. (2011) The Indian Council of Medical Research-India Diabetes (ICMR-INDIAB) study: methodological details. *Journal of Diabetes Science and Technology* 5, 906–914.

138. Anjana, R.M., Pradeepa, R., Deepa, M., Datta, M., Sudha, V., Unnikrishnan, R., Bhansali, A., Joshi, S.R., Joshi, P.P., Yajnik, C.S., Dhandhania, V.K., Nath, L.M., Das, A.K., Rao, P.V., Madhu, S.V., Shukla, D.K., Kaur, T., Priya, M., Nirmal, E., Parvathi, S.J., Subhashini, S., Subashini, R., Ali, M.K., Mohan, V. and the ICMR–INDIAB Collaborative Study Group (2011) Prevalence of diabetes and prediabetes (impaired fasting glucose and/or impaired glucose tolerance) in urban and rural India: phase I results of the Indian Council of Medical Research-INdia DIABetes (ICMR-INDIAB) study. *Diabetologia* 54, 3022–3027.
139. Narayan, K.M. and Echouffo-Tcheugui, J.B. (2011) Analysis of the Indian Council of Medical Research-India Diabetes (ICMR-INDIAB) study. *Journal of Diabetes Science and Technology* 5, 915–917.
140. Nair, M., Ali, M.K., Ajay, V.S., Shivashankar, R., Mohan, V., Pradeepa, R., Deepa, M., Khan, H.M., Kadir, M.M., Fatmi, Z.A., Reddy, K.S., Tandon, N., Narayan, K.M.V. and Prabhakaran, D. (2012) CARRS Surveillance study: design and methods to assess burdens from multiple perspectives. *BMC Public Health* 12, 701.
141. Li, Y., Jiang, Y., Zhang, M., Yin, P., Wu, F. and Zhao, W. (2011) Drinking behaviour among men and women in China: the 2007 China Chronic Disease and Risk Factor Surveillance. *Addiction* 106, 1946–1956.
142. Li, Y., Zhang, M., Jiang, Y. and Wu, F. (2012) Co-variations and clustering of chronic disease behavioral risk factors in China: China Chronic Disease and Risk Factor Surveillance, 2007. *PloS One* 7, e33881.
143. Yin, P., Zhang, M., Li, Y., Jiang, Y. and Zhao, W. (2011) Prevalence of COPD and its association with socioeconomic status in China: findings from China Chronic Disease Risk Factor Surveillance 2007. *BMC Public Health* 11, 586.
144. World Bank (1993) *World Development Report 1993 – Investing in Health.* Oxford University Press Oxford, UK.
145. Murray, C.J.L. (1996) Rethinking DALYs. In: Murray, C.J.L. and Lopez, A.D. (eds) *Global Burden of Disease – a Comprehensive Assessment of Mortality and Disability From Diseases, Injuries, and Risk Factors in 1990 and Projected to 2020.* Harvard School of Public Health on behalf of the World Health Organization and the World Bank. Cambridge, UK.
146. Murray, C.J.L. and Lopez, A.D. (eds) (1996) *Global Burden of Disease – A Comprehensive Assessment of Mortality and Disability From Diseases, Injuries, and Risk Factors in 1990 and Projected to 2020.* Harvard School of Public Health on behalf of the World Health Organization and the World Bank. Cambridge, UK.
147. Wang, H., Dwyer-Lindgren, L., Lofgren, K.T., Rajaratnam, J.K., Marcus, J.R., Levin-Rector, A., Levitz, C.E., Lopez, A.D. and Murray, C.J. (2012) Age-specific and sex specific mortality in 187 countries, 1970–2010, a systematic analysis for the Global Burden of Disease Study 2010. *Lancet* 380, 2071–2094.
148. Thacker, S.B., Qualters, J.R., Lee, L.M. and the Centers for Disease Control and Prevention (2012) Public health surveillance in the United States: evolution and challenges. *MMWR Surveillance Summaries* 61, 3–9.

8 Community-based Interventions for Preventing Chronic Non-communicable diseases in Low- and Middle-income Countries

JULIET ADDO[1]* AND STEVEN VAN DE VIJVER[2]

[1]*London School of Hygiene and Tropical Medicine, London, UK;* [2]*African Population and Health Research Centre, Nairobi, Kenya*

8.1 Introduction

Chronic non-communicable diseases (NCDs) are a significant cause of premature morbidity and mortality globally. They have a huge impact on low- and middle-income countries (LMICs), where they often strike at younger ages and with more severe consequences. Current evidence points to a growing burden of NCDs in LMICs with serious implications for economic development and growth [1]. The increasing burden of NCDs often disproportionately affects poorer populations, thereby widening health inequalities between and within populations. The principal NCDs contributing to the greatest burden of mortality globally are cardiovascular disease, cancer, chronic obstructive pulmonary disease and diabetes. These conditions generally share modifiable and preventable lifestyle-related risk factors including unhealthy nutrition over a prolonged period, tobacco use, physical inactivity and excessive use of alcohol [2]. Effective strategies to prevent NCDs need to address these risk factors and the adverse social and physical environments in which they thrive. Such public health strategies can either target entire populations or high-risk individuals in the population, or a combination of both. The primary tool for implementing population strategies of prevention is a community-based programme where community interventions use education or environmental change to promote and facilitate lifestyle and behaviour changes needed to address a particular problem [3].

Previous studies have shown the need for interventions to be delivered with an appropriate intensity and sustained over extended periods of time to achieve

*E-mail: juliet.addo@lshtm.ac.uk

substantial reductions in the levels of risk factors [2]. However, even modest changes in risk factor levels have been shown to be of significant public health benefit [2].

The aim of this chapter is to examine some of the community-based NCD interventions conducted in LMICs, specifically interventions from sub-Saharan Africa, Asia and Latin America, and to examine the components of interventions that promote uptake and successful implementation, the cost-effectiveness of such programmes and the sustainability of the health gains achieved.

8.2 Why Community-based Interventions?

The main pillars of the World Health Organization (WHO)'s Action Plan for NCD prevention include: risk factor surveillance, multi-sector policies aimed at creating an environment that enhances healthy behaviour, programmes targeting both the general population and high-risk groups, and integrated cost-effective case management at the primary healthcare level [4]. There are several ways to describe community-based interventions for prevention of NCDs, but an overview is given in the American Heart Association Framework for public health practice

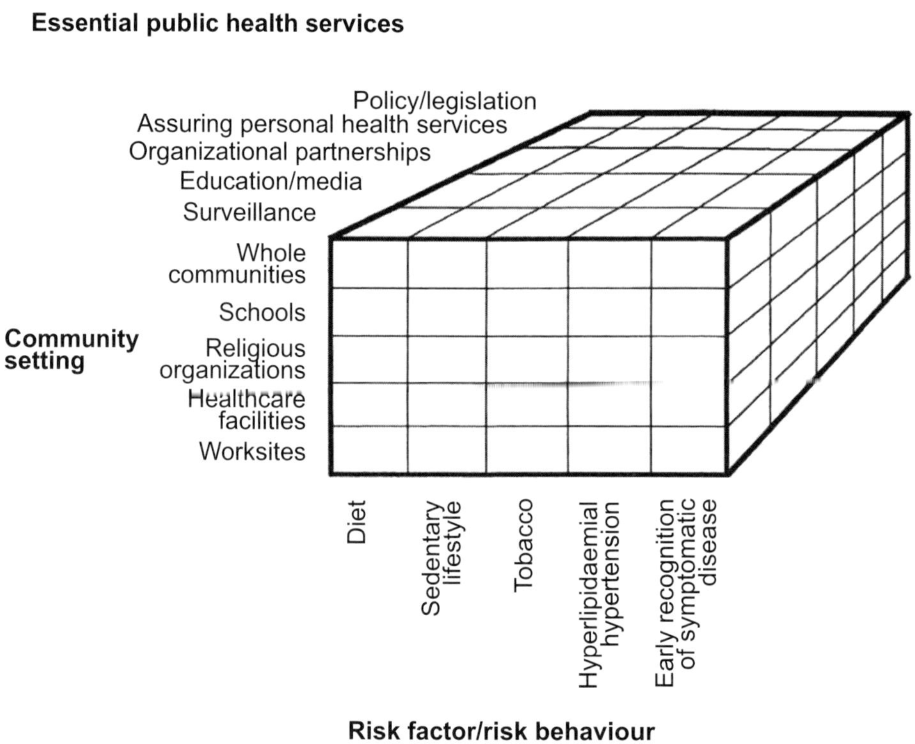

Fig. 8.1. American Heart Association Framework for public health practice for cardiovascular disease prevention. (Reproduced from [5] with permission of the American Heart Association.)

for cardiovascular disease prevention (Fig. 8.1), which includes involvement through different channels such as worksites, schools and religious organizations. These strategies may be applicable for use with other NCDs apart from cardiovascular disease.

The prevention strategies targeting entire communities aim to lower the mean level of risk factors in populations through lifestyle and environmental changes without necessarily requiring health screening of high-risk individuals in the populations. Such strategies generally use mass education or policy interventions directed at the entire population to reduce the overall level of risk factors [6]. The success of community-based interventions requires community participation, supportive policy decisions, intersectoral action, legislation and collaboration with non-governmental organizations and the private sector [1]. Community-based intervention strategies are undoubtedly important for LMIC settings where existing health systems often lack the capacity to deal with chronic NCDs at the same time as they struggle to cope with communicable diseases and other pressing health issues. Community-wide strategies generally target a large number of people at small risk with the assumption that these people may give rise to more cases of disease than a small number at high risk [7]. Targeting an entire population with an intervention is also behaviourally more appropriate, and once a social norm has become accepted and widely adopted, it is easier to maintain in the long term [7]. The community-based intervention strategy recognizes that individual behaviour is greatly influenced by societal factors, and that considerable reductions in risk factors for a disease are more likely to be attained at the population rather than the individual level.

There have been previous community-based health interventions in high-income countries aimed at promoting risk-reducing lifestyle changes in response to the high and increasing burden of NCDs, particularly cardiovascular disease (see also Agyemang *et al.*, Chapter 11, this volume). Examples of these include the North Karelia Project in Finland [8] and the Stanford Five-City Project [9] and Minnesota Heart Health Program (MHHP) in the USA [10]. The experience gained from these previous community-based interventions is important in planning and implementing NCD prevention and control activities in LMICs [11]. However, it is known that the gap between existing medical knowledge and effective real-life NCD preventive strategies is often due to obstacles including cultural, political, economic and psychological barriers, which prevent healthy choices being made [11, 12]. Experience gained from community-based interventions conducted in LMICs is important in helping communities with similar characteristics bridge the gap between knowledge and practice.

8.3 Examples of Community-based Interventions in LMICs

One of the first community-based NCD prevention programmes in LMICs was the Coronary Risk Factor Study (CORIS), which was conducted in South Africa over three decades ago [13]. This paved the way for other NCD intervention programmes in LMICs. Different strategies were used in the different settings as part of the community-based intervention and generally involved mass campaigns with health promotion messages that were either national programmes as in the case of Mauritius [14], or comprehensive regional projects as in the area of Isfahan in Iran [5] and Ballabgarh in India [16]. Some of these interventions were directed at employers at working sites [17, 18] and focused on a specific risk factor such as salt reduction [19], diet adjustments [20] and improving physical activity [17], or involved programmes targeting several risk factors as outlined in a few examples of interventions described below.

8.3.1 The Coronary Risk Factor Study (CORIS) in South Africa

During the 1980s, the Afrikaans-speaking South African population had been shown to have a high coronary heart disease mortality and a high prevalence of coronary heart disease risk factors [21]. CORIS examined the feasibility and effectiveness of a multi-factorial community intervention programme to reduce coronary heart disease risk factor levels in three Afrikaner communities – two intervention communities and one control. Intervention communities received a mass media programme in the form of posters, bill boards, mailings and items in local newspapers [13]. Community-initiated activities included fun runs and family walks, and local food suppliers and restaurants were encouraged to provide low-fat, low-cholesterol and low-salt foods. A blood pressure station offering free blood pressure screening and educational materials was established in both intervention areas. After 4 years of intervention, a significant reduction in blood pressure and smoking was observed in the intervention communities. Although total cholesterol decreased by 10–12%, there was no net reduction in favour of the intervention communities. There was little change in body mass index in all three communities. Women engaged more with the intervention activities and interestingly, with the exception of body mass index, risk factor change was consistently higher in women than in men in the intervention communities. As the intervention was multi-factorial and integrated, it was difficult to identify the most successful elements. However, in terms of having the largest degree of continuing contact with the communities, the blood pressure station could be considered to be the most successful and, interestingly, blood pressure showed the most consistent and significant net reductions. During an additional 8 years of follow-up, the risk factor profile of all three study communities improved despite less active intervention, possibly due to regional and national secular trends occurring at the same time [22]. The main lesson from CORIS was that a comprehensive approach including broad-based media and education interventions is effective.

8.3.2 NCD intervention programme in Mauritius

The government of Mauritius instituted a national NCD intervention programme after a baseline survey of the distribution of disease and risk factors confirmed a high prevalence of diabetes, hypertension and coronary heart disease [23]. A dedicated NCD unit was created within the Ministry of Health, which coordinated an intensive national programme aimed at modifying levels of risk factors related to lifestyle, including glucose intolerance, hypertension, hyperlipidaemia, obesity, cigarette smoking, alcohol misuse and physical inactivity [14]. Components of the intervention included extensive use of the mass media; fiscal and legislative measures; and widespread community, school and workplace health education activities. There was a comprehensive anti-tobacco campaign using the mass media, advertising bans and increased taxation. As well as promoting healthy lifestyles, the government also limited the content of palm oil in the cooking oil used almost universally in Mauritius ('ration oil'), which is high in saturated fatty acids and which was then the main component of ration oil. After 5 years, the estimated intake of saturated fatty acids decreased and the intake of polyunsaturated fatty acids increased significantly. Mean serum cholesterol concentration decreased by 15% after the cooking oil intervention was introduced nationwide [24]. There were also significant reductions in population blood pressure, increased leisure exercise, and decreased smoking and alcohol consumption. The health knowledge about NCDs and their risk factors also increased significantly in the Mauritian public over the intervention period. The prevalence of overweight or obesity, however, increased, and the rates of glucose intolerance changed little [14]. The NCD project in Mauritius shows how lifestyle intervention programmes can be implemented with positive effects in developing countries.

8.3.3 Community-based intervention project in China: the Tianjin Project

The State Council of China issued the National Plan of Action for Nutrition in 1997 in response to a shift in nutrition towards a high intake of fat and animal food and an increase in the prevalence of diet-related NCDs [25]. One of the goals was to improve the general nutritional status of the people and prevent diet-related NCDs through proper guidance on food consumption, improvement of dietary patterns and promotion of healthy lifestyles. The Ministries of Health, Agriculture and Education got involved and various activities were included such as subsidization of vegetables, promotion of soybean consumption, efforts to promote smoking cessation such as bans on smoking in schools and on tobacco advertisements via mass media, and promotion of physical activity in schools.

A major community-based programme for the prevention of NCDs, especially stroke, coronary heart disease and cancer, through lifestyle and risk factor changes was initiated in Tianjin, China [26]. Community-level efforts to control and prevent high blood pressure focused on a reduction in salt intake, control of body weight in the community and appropriate antihypertensive therapy for patients with hypertension. There was a significant net reduction in sodium intake in men in the intervention area after 3 years of intervention [27]. The prevalence of hypertension and obesity decreased among men and women aged between 45 and 64 years over a 7-year period [26]. Stroke mortality rates also decreased significantly in the intervention sites [25]. Body mass index remained unchanged, and there were no changes in salt consumption at household levels after 7 years. The investigators concluded that influencing obesity and salt consumption at the community level was challenging, particularly among younger people.

8.3.4 Community-based intervention in Ballabgarh, India, and Depok, Indonesia

A community-based intervention for NCD prevention and control was conducted in urban populations of India and Indonesia where baseline assessments had shown a high prevalence of tobacco use, obesity, low levels of physical activity, and low intake of fruit and vegetables [16].

The intervention consisted of advocacy and mediation with stakeholders including policy makers, programme managers, and school and industry administrators, training of volunteers and school teachers, communication campaigns, risk assessment camps and reorientation of health services. Specific interventions included policies establishing tobacco-free areas, provision of cycling and pedestrian areas, community empowerment activities that included communication campaigns to increase awareness and healthy lifestyle camps. There was a small decline in smoking and alcohol use at both sites, whereas obesity levels decreased significantly in Indonesia, especially among females, but increased marginally in India. The use of mass media was limited at both sites, and the focus was more on interpersonal communication, which possibly compromised the reach of the campaign. The intervention also included reorientation of health services, which included strengthening of health facilities with equipment and drugs, and providing tobacco and nutritional counselling services [16].

8.3.5 Promoting healthy diets and active lifestyles in Brazil

In response to an increasing pattern of diet and sedentary lifestyle-related NCDs, the Brazilian government introduced a series of innovative policies and initiatives at national, state and local levels to promote healthy food habits and encourage physical activity as part of the efforts to prevent NCDs [28]. Innovative legislative and regulatory actions, mass communications and capacity building were combined to create a comprehensive approach for addressing poor dietary and activity patterns that were leading to obesity and NCDs. Legislative action mandated that manufacturers of packaged foods listed their content in calories, protein, carbohydrates, total fats, saturated fats, cholesterol, calcium, iron, sodium and dietary fibre in standardized, consumer-friendly tables. This packaged-food information regulation process was constructed with intense participation of the Brazilian academic community and the food industry in a series of workshops. Such initiatives allowed people to make better food choices. Another key step was the provision of government-funded healthy school meals using locally grown and minimally processed foods. Other components included training of teachers on healthy nutrition via television, videos, posters and magazines with information on the richness of cultural foods. Another initiative was the 'healthy streets' in Rio de Janeiro, which allow traffic to be interrupted during certain hours during the day or at night so that people can exercise safely.

8.3.6 Community-based interventions for the prevention of cancers

Most of the community-based interventions described above have targeted the common modifiable risk factors for the four types of NCDs that make the largest contribution to mortality in the majority of LMICs such as cardiovascular disease, cancer, chronic respiratory disease and diabetes [2]. In the case of cancer, however, it is important to additionally consider the substantial burden related to infections in LMICs where they explain 22.9% of cancers [29] (see also Adeloye and Grant, Chapter 2; Oni and Unwin, Chapter 3, both this volume). Examples are infections with hepatitis B virus in liver cancer, human papillomavirus (HPV) in cervical cancer, and *Helicobacter pylori* infections in stomach cancer [30]. The WHO recommends infant HPV vaccination including a birth dose, and HPV vaccination targeting adolescent girls before the onset of sexual activity. Hepatitis B virus vaccination has consequently been incorporated into the national immunization programmes of many LMICs and has been demonstrated to be highly effective [31, 32]. Peru has introduced HPV prophylactic vaccination in the national immunization programme for 11-year-old girls, and the feasibility of delivering vaccines through schools and health systems has been demonstrated in other LMICs such as India, Uganda and Vietnam [33, 34]. HPV vaccination in most LMICs is, however, currently limited, and many countries have still not conducted research to establish its cost-effectiveness [35].

8.4 Cost-effectiveness of Community-based NCD Interventions

Considering the limited resources available in LMICs, it is important for prevention strategies to be cost-effective and sustainable. Interventions to prevent NCDs on a population-wide basis have been shown not only to be achievable but also cost-effective, irrespective of the income level of the population [2]. The cost of implementing a set of evidence-based NCD interventions addressing tobacco and harmful alcohol use, as well as unhealthy diet and physical inactivity, across LMICs is projected to be US$2 billion per year amounting to US$0.20 per head of population [36]. While many of the interventions discussed are considered to be cost-effective, some are considered 'best buys', referring to actions that require immediate attention to produce accelerated results in terms of lives saved, diseases prevented and costs avoided [2]. These include protection of people from tobacco smoke and banning smoking in public places; warnings about the dangers of tobacco use; enforcement of bans against tobacco advertising, promotion and sponsorship; raising taxes on tobacco; restricted access to retailed alcohol; enforcing bans on alcohol advertising; raising taxes on alcohol; reducing salt intake and salt content of food; replacing *trans*-fat in food with polyunsaturated fat; and promoting public awareness about diet and physical activity, including through mass media [2]. Legislative changes, food subsidies and the involvement of private industry can be effective without incurring many direct costs [11].

A summary of costs benefits and cost-effectiveness of population-wide interventions to reduce exposure to NCD risk factors has been previously reported [37]. There is limited information on the cost-effectiveness of the population-based interventions from LMICs, despite many of the previous examples employing these suggested interventions. Such information is important in informing policy makers and governments of LMICs of the possibility of implementing effective strategies, even with limited resources.

8.5 Determinants of Successful Implementation

Success in the implementation of prevention strategies may be improved if potential barriers are identified and addressed. Barriers to prevention include cultural norms, insufficient attention to health education from healthcare practitioners, lack of reimbursement for health education services and economic disincentives to healthier lifestyles [38]. Overcoming these barriers requires the involvement of governments, industry, national health authorities, health professionals and society [39, 40].

The results of the various population-wide strategies conducted in LMICs have generally been positive. Community-based interventions such as the national programme in Mauritius and the regional programmes in Iran, Indonesia, India, China and South Africa showed significant reductions in NCD risk factors, demonstrating the effectiveness of comprehensive programmes in LMICs. Many of these programmes targeted various risk factors using multiple strategies, thus limiting the ability to identify the most effective components. Interventions used in the different programmes include health education and mass media campaigns, fiscal and legislative measures, advocacy and mediation with stakeholders including policy makers and industry, capacity building and provision of health-promoting environments. Successful intervention programmes combined well-organized mass media campaigns and health education with legislative action, and involved various stakeholders such as the Ministries of Health, Agriculture and Education in the planning and implementation of various activities. Most were sustained over significant periods and established mechanisms to be in regular contact with the participating communities. Involvement of national and local governments influenced the uptake and sustainability of the programmes significantly. The experience of Mauritius illustrates the important role of national policies in supporting lifestyle changes in NCD prevention and the longer-term benefits of such measures. Active engagement of community organizations and their leaders in the planning and implementation of preventive strategies, and tailoring interventions to address the specific needs and characteristics of different sectors of the population, ultimately encourages participation and uptake of the prevention strategy as observed in Brazil.

Interestingly, most of the community-based interventions discussed above observed little or no change in body mass index and obesity levels in the populations, despite significant changes in other NCD risk factors. The reasons for the seeming lack of effect on body mass index remain unclear, and it is important to identify effective strategies that promote favourable changes in all NCD risk factors including obesity.

8.6 Conclusion

The burden of NCDs in LMICs is currently huge and is projected to increase further. Cost-effective community-based interventions targeting key NCD risk factors and the adverse social and physical environments in the population are feasible and have been implemented successfully in LMICs. These interventions have often combined mass media campaigns with a broad range of health-promoting community activities and have involved various sectors and stakeholders including community organizations and their leaders. Involvement of local and national governments is important for incorporating legislative and regulatory actions and creating supportive physical and social environments that enhance uptake of the interventions.

References

1. Alwan, A. and Maclean, D.R. (2009) A review of non-communicable disease in low- and middle-income countries. *International Health* 1, 3–9.
2. WHO (2009) *2008–2013 Action Plan for the Global Strategy for the Prevention and Control of Non-communicable Diseases*. World Health Organization, Geneva, Switzerland <http://www.who.int/nmh/publications/ncd_action_plan_en.pdf>.
3. WHO (2009) *Integrated Chronic Disease Prevention and Control*. World Health Organization, Geneva, Switzerland <http://wwwwhoint/chp/about/integrated_cd/en/index2.html>.
4. World Health Organization (2008) *Action Plan for the Global Strategy for the Prevention and Control of Non Communicable Diseases, 2008–2012*. World Health Organization, Geneva, Switzerland.
5. Pearson, T.A., Palaniappan, L.P., Artinian, N.T., Carnethon, M.R., Criqui, M.H., Daniels, S.R., Fonarow, G.C., Fortmann, S.P., Franklin, B.A., Galloway, J.M., Goff, D.C. Jr, Heath, G.W., Frank, A.T., Kris-Etherton, P.M., Labarthe, D.R., Murabito, J.M., Sacco, R.L., Sasson, C., Turner, M.B. and the American Heart Association Council on Epidemiology and Prevention (2013) American Heart Association Guide for Improving Cardiovascular Health at the Community Level, 2013 update: a scientific statement for public health practitioners, healthcare providers, and health policy makers. *Circulation* 127, 1730–1753.
6. Gaziano, T.A. and Pagidipati, N. (2013) Scaling up chronic disease prevention interventions in lower- and middle-income countries. *Annual Review of Public Health* 34, 317–335.
7. Rose, G. (1985) Sick individuals and sick populations. *International Journal of Epidemiology* 14, 32–38.
8. Puska, P., Tuomilehto, J., Salonen, J., Nissinen, A., Virtamo, J., Björkqvist, S., Koskela, K., Neittaanmäki, L., Takalo, L. and Kottke, T.E. (1981) *Community Control of Cardiovascular Diseases: Evaluation of a Comprehensive Community Programme for Control of Cardiovascular Diseases in North Karelia, Finland, 1972–1977*. Published on behalf of the National Public Health Laboratory of Finland by the World Health Organization, Regional Office for Europe, Geneva, Switzerland.
9. Farquhar, J.W., Fortmann, S.P., Flora, J.A., Taylor, C.B., Haskell, W.L., Williams, P.T., Maccoby, N. and Wood, P.D. (1990) Effects of communitywide education on cardiovascular disease risk factors. The Stanford Five-City Project. *Journal of the American Medical Association* 264, 359–365.
10. Flora, J.A., Lefebvre, R.C., Murray, D.M., Stone, E.J., Assaf, A., Mittelmark, M.B. and Finnegan, J.R. Jr (1993) A community education monitoring system: methods from the Stanford Five-City

Project, the Minnesota Heart Health Program and the Pawtucket Heart Health Program. *Health Education Research* 8, 81–95.
11. Nissinen, A., Berrios, X. and Puska, P. (2001) Community-based noncommunicable disease interventions: lessons from developed countries for developing ones. *Bulletin of the World Health Organization* 79, 963–970.
12. Puska, P. (2002) Successful prevention of non-communicable diseases: 25 year experiences with North Karelia Project in Finland. *Public Health Medicine* 4, 5–7.
13. Rossouw, J.E., Jooste, P.L., Chalton, D.O., Jordaan, E.R., Langenhoven, M.L., Jordaan, P.C., Steyn, M., Swanepoel, A.S. and Rossouw, L.J. (1993) Community-based intervention: the Coronary Risk Factor Study (CORIS). *International Journal of Epidemiology* 22, 428–438.
14. Dowse, G.K., Gareeboo, H., Alberti, K.G., Zimmet, P., Tuomilehto, J., Purran, A., Fareed, D., Chitson, P. and Collins, V.R. (1995) Changes in population cholesterol concentrations and other cardiovascular risk factor levels after five years of the non-communicable disease intervention programme in Mauritius. Mauritius Non-communicable Disease Study Group. *British Medical Journal* 311, 1255–1259.
15. Khosravi, A., Mehr, G.K., Kelishadi, R., Shirani, S., Gharipour, M., Tavassoli, A., Noori, F. and Sarrafzadegan, N. (2010) The impact of a 6-year comprehensive community trial on the awareness, treatment and control rates of hypertension in Iran: experiences from the Isfahan healthy heart program. *BMC Cardiovascular Disorders* 10, 61.
16. Krishnan, A., Ekowati, R., Baridalyne, N., Kusumawardani, N., Suhardi, Kapoor, S.K. and Leowski, J. (2011) Evaluation of community-based interventions for non-communicable diseases: experiences from India and Indonesia. *Health Promotion International* 26, 276–289.
17. Lara, A., Yancey, A.K., Tapia-Conye, R., Flores, Y., Kuri-Morales, P., Mistry, R., Subirats, E. and McCarthy, W.J. (2008) Pausa para tu Salud: reduction of weight and waistlines by integrating exercise breaks into workplace organizational routine. *Preventing Chronic Disease* 5, A12.
18. Chen, J., Wu, X. and Gu, D. (2008) Hypertension and cardiovascular diseases intervention in the capital steel and iron company and Beijing Fangshan community. *Obesity Reviews* 9 (Suppl. 1), 142–145.
19. Forrester, T., Adeyemo, A., Soarres-Wynter, S., Sargent, L., Bennett, F., Wilks, R., Luke, A., Prewitt, E., Kramer, H. and Cooper, R.S. (2005) A randomized trial on sodium reduction in two developing countries. *Journal of Human Hypertension* 19, 55–60.
20. Almeida-Pittito, B., Hirai, A.T., Sartorelli, D.S., Gimeno, S.G.A. and Ferreira, S.R.G. (2010) Impact of a 2-year intervention program on cardiometabolic profile according to the number of goals achieved. *Brazilian Journal of Medical and Biological Research* 43, 1088–1094.
21. Rossouw, J.E., Du Plessis, J.P., Benade, A.J., Jordaan, P.C., Kotze, J.P., Jooste, P.L. and Ferreira, J.J. (1983) Coronary risk factor screening in three rural communities. The CORIS baseline study. *South African Medical Journal* 64, 430–436.
22. Steyn, K., Steyn, M., Swanepoel, A.S., Jordaan, P.C., Jooste, P.L., Fourie, J.M. and Rossouw, J.E. (1997) Twelve-year results of the Coronary Risk Factor Study (CORIS). *International Journal of Epidemiology* 26, 964–971.
23. Tuomilehto, J., Li, N., Dowse, G., Gareeboo, H., Chitson, P., Fareed, D., Min, Z., Alberti, K.G. and Zimmet, P. (1993) The prevalence of coronary heart disease in the multi-ethnic and high diabetes prevalence population of Mauritius. *Journal of Internal Medicine* 233, 187–194.
24. Uusitalo, U., Feskens, E.J., Tuomilehto, J., Dowse, G., Haw, U., Fareed, D., Hemraj, F., Gareeboo, H., Alberti, K.G. and Zimmet, P. (1996) Fall in total cholesterol concentration over five years in association with changes in fatty acid composition of cooking oil in Mauritius: cross sectional survey. *British Medical Journal* 313, 1044–1046.
25. Zhai, F., Fu, D., Du, S., Ge, K., Chen, C. and Popkin, B.M. (2002) What is China doing in policy-making to push back the negative aspects of the nutrition transition? *Public Health Nutrition* 5, 269–273.

26. Yu, Z., Song, G., Guo, Z., Zheng, G., Tian, H., Vartiainen, E., Puska, P. and Nissinen, A. (1999) Changes in blood pressure, body mass index, and salt consumption in a Chinese population. *Preventive Medicine* 29, 165–172.
27. Tian, H.G., Guo, Z.Y., Hu, G., Yu, S.J., Sun, W., Pietinen, P. and Nissinen, A. (1995) Changes in sodium intake and blood pressure in a community-based intervention project in China. *Journal of Human Hypertension* 9, 959–968.
28. Coitinho, D., Monteiro, C.A. and Popkin, B.M. (2002) What Brazil is doing to promote healthy diets and active lifestyles. *Public Health Nutrition* 5, 263–267.
29. de Martel, C., Ferlay, J., Franceschi, S., Vignat, J., Bray, F., Forman, D. and Plummer, M. (2012) Global burden of cancers attributable to infections in 2008, a review and synthetic analysis. *Lancet Oncology* 13, 607–615.
30. Wild, C.P. (2012) The role of cancer research in noncommunicable disease control. *Journal of the National Cancer Institute* 104, 1051–1058.
31. Tsebe, K.V., Burnett, R.J., Hlungwani, N.P., Sibara, M.M., Venter, P.A. and Mphahlele, M.J. (2001) The first five years of universal hepatitis B vaccination in South Africa: evidence for elimination of HBsAg carriage in under 5-year-olds. *Vaccine* 19, 3919–3926.
32. Fortuin, M., Chotard, J., Jack, A.D., Maine, N.P., Mendy, M., Hall, A.J., Inskip, H.M., George, M.O. and Whittle, H.C. (1993) Efficacy of hepatitis B vaccine in the Gambian expanded programme on immunisation. *Lancet* 341, 1129–1131.
33. LaMontagne, D.S., Barge, S., Le, N.T., Mugisha, E., Penny, M.E., Gandhi, S., Janmohamed, A., Kumakech, E., Mosqueira, N.R., Nguyen, N.Q., Paul, P., Tang, Y., Minh, T.H., Uttekar, B.P. and Jumaan, A.O. (2011) Human papillomavirus vaccine delivery strategies that achieved high coverage in low- and middle-income countries. *Bulletin of the World Health Organization* 89, 821–830B.
34. Penny, M., Bartolini, R., Mosqueira, N.R., LaMontagne, D.S., Mendoza, M.A., Ramos, I., Winkler, J.L., Villafana, J., Janmohamed, A. and Jumaan, A.O. (2011) Strategies to vaccinate against cancer of the cervix: feasibility of a school-based HPV vaccination program in Peru. *Vaccine* 29, 5022–5030.
35. Fesenfeld, M., Hutubessy, R. and Jit, M. (2013) Cost-effectiveness of human papillomavirus vaccination in low and middle income countries: a systematic review. *Vaccine* 31, 3786–3804.
36. WHO (2011) *Scaling Up Action against Noncommunicable Disease: How Much Will It Cost?* World Health Organization, Geneva, Switzerland <http://www.who.int/nmh/publications/cost_of_inaction/en>.
37. Mendis, S. and Chestnov, O. (2013) Costs, benefits, and effectiveness of interventions for the prevention, treatment, and control of cardiovascular diseases and diabetes in Africa. *Progress in Cardiovascular Diseases* 56, 314–321.
38. Whelton, P.K., He, J., Appel, L.J., Cutler, J.A., Havas, S., Kotchen, T.A., Roccella, E.J., Stout, R., Vallbona, C., Winston, M.C., Karimbakas, J. and the National High Blood Pressure Education Program Coordinating Committee (2002) Primary prevention of hypertension: clinical and public health advisory from The National High Blood Pressure Education Program. *Journal of the American Medical Association* 288, 1882–1888.
39. Beaglehole, R., Ebrahim, S., Reddy, S., Voute, J., Leeder, S. and the Chronic Disease Action Group (2007) Prevention of chronic diseases: a call to action. *Lancet* 370, 2152–2157.
40. Bonita, R., Mendis, S., Truelsen, T., Bogousslavsky, J., Toole, J. and Yatsu, F. (2004) The global stroke initiative. *Lancet Neurology* 3, 391–393.

9 Self-help and Chronic Non-communicable Disease Care: a Preliminary Review of Existing Models in Low- and Middle-income Countries

Ama de-Graft Aikins[1]*, Pascale Allotey[2] and Lilian Lem Atanga[3]

[1]*Regional Institute for Population Studies, University of Ghana;* [2]*Monash University, Malaysia;* [3]*University of Bamenda, Cameroon*

9.1 Introduction

Individuals living with chronic non-communicable diseases (NCDs) in many low- and middle-income countries (LMICs) experience multiple challenges. The quality of medical care is poor, as health systems resources focus on a complex burden of infectious and chronic conditions, and minimal investments are made in chronic disease management [1, 2]. Continuity of medical care is affected by the existence of traditional and complementary medical systems, which are more readily accessible and have cultural legitimacy for a number of populations [3–5]. Public health education about NCDs is limited. as a result there is poor knowledge of the common NCDs, their risk factors, and their medical and psychosocial impact among lay society, patients and non-specialist healthcare providers. NCDs present major financial and psychosocial challenges for affected individuals, families, households and communities (hereafter referred to as NCD-affected communities) [1, 2]. This has implications for the quality and sustainability of social support for individuals living with NCDs and their caregivers. Discrimination, stigma and related psychosocial problems emerge for individuals living with conditions that are negatively perceived and/or lead to culturally devalued disabilities such as blindness, loss of limbs and sexual dysfunction [4, 6].

One major recommendation by experts has been to empower NCD-affected communities to participate in developing solutions to the rising NCD burden. There have been two aspects to this recommendation. Some experts argue that

*E-mail: adaikins@ug.edu.gh

given the significant and long-term burden NCDs pose for weak health systems, there is an urgent need for supporting patients towards full self-management of chronic life-long conditions in order to prevent avoidable complications and premature deaths [2, 7]. Other experts recommend the need for patient-led advocacy to change the political and financial landscape of NCD care [8, 9]. These experts argue that the lack of action on NCDs, in terms of allocation of resources and the implementation of globally accepted policies, is partly due to the lack of community and civil society pressure on politicians and policy makers to address the growing NCD burden in their countries (see also Koram and Nimako, Chapter 10, and Mendis and Chestnov, Chapter 12, this volume). Health systems improvements for the care of conditions such as human immunodeficiency virus (HIV)/AIDS and tuberculosis have occurred because of grassroots and civil society advocacy for concrete changes in policies and resource allocations. These provide important lessons for developing frameworks for community-led NCD advocacy.

In this chapter, we focus on the role of NCD-affected communities in improving NCD care through the lens of empowerment and the action of 'self-help groups', and we draw on the World Health Organization (WHO)'s building blocks as an overarching framework.

The recommendations on community empowerment dovetail into broader discussions on health systems strengthening, which place people at the centre of reforms. The WHO has proposed six building blocks of health systems, which comprise service delivery, health workforce, information systems, medicines and technologies, financing, and leadership and governance (see Coast *et al.*, Chapter 6, this volume, for a comprehensive review). The central argument is that a health system can achieve the goal of universal health coverage if these building blocks are present and are working synergistically [10] (Coast *et al.*, Chapter 6, this volume). One important aspect of the building blocks model is the role of people, as both recipients and producers of healthcare (Fig. 9.1).

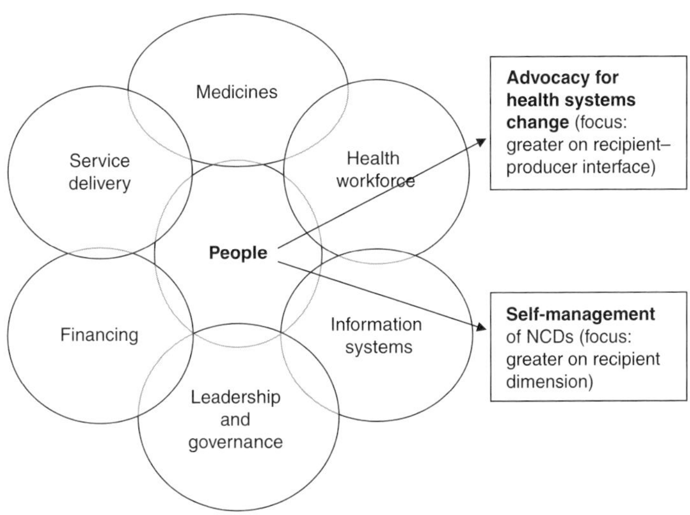

Fig. 9.1. Health systems, NCDs and the central role of people. (Adapted from [11] and [12].)

Patient empowerment is typically defined as a process through which patients, as individuals or members of a group, gain control of their health and lives [13]. Control can be gained through patients' access to the right health information, care and products and involvement in decision making about their healthcare and the broader systems structuring healthcare. Therefore, the emphasis on empowering NCD-affected communities underscores the idea of people as both recipients and producers of healthcare. The focus on patient-led advocacy in principle provides a strong framework for developing reciprocal and mutually influential relationships between NCD-affected communities and their health systems (Fig. 9.1).

Katz [14] offered one of the earliest definitions of the self-help group as follows:

> Self-help groups are voluntary small group structures for mutual aid and the accomplishment of a special purpose. They are usually formed by peers who have come together for mutual assistance in satisfying a common need, overcoming a common handicap of life-disrupting problem, and bringing about desired social and/or personal change. The initiators and members of such groups perceive that their needs are not, or cannot be, met by or through existing social institutions.

There are two dominant forms of self-help groups: (i) the peer participatory model, which is managed by a group of peers with the same condition or problem, who inform the formation of the group; and (ii) the professional expert model in which the group is led by a specialist professional or for which additional resources are provided through professional sources. Some groups may evolve from the peer participatory model into the professional expert model, or vice versa, or they may blend both approaches depending on the nature of their problem and the resources available [15, 16].

We present a preliminary review of existing models of self-help within the context of NCDs in LMICs. In the next section we present a brief review of the socio-cultural and ideological context of self-help and advocacy in Africa, Asia and Latin America to underscore the feasibility of developing productive and sustainable NCD advocacy movements in LMICs. We then present the results of a preliminary review of the types of NCD self-help groups that exist and the emerging studies on a limited number of these groups. We focus on the conditions, the types of self-help groups, and the reported functions and impact of the groups, where this information exists. We conclude by discussing the future prospects and challenges for self-help groups in strengthening NCD care in resource-poor settings.

9.2 Advocacy and Self-help in Africa, Asia and Latin America

The ideology of self-help and its evolution in healthcare is reported to have European and North American roots [17]. However, the concept of self-help is ideologically and functionally compatible with grassroots movements in Africa, Asia and Latin America aimed at improving healthcare or broader developmental needs.

In Africa, there is a wide range of grassroots and community-based groups that perform a variety of developmental functions. The traditional groups included women's groups, youth groups and indigenous professional groups (such as market women and healers). Some of these long-existing community movements played important roles in the independence struggles of their countries, some have restructured their functions in response to new forms of structural crises and newer groups have emerged through a rising dominance of civil society action [18]. For example, chronic weaknesses in African health systems have typically driven individuals to treat various conditions in the informal sector of traditional medicine and faith healing, and to rely on family and social networks for diagnosis, treatment and care [4]. Contemporary health-oriented self-help groups have developed from this context of social networking and community support. When Africa encountered the HIV/AIDS crisis, community-based groups grew exponentially in countries like Kenya, South Africa and Uganda [19]. These groups provided essential care, particularly in remote areas not covered by formal healthcare services, and in Uganda, community-based action was credited for reducing the incidence and prevalence of HIV in the early years [20]. Mental health non-governmental organizations (NGOs) are a more recent form of health-focused self-help group. However, they have a longer history, as the village settlements developed in Nigeria, Ghana and other African countries before the introduction of colonial mental health services, to address the treatment and rehabilitation of the mentally ill within the community [21, 22].

In Asia, self-help and advocacy movements have focused on broader developmental needs, including poverty alleviation and women's empowerment, particularly in rural areas [17, 23]. Some of the Asian self-help models, such as initiatives on savings and loans for rural women and farmers, have been applied in other LMIC regions with mixed success. These models have been supported by the development agenda of governments and their development partners [23]. However, they have historical roots in the colonial-era Gandhian philosophy of self-reliance [17]. Like other LMIC regions, the focus of Asian advocacy groups has expanded to include addressing new public health threats such as HIV/AIDS and substance abuse disorders [24–26].

In Latin America, grassroots movements and community advocacy exist for a wide range of developmental, social and health problems including the regeneration of slum communities, women's empowerment and improving the health of communities [27–29]. The goals and impact of these movements have been critically evaluated through the lens of Paulo Freire's (1973) notion of conscientization [30]. Guareschi and Jovchelovitch [27] defined conscientization as a 'process through which critical thinking develops' and in terms of 'a politics and a psychology of recognition where otherwise socially excluded subjects come into the public arena to state who they are, what they know and what they want'. Power between groups can be 'relational and productive . . . coercive and possessive' [31]. Implementers of interventions and programmes that seek to facilitate social change through community participation or advocacy have to recognize the ambiguous and double-edged nature of power. Theorists such as Fraser [31] suggest that this recognition offers scope for developing and/or facilitating 'more "creative" and "lateral" connections' essential for developing and sustaining 'unorthodox alliances across groups that otherwise are not seen to have much in common' [31]. It also underscores the need for moving beyond either 'top-down' (e.g. professional led) or 'bottom-up' (e.g. peer led) participatory approaches to recognize the role of multi-level mutually influential approaches to participation. A number of successful infectious disease initiatives that built on community empowerment and participation have benefited from such an approach (see Koram and Nimako, Chapter 10, this volume).

At least two cross-cutting themes emerge from existing grassroots and community-led movements in Africa, Asia and Latin America that provide locally relevant context to embed NCD self-help groups. First, communities (can) participate in their own development, alone or with the assistance of external experts, particularly when resources are limited and during times of crises. Secondly, under resource-poor conditions, the long-term impact of advocacy movements depends on a creative mix of top-down and bottom-up approaches to participation. This requires developing productive alliances between various actors, a recognition of the skewed power relationships and distribution of resources between actors, and an understanding that the potential strengths and limitations of participation depend on the structure and dynamics of specific alliances.

9.3 NCD Self-help Groups: a Preliminary Review of What Exists and What Works in LMICs

We conducted two sets of searches to identify the types of NCD self-help groups in LMICs. The first search focused on the database of the NCD Alliance. The NCD Alliance was established in May 2010 as a consortium of the four major international NCD NGO federations: the International Diabetes Federation, the World Heart Federation, the Union for International Cancer Control and the International Union Against TB and Lung Disease. Currently, the NCD Alliance brings together a global network of over 2000 NCD civil society organizations from 170 countries, which are categorized under seven groups: federation member associations, NGOs, academic institutions, research institutes, patient support organizations, scientific associations and professional societies.

The NCD Alliance website profiles this global network of NCD civil society organizations under its Common Interest Group (CIG). We reviewed the profiles of these NCD civil society organizations to identify the number of LMICs with NCD associations that could be characterized as self-help groups and the types of associations in terms of condition focus and target members (e.g. adult, children, elderly).

In total, 105 LMICs in Africa, Asia, Latin America and the Caribbean, the Middle East and the Pacific were listed as CIG members. Of this total, 92 (approximately 88%) had NCD associations for the following conditions: Alzheimer's disease, cancers, cardiovascular diseases (CVDs), diabetes and respiratory diseases.

The second search focused on published studies on NCD self-help groups, using the databases PubMed and PsycINFO and simple search terms of 'self-help groups' and a combination of 'Africa', 'Asia' and 'Latin America'. Eight relevant studies focusing on six African countries, six Asian countries and one Latin

American country were selected for review. The reports focused on self-help groups for six conditions: cancer, dementia, diabetes, health problems of the elderly (including NCDs), mental health disorders and stroke.

First, we provide an overview of what exists in terms of a simple count of which conditions have reported self-help groups and in which countries these self-help groups have a presence. Secondly, we outline the preliminary insights on the types of groups, their functions and their reported impact. We limit attention to self-help groups in Africa, Asia, and Latin America and the Caribbean.

9.3.1 NCD self-help groups: what exists in LMICs

NCD self-help groups exist in a number of LMICs and focus on eight key conditions: Alzheimer's disease, cancer, CVDs, dementia, diabetes, health problems related to ageing (including NCDs), mental health disorders and respiratory diseases. The distribution of five types of NCD self-help groups across countries registered on the NCD Alliance database is presented in Fig. 9.2.

Ninety-five countries have at least one association or group for the four major NCDs: cardiovascular disease, cancers, respiratory disease and diabetes. Thirty countries have additional groups for Alzheimer's disease and related dementias. Across the three regions, diabetes associations are the most prominent, and associations for respiratory diseases the least prominent. The kinds and dominance of self-help groups do not correspond to the epidemiological profile of NCDs across the affected regions. For example, most countries have more diabetes associations compared with CVD associations, although CVD causes the majority of deaths in LMICs (see Awuah *et al.*, Chapter 1, this volume).

Inter-regional differences occur for neurodegenerative diseases. There are higher numbers of Alzheimer's disease and dementia groups in Asian and Latin American countries (compared with the total number of countries with NCD self-help groups) compared with African countries. Finally, most NCD groups and associations are adult focused. Only three groups are reported for children living with type 1 diabetes (Brazil and Ghana) and cancers (Pakistan). Some groups focus on caregivers of people living with NCDs, particularly mental health disorders and neurodegenerative diseases.

9.3.2 NCD self-help groups in LMICs: functions and impact

The NCD Alliance database suggests the existence of three types of NCD self-help groups: (i) federation member associations (e.g. national diabetes associations and national heart foundations); (ii) NGOs (e.g. women's health and development groups); and (iii) patient support organizations (e.g. cancer groups such as Reach to Recovery). The federation member associations follow the professional expert model and are in the majority. The NGOs and some patient support organizations follow the peer participatory model and are in the minority. These categories of self-help groups and associations also emerge in the published studies on NCD self-help groups.

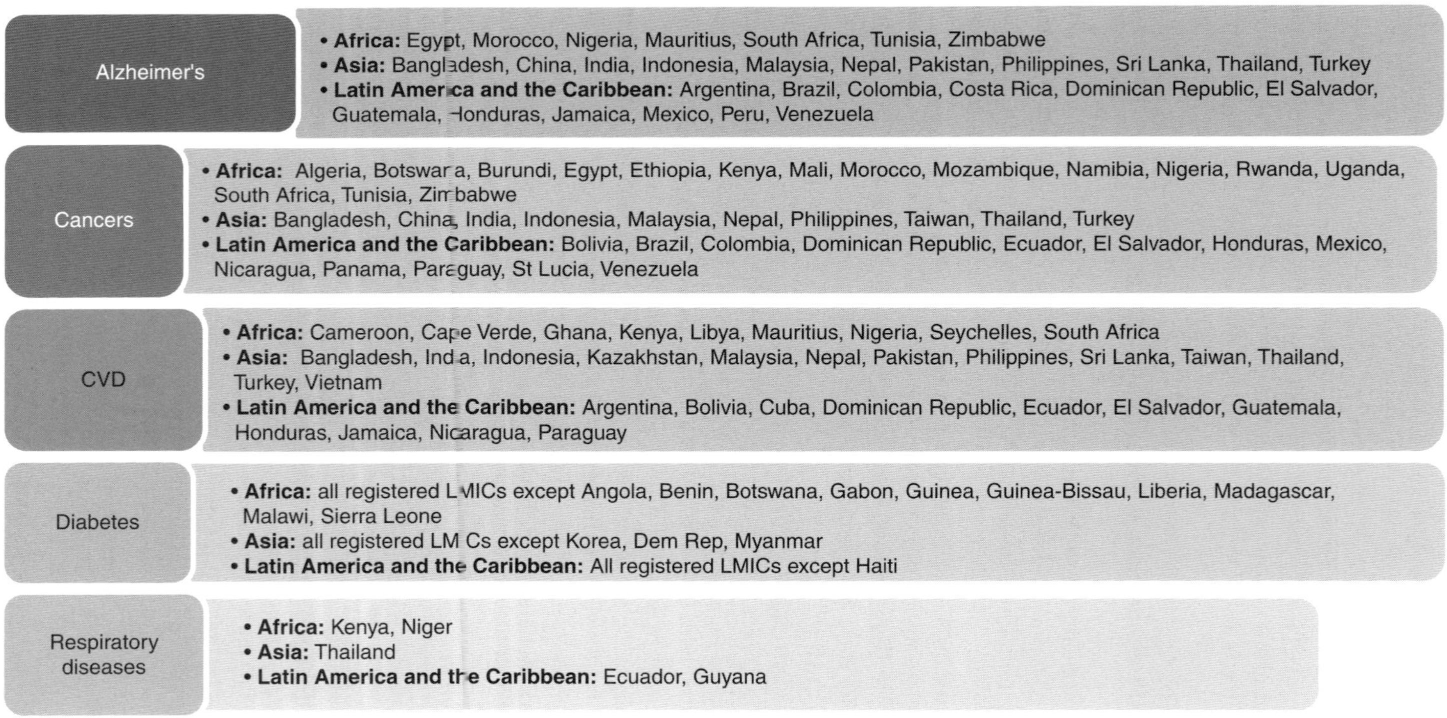

Fig. 9.2. African, Asian and Latin American/Caribbean LMICs with NCD self-help groups registered on the NCD Alliance Database.

Preliminary analysis of the information offered on the NCD Alliance self-help group suggests that members and associations serve one or more of three functions. Some groups focus on education and NCD literacy. For example, a number of the respiratory disease groups, whether led by professionals or peers, prioritize education on smoking and related lifestyles. The diabetes associations, most of which are national members of the International Diabetes Federation, offer a range of services to members including diabetes education and marking annual diabetes days with public advocacy.

A second set of groups focuses on psychosocial support, in addition to providing education. The cancer groups prioritize this goal, for example providing psychosocial support services to women newly diagnosed with breast cancer or women undergoing debilitating treatment.

A third set of groups focuses on advocacy, including lobbying government for policy change and implementation or lobbying the private sector for funds to support NCD initiatives. The national diabetes associations and heart foundations for example fall under this category. In many countries, these national associations are led by doctors, but some countries have nurse leaders. They blend a focus on improving medical care with improving the life circumstances of individuals living with the target condition.

Studies of self-help groups are reported to apply two main methods [32]. The single-group cross-sectional survey method engages with self-help group members, using either qualitative, quantitative or mixed methods, to examine experiences of membership at a given time. It offers a snapshot of members' narratives of experiences but does not provide insight into changing experiences over time. The longitudinal study method gathers data from self-help group members over time and offers more in-depth evidence of experiences and impact over time. The majority of studies on the existing NCD self-help groups applied the single-group cross-sectional survey method to evaluate the benefits of self-advocacy for cancer experiences in Taiwan [33], mental health in South Africa [34, 35], addressing health problems of the elderly in Egypt and Thailand [36, 37] and understanding inflammatory bowel disease in Iran [38]. Two studies applied the cross-sectional survey method but conducted an analysis of multiple cancer support groups in six LMICs (Brazil, China, Ghana, India, Kenya and Malaysia) [39] and multiple mental health groups in seven African countries (Ghana, Kenya, Rwanda, South Africa, Tanzania, Uganda and Zambia) [40]. One study examined the impact of a public awareness campaign informed by longitudinal research conducted by a cancer support group in Pakistan [41].

The studies, including the one employing the longitudinal approach, suggested that self-help groups provide important benefits for group members including access to health and disease-specific information [38, 39], social support [36, 37] and improved health and psychological outcomes [33, 36, 37, 39]. The activities of a smaller set of groups engaged in broader advocacy benefit the general population beyond the group [39–41]. This suggests that, at present, most NCD self-help groups focus on improving the self-management and coping aspects of NCD experiences. A restricted set of groups for mental health and cancers lead the effort to advocate for broader health systems change at the national level. The activities of these groups embody the expected role of the empowered

NCD-affected community as 'both recipient and producer' of their health system. These groups are also members of international associations or federations that provide standardized resources for education, social support and advocacy.

9.4 NCD Self-help Groups in LMICs: Understanding Future Trends

This preliminary review of NCD self-help groups in LMICs suggests that most LMICs in Africa, Asia, and Latin America and the Caribbean have at least one NCD self-help group. National diabetes associations are the most dominant groups across many countries. A small number of countries have self-help groups representing the major NCDs as well as neurodegenerative diseases. The majority of groups are professionally led groups and are associated with international NCD associations and federations. Most groups serve an educational function. Some groups serve additional functions including providing psychosocial support to members and advocating for change at the national level and/or beyond. Cancer and mental health groups are more likely to be engaged in advocacy. These groups are also more likely to be affiliated with international associations and federations that provide support for group activities.

The limited evidence available suggests that the multi-level participatory approach appears to be the most feasible for empowering NCD-communities to become both 'recipients and producers' of their health systems. In a previous review of participatory NCD prevention approaches in Ghana and Cameroon, we outlined the dominance of a bottom-up approach to NCD care in Ghana (with a wide range of NCD self-help groups and other community-based resources) and a top-down approach in Cameroon (with an emphasis on government-led prevention and treatment initiatives) [42]. We argued that neither approach offered a model for sustained nationwide NCD prevention and suggested that 'a multi-level framework that encompasses top-down and bottom-up responses will offer a more successful model for prevention' [42].

More research is required to examine and track the trends in the formation, organization, functions and impact of NCD self-help groups. To gain a deeper understanding of how the structure and functions of groups evolve over time, it will be important to consider the complex medical, psychological, psychosocial and political profile of NCDs. Some NCDs are disabling and psychologically disruptive. Some conditions place a considerable long-term burden on relationships in the real world and disrupt social identities and wider social relationships. The long-term and complex nature of treatment and management undermines professional and client relationships and fuels professional antagonism between medical, allied and traditional medical systems. The competing demands of complex public health challenges have led to the marginalization of NCDs by policy makers. Structural (e.g. poverty) and demographic (e.g. ageing) challenges are implicated in the rising trend of co-morbidity and multi-morbidity (of NCDs, mental health disorders and infectious diseases), especially among the elderly and the urban poor (see Oni and Unwin, Chapter 3, de-Graft Aikins *et al.*, Chapter 4, and Huang *et al.*, Chapter 5, this volume). Therefore, the successes or failures of NCD self-help groups will depend on the nature of the NCD, the groups the condition directly affects and groups who will benefit from membership in self-help groups. It will also depend on the groups who can participate, the capabilities they possess, the internal or external resources available to them, and to what extent and for how long they can participate. Understanding these dynamics will provide important insights into whether and how NCD self-help groups offer long-term sustainable changes for individual health outcomes, community well-being and health systems strengthening.

References

1. Beaglehole, R., Bonita, R., Horton, R., Adams, C., Alleyne, G., Asaria, P., Baugh, V., Bekedam, H., Billo, N., Casswell, S., Cecchini, M., Colagiuri, R., Colagiuri, S., Collins, T., Ebrahim, S., Engelgau, M., Galea, G., Gaziano, T., Geneau, R., Haines, A., Hospedales, J., Jha, P., Keeling, A., Leeder, S., Lincoln, P., McKee, M., Mackay, J., Magnusson, R., Moodie, R., Mwatsama, M., Nishtar, S., Norrving, B., Patterson, D., Piot, P., Ralston, J., Rani, M., Reddy, K.S., Sassi, F., Sheron, N., Stuckler, D., Suh, I., Torode, J., Varghese, C., Watt, J., the Lancet NCD Action Group and the NCD Alliance (2011) Priority actions for the non-communicable disease crisis. *Lancet* 377, 1438–1447.
2. Allotey, P., Reidpath, D.D., Yasin, S., Chan, C. and de-Graft Aikins, A. (2010) Rethinking health systems: a focus on chronicity. *Lancet* 377, 450–451.
3. Awah, P.K., Unwin, N. and Phillimore, P. (2008) Cure or control: complying with biomedical regime of diabetes in Cameroon. *BMC Health Services Research* 8, 43.
4. de-Graft Aikins, A., Unwin, N., Agyemang, C. Allotey, P., Campbell, C. and Arhinful, D.K. (2010) Tackling Africa's chronic disease burden: from the local to the global. *Globalization and Health* 6, 5.
5. Marshall, I., Wolfe, C.D.A. and McKevitt, C. (2012) Lay perspectives on hypertension and drug adherence: a systematic review of qualitative research. *British Medical Journal* 344, e3953.
6. Read, U.M., Adiibokah, E. and Nyame, S. (2009) Local suffering and the global discourse of mental health and human rights: an ethnographic study of responses to mental illness in rural Ghana. *Globalization and Health* 5, 13.
7. Van Olmen, J., Ku, G., Bermejo, R., Kegels, G., Hermann, K. and van Damme, W. (2011) The growing caseload of chronic life-long conditions calls for a move towards full self-management in low-income countries. *Globalization and Health* 7, 38.
8. Clarke, J. (2014) Medicalization of global health. 3: The medicalization of the non-communicable diseases agenda. *Global Health Action* 7, 24002.
9. Wong, D.K. and Chow, S.F. (2006) Beyond clinical trials and narratives: a participatory action research with cancer patient self-help groups. *Patient Education and Counseling* 60, 201–205.
10. Gonzáles-Block, M.A., Akisa, A.B. and Chowdhury, A. (2012) Health systems research and infectious diseases of poverty: from the margins to the mainstream. In: *Global Report for Research on Infectious Diseases of Poverty*. World Health Organization, Geneva, Switzerland, pp. 67–93.
11. de Savigny, D. and Adam, T. (2009) *Systems Thinking for Health Systems Strengthening*. World Health Organization, Geneva, Switzerland.
12. de-Graft Aikins, A., Kushitor, M., Koram, K., Gyamfi, S. and Ogedegbe. G. (2014) Chronic non-communicable diseases and the challenge of universal health coverage. Insights from community-based cardiovascular disease research in urban poor communities in Accra, Ghana. *BMC Public Health* 14 (Suppl. 2), S3.
13. O'Cathain, A., Goode, J., Luffa, D., Strangleman, T., Hanlon, G. and Greatbatch, D. (2005) Does NHS Direct empower patients? *Social Science & Medicine* 61, 1761–1771.

14. Katz, A.H. (1981) Self-help and mutual aid: an emerging social movement? *Annual Review of Sociology* 7, 129–155.
15. Ben-Ari, A.T. (2002) Dimensions and predictions of professional involvement in self-help groups: a view from within. *Health and Social Work* 27, 95–103.
16. Bell, K., Lee, J., Foran, S., Kwong, S. and Christopherson, J. (2010) Is there an "ideal cancer" support group? Key findings from a qualitative study of three groups. *Journal of Psychosocial Oncology* 28, 432–449.
17. Nayar, K.R., Kyobotungi, C. and Razum, O. (2004) Self-help: what future role in healthcare for low and middle income countries? *International Journal for Equity in Health* 3, 1.
18. Aryeetey, E. and de-Graft Aikins, A. (2013) Ethnicity, social development and wellbeing in sub-Saharan Africa: a conceptual review. In: Agyemang, C., Airhenbuwa, C. and de-Graft Aikins, A. (eds) *Ethnicity: Theories, International Perspectives and Challenges.* Nova Science Publishers, New York.
19. Iliffe, J. (2006) *The African Aids Epidemic: A History*. James Currey, Oxford, UK.
20. Low-Beer, D. and Stoneburner, R.L. (2003) Behaviour and communication change in reducing HIV: Is Uganda unique? *African Journal of AIDS Research* 2, 9–21.
21. de-Graft Aikins, A. (2015) Mental illness and destitution in Ghana: a social psychological perspective. In: Akyeampong, E., Hill, A. and Kleinman, A. (eds) *Culture, Mental Illness and Psychiatric Practice in Africa.* Indiana University Press, Bloomington, Indiana.
22. Read, U.M., Doku, V. and de-Graft Aikins, A. (2015) Schizophrenia and psychosis in West Africa from the colonial era to the present. In: Akyeampong, E., Hill, A. and Kleinman, A. (eds) *Culture, Mental Illness and Psychiatric Practice in Africa.* Indiana University Press, Bloomington, Indiana.
23. Pattenden, J. (2010) A neoliberalisation of civil society? Self-help groups and the labouring class poor in rural South India. *Journal of Peasant Studies* 37, 485–512.
24. Deshpande, K., Shivaswamy, M.S., Diwan, V., De Costa, A., Bhattacharya, A. and Mahadik, V.K. (2013) Establishment of social club for adolescents living in urban slums: a potential tool to impart HIV/AIDS *education. Journal of the Indian Medical Association* 111, 320–323.
25. Hayes-Larson, E., Grau, L.E., Khoshnood, K., Barbour, R., Khuat, O.T. and Heimer, R. (2013) Drug users in Hanoi, Vietnam: factors associated with membership in community-based drug user groups. *Harm Reduction Journal* 10, 33.
26. Jhirwal, O.P. and Basu, D. (2005) Involvement of Alcoholics Anonymous and other self-help groups in professional treatment of substance abusers: an Indian perspective. *Journal of Substance Abuse Treatment* 29, 65.
27. Guareschi, P.A. and Jovchelovitch, S. (2004) Participation, health and the development of community resources in southern Brazil. *Journal of Health Psychology* 9, 311–322.
28. Guthmann, J.P., Calmet, J., Rosales, E., Cruz, M., Chang, J. and Dedet, J.P. (1997) Patients' associations and the control of leishmaniasis in Peru. *Bulletin of the World Health Organization* 75, 39–44.
29. Ferguson, B.W. (1992) From protest to programs: neighborhood associations in a Brazilian municipality. *Grassroots Development* 16, 12–21.
30. Freire, P. (1973) *Education for Critical Consciousness*. Continuum, New York.
31. Fraser, H. (2005) Four different approaches to community participation. *Community Development Journal* 40, 286–300.
32. Kyrouz, E. and Humphreys, K. (1997) A review of research on the effectiveness of self-help mutual aid groups. *International Journal of Psychosocial Rehabilitation* 2, 64–68.
33. Chien, T.W., Wang, W.C., Chien, C.C. and Hwang, W.S. (2011) Rasch analysis of positive changes following adversity in cancer patients attending community support groups. *Psychooncology* 20, 98–105.
34. Seedat, S., Stein, D.J., Berk, M. and Wilson, Z. (2002) Barriers to treatment among members of a mental health advocacy group in South Africa. *Social Psychiatry and Psychiatric Epidemiology* 37, 483–487.

35. Lustig, S.L., Malomane, E. and Tollman, S. (1997) A support group for mentally ill people. *World Health Forum* 18, 319–322.
36. Mitwally, H.H. and Mahmoud, N.M. (1999) Do elderly clubs in Alexandria meet the needs of their consumers? *Journal of the Egyptian Public Health Association* 74, 601–626.
37. Taboonpong, N., Thaniwattananon, P. and Chailungka, P. (1996) Thailand: participation in an elderly club designed to promote health. *International Journal of Nursing Practice* 2, 50.
38. Rezailashkajani, M., Roshandel, D., Ansari, S. and Zali, M.R. (2008) A web-based patient education system and self-help group in Persian language for inflammatory bowel disease patients. *International Journal of Medical Informatics* 77, 122–128.
39. Errico, K.M. and Rowden, D. (2006) Experiences of breast cancer survivor-advocates and advocates in countries with limited resources: a shared journey in breast cancer advocacy. *Breast Journal* 12 (Suppl. 1), S111–S116.
40. Kleintjes, S., Lund, C. and Swartz, L. (2013) Organising for self-advocacy in mental health: experiences from seven African countries. *African Journal of Psychiatry* 16, 187–195.
41. Ali, T.S. and Baig, S. (2006) Evaluation of a cancer awareness campaign: experience with a selected population in Karachi. *Asian Pacific Journal of Cancer Prevention* 7, 391–395.
42. de-Graft Aikins, A., Boynton, P. and Atanga, L.L. (2010) Developing effective chronic disease prevention in Africa: insights from Ghana and Cameroon. *Globalization and Health* 6, 6.

10 Prevention and Control of Chronic Non-communicable Diseases: Lessons from Infectious Disease Control

KWADWO ANSAH KORAM[1*] AND BELINDA AFRIYIE NIMAKO[2]

[1]*Noguchi Memorial Institute for Medical Research, University of Ghana, Ghana;* [2]*Volta Regional Hospital, Ghana Health Service, Ho, Ghana*

10.1 Introduction

Low- and middle-income countries (LMICs) continue to grapple with infectious diseases (IDs) alongside the emerging threat posed by non-communicable diseases (NCDs), aptly described as a double burden of disease [1, 2]. ID control has been influenced remarkably by the recognition of the role of environmental determinants such as sanitation, development of vaccines and antimicrobials over the centuries. ID control has resulted in varied levels of success, with some controls being very successful, others moderately successful and a number considered failures when considering the incidence and burden of specific diseases. This is true even for countries with a double burden of disease.

NCDs, once thought to be a challenge for high-income countries, are now recognized as a global challenge extending also to LMICs. Indeed, the burden is reported to be disproportionately higher in LMICs, with more people affected and at younger ages, and with poorer outcomes including a higher burden of disability and deaths. Chronic diseases account for 60% of all deaths worldwide, and 80% of these deaths occur in LMICs, where the toll is heaviest during the prime productive years of youth and middle age [3, 4]. Trends also suggest that the major risk factors for NCDs including obesity and inactivity are on the rise, especially in developing countries [5, 6] (see Awuah *et al.*, Chapter 1, this volume).

Consequently, it is clear that it is essential for LMICs to tackle NCDs alongside ID control. Doing this effectively will require specific control measures for NCDs stemming from policies that are result oriented. The centuries of experience with ID control, irrespective of the outcome of the efforts as related to the disease entity, have many lessons that could be applied to NCD control. These lessons may be due

*E-mail: kkoram@noguchi.ug.edu.gh

to interactions between NCDs and IDs and the resulting synergies (discussed in detail by Oni and Uwin, Chapter 3, this volume), to risk factors that are common to the two, or other factors.

In various discussions to consider the options available to control NCDs, there appears to be a consensus on the need for an approach that takes into consideration the total health system rather than focusing solely on the health condition per se (see Coast *et al.*, Chapter 6, this volume).

What this chapter does is to consider the various lessons from ID control that may be applicable to NCDs using the World Health Organization (WHO) building blocks [7] as the framework. As the health system is discussed elsewhere in this volume, the aim will be to focus on lessons from ID control that may be relevant to policies targeted at each block.

In doing this, we recognize that the building blocks in themselves are not exhaustive with respect to disease control. Critical considerations need to be given to overarching elements such as research and development, partnerships, advocacy, and individual and community empowerment, which in synergy with a functioning health system will yield the anticipated results.

Infectious disease control has evolved over the years in tandem with scientific advancement. Prior to John Snow's classic epidemiological approach of controlling disease, ID control was carried out in various forms, such as using isolation for persons with Hansen's disease and vaccination. The role of the environment has always been appreciated [8, 9]. The British Act of 1860, which was influenced by the typhus outbreaks in 1817–1819, 1826–1827 and 1831–1832, recognized the role that the environment played in disease causation and sought to provide a policy to address this [10]. Edward Jenner's experiment on the use of vaccines introduced a new era to ID control offering the opportunity to prevent the occurrence of diseases [11]. Today, vaccines have been instrumental in saving lives worldwide across the lifespan, for diseases as age old as measles, emerging ones such as avian influenza and even NCDs such as cervical and hepatocellular malignancies.

The most remarkable scientific development of this century arguably has been the development of antimicrobials. Antibiotics in particular have been critical in saving lives that may have been lost to IDs.

The attempt, successful or otherwise, to keep up with IDs whether age old or emerging, localized or global, provides useful lessons for NCDs. This is particularly relevant to LMICs considering the centuries of experience with ID control and the continued significant presence of IDs in these regions.

NCDs are a shared threat. The known modifiable and non-modifiable risk factors are common to a subset of conditions (see Awuah *et al.*, Chapter 1, this volume). In very recent history, one infectious condition that has mimicked the NCD profile is human immunodeficiency virus (HIV). There are significant lessons to be learnt from HIV and other diseases such as tuberculosis, which are a shared global threat similar to the shared threat of NCDs. This chapter will draw lessons extensively from the control of these diseases as well as other IDs.

10.2 ID Control and the Health System Building Blocks

NCD control requires both population- and individual-level efforts to be successful in disease prevention and treatment measures. This will require a robust health system as the critical component to yield results. The WHO recognizes some essential components of the health system, primarily the six building blocks needed for the system to function effectively [7]. These comprise: leadership/governance, service delivery, health workforce, health information, access to essential medicines and financing. This section will explore some critical lessons that ID control has to offer in terms of these building blocks (summarized in Box 10.1). We focus on leadership/governance, service delivery, health information, access to essential medicines and financing. The challenges and opportunities relating to the health workforce are dealt with extensively by Huang *et al.*, Chapter 5, and Coast *et al.*, Chapter 6 (this volume).

10.2.1 Leadership and governance

Global interest is essential for NCDs to be prioritized, but local commitment is critical to sustain prevention and control measures. ID prevention and control

Box 10.1. Lessons from ID control for NCDs using the WHO health systems framework.

Leadership/governance
1. A global initiative that is locally driven
2. Multi-sectorial collaboration

Service delivery
1. Prevention–treatment balance is critical
2. Primary healthcare is required for sustainability
3. Prioritization of major conditions
4. Integrated control initiatives

Health workforce
1. Multi-disciplinary cadre of staff
2. Equitable distribution of well-motivated health workers
3. Task shifting

Health information
1. Disease surveillance
2. Monitoring and evaluation

Access to essential medicines
1. Local development of drugs and diagnostics
2. Supply chain

Financing
1. Universal healthcare
2. Cost-effective interventions

history is replete with examples where otherwise laudable initiatives have failed because they could not garner the needed international attention and/or local support. The successes in ID prevention and control of smallpox eradication, guinea worm eradication and polio eradication measures have been attributed to extensive global attention and local support. Malaria eradication efforts in the 1950s and 1960s failed largely because of inadequate international and local support, among other factors. Recently, malaria, tuberculosis and HIV/AIDS have enjoyed immense global support, which is seen in the increased funding for research and development of new tools and technology for the control of these diseases [12, 13]. For others that have not enjoyed similar success, such as neglected tropical diseases, there has been a demonstrable lack of global attention possibly because of the limited geographical spread of the disease or its risk factors, among other reasons.

Global attention on NCDs and the additional threat they pose to LMICs should make it relatively easier for funds to be allocated to NCD control and research by governments, donor organizations and research institutions.

Despite the need for NCDs to be a global priority coordinated at the global level with consensus on management guidelines and broad objectives, the responsibility of NCD control must rest with nations and affected communities. Various ID control programmes have been successful because of the kind of commitment that nations provided. Current efforts at polio eradication constitute a good example. The countries where there has been lack of local support or outright opposition to the programme have not been able to bring cases down to zero as required for eradication [14]. In some instances where the external effort was disproportionate to the national effort, anticipated outcomes were not realized. Relatively successful ID control programmes such as those for malaria and HIV have enjoyed both international and local support.

The NCD profile varies in different countries and even within communities with slight variations in risk factors, manifestation and outcomes of NCDs and will require local commitment and context in addition to international initiatives to achieve the desired results. This is expected to translate into locally relevant and appropriate policies and actions intended to support NCD control.

Multi-sectorial collaboration

Our environment influences the incidence and prevalence of many IDs. Making the necessary changes in the environment has been one of the measures used in various ID control programmes. In their study, Uchoa *et al.* [15] attributed the reduction in the prevalence of schistosomiasis in Brazil to improved access to clean water and sanitation among other measures such as mass treatment. The guinea worm eradication programme has also been successful, largely as a result of measures to ensure access to potable drinking water.

These ID policies recognize that the causes of IDs are multiple, comprising complex biological, social and behavioural factors. These factors must be catered for in any attempt to control disease. HIV control exemplifies the extensive use of cross-disciplinary personnel and a multi-disciplinary approach in disease control. In disease prevention, disciplines that contributed to HIV control included sociology, epidemiology, gender studies, psychology, religion, economics, politics/policy and communication. Similarly, management of the disease has made use of a host of disciplines including medicine and allied health, nursing, social work, psychology and nutrition. Indeed the broad-based governance in identifying the problems and responses to the HIV/AIDS epidemic has been described as a key lesson inherent in the AIDS response [16].

Conversely, there have been instances, for example in the control of lymphatic filariasis and onchocerciasis, where an over-reliance on drugs and neglect of the broader determinants of the diseases, have led to failed control measures [17].

Any credible discussion on reduction of the NCD threat must likewise focus on the complex determinants of NCDs. In additional to the known modifiable and non-modifiable risks, broader structural determinants such as air pollution, transport infrastructure and trade policies must be factored into the development of NCD control strategies.

10.2.2 Service delivery

Prevention–treatment balance

The limited health systems resources in LMICs require that a balance is struck between prevention and cure. This is one instance where the long-standing efforts to control IDs have important lessons to teach. While disease incidence can be reduced particularly through prevention and policies aimed at cutting transmission, disease morbidity and mortality require optimum treatment. In outlining the lessons learnt from scaling up of the HIV programme, Atun *et al.* [18] proposed that NCD prevention is likely to be suboptimal without treatment, and treatment without effective prevention is unlikely to be associated with a significant sustained effect.

The decline seen in the incidence of diseases such as bacterial diarrhoeal and vaccine-preventable diseases such as measles has been attributed to the implementation of policies to prevent these diseases, such as the provision of safe water and adequate health education [19]. Malaria control is a classic example of the usefulness of ensuring optimum levels of both prevention and treatment. Interventions such as indoor residual spraying, use of insecticide-treated nets and even intermittent treatment therapy for pregnant women have led to a remarkable decrease in the incidence of malaria. However, in order to improve the associated morbidity and mortality, there have been continued improvements in case management including diagnostics, surveillance for resistance and the introduction of artemisinin combination therapy among other measures. The United States Centers for Disease Control and Prevention (CDC), for instance, in its framework for preventing IDs suggests strong public health fundamentals such as surveillance and epidemiological investigation as the basis for the USA's ability to protect the public from IDs [20].

A major objective of any strategy to prevent and control NCDs will be to reduce the level of exposure of individuals and populations to the common risk factors and their determinants.

A worldwide goal for the prevention and control of NCDs has been proposed to complement existing Millennium Development Goal targets for communicable disease control, with the accompanying target of an additional 2% per year reduction in death rates attributable to the main chronic diseases (heart disease, stroke, cancer, diabetes and chronic respiratory diseases) [21]. Achieving this goal will require comprehensive action covering the range of diseases and risk factors through a two-pronged approach: (i) implementation of multi-sectorial policies aimed at decreasing population-level risks for NCDs; and (ii) effective and affordable delivery of health sector interventions for patients with NCDs, as spelt out in the WHO's action plan on NCDs.

Importance of primary healthcare

One of the criticisms of the NCD Alliance is that it seems to be lobbying for a vertical approach to NCD control [22]. The vertical approach is useful in focusing attention on accompanying resources such as funding, highly skilled personal and increased research interest. A number of ID control programmes have used a vertical approach with varied outcomes.

Smallpox eradication used a vertical approach and succeeded in eradication. Malaria eradication efforts, however, yielded a mixed bag of outcomes even when it was managed vertically. Additionally, with the vertical approach, some otherwise successful programmes have faced challenges because funds run out.

In NCDs, the factors influencing the challenge are numerous and complex, spanning individual behaviours through cultural practices to global trade policies. It is imperative that these complex factors are carefully considered in the formulation of NCD policies. Should there be an initial vertical response? Should the strategy be integrated into the primary healthcare system? Or alternatively should the strategy be a blend – a diagonal approach? There are various schools of thought on this, with some calling for the initial approach to be vertical [23].

What primary healthcare does is to afford the opportunity to integrate the control of NCD with other disease control programmes such as HIV/AIDs [24] and reproductive health services.

Primary healthcare is more relevant in the context of LMICs because of the limited availability of resources. In addition, because of the nature of NCDs including their dependency on human behaviour, the broad base required for primary prevention and the heavy reliance and chronicity of the required clinical care for affected persons, primary healthcare appears to be a promising approach.

In LMICs, the existing health systems have been designed for single episodes of care or long-term prevention and control of IDs such as HIV and tuberculosis, with fragmented healthcare services unsuitable for NCDs [25–27], leading to a call for integrated health services with anticipated health and economic gains [28].

Diagnosis, treatment and prevention are most likely to succeed when delivered at the community level. In LMICs, it may be helpful to keep the package simple and, where necessary, to minimize the use of clinicians, as they are in short supply. This approach has been used by Malawi to achieve high coverage of antiretroviral therapy [29, 30]. The success of smallpox eradication has often been attributed to the availability and use of vaccines, as well as other health systems factors [31, 32].

Prioritization of major conditions

NCDs constitute a group of varied conditions. The priority focus at present is on chronic NCDs, defined by the WHO as cardiovascular diseases, diabetes, chronic respiratory diseases and cancer [26, 27]. These share modifiable and preventable risk factors related to lifestyle. These lifestyle factors are predominantly tobacco use, an unhealthy diet, physical inactivity and the harmful use of alcohol (see Awuah *et al.*, Chapter 1, this volume).

By being grouped as priority diseases of poverty, HIV, tuberculosis and malaria have been able to attract phenomenal funding from governments [33] and charity organizations, particularly through the establishment of the Global Fund to Fight AIDS, Tuberculosis and Malaria. Similarly, grouping and prioritization of NCDs, whether based on the burden associated with them or the shared risk factors mentioned previously, can be expected to help focus funding, research and innovation to achieve maximum impact. A note of caution, however, is that this should not lead to the neglect of other NCDs. Already, some chronic conditions such as asthma are being described as 'neglected' [34]. Other conditions, particularly genetic NCDs such as sickle cell disease, will need to be prioritized perhaps at a national or subregional level depending on the associated burden.

Even the risk factors may need to be prioritized, as the set of predisposing factors may have marginal or significant variations, which will need to be fully considered when designing any intervention. Maximum returns will be achieved when the effort is made to prioritize NCDs and associated risk factors locally to inform policy.

Integrated control initiatives

Behavioural change is a complex phenomenon requiring patience and a variety of approaches. This is yet one other lesson that can be learnt from ID control. Malaria intervention has benefited from a number of interventions including environmental measures such as mass spraying exercises, vector control measures such as the use of insecticide-treated nets and interventions targeting the host such as intermittent preventative treatment. The usefulness of these multiple interventions has been documented [35, 36]. Similarly, in the guinea worm eradication programme, a variety of interventions such the use of ABATE® targeting the vector, provision of good drinking water, early case detection and containment, and health education have been used [37].

For many years, polio, a vaccine-preventable disease, has plagued the world despite the availability of vaccines. Socio-cultural challenges, failed social mobilization and insecurity led to a derailment of the gains of polio immunization and the potential elimination of polio in the sub-Saharan region [38–41]. Clearly, over-reliance on pharmacological treatment is not enough – other tools and a robust health system are just as important.

Given the multi-factorial nature of the NCDs, LMICs need to recognize and adopt multiple interventions that can be deployed simultaneously. Admittedly, this seems to be the path that NCD control is taking – with interventions ranging from healthy diets to exercise, cessation of smoking and the use of statins. In the wake of developments such as the polypill Polycap, it is essential to realize that, in dealing with such a group of diseases arising as a result of multiple factors, over-reliance on a so-called 'magic bullet' may be ill informed.

10.2.3 Health information

To be able to plan and effectively control NCDs, a strong and well-functioning surveillance system for the programme is needed (see Kengne *et al.*, Chapter 7, this volume). Data are needed on exposure risks and outcome indicators as well as the health system response. Currently, the capacity for such a surveillance system is either inadequate or non-existent in the countries with the greatest needs [3]. However, even in low-resourced LMICs, one can establish robust systems using the structures on the ground. For example, the Community-Based Health Planning and Services (CHPS) programme in Ghana has the potential to provide data on the household prevalence of hypertension as the community health nurses visit the households. An integration of their daily routine with current electronic communication systems should enable us obtain values for blood pressure by linking to a central database. Although it is essential to keep such platforms as simple as possible, they provide myriad opportunities for data collection at the household level that need to be exploited.

The civil registration systems need to be improved and strengthened to ensure that all vital statistics are captured as much as possible. This will be essential in monitoring the effects of any interventions (morbidity and mortality statistics). In addition, a surveillance system should attempt to monitor exposures (risk factors and determinants) and also what interventions are applied by the health system. A well-structured, adequately supported and resilient surveillance system that is integrated into the national health information system will be essential to monitor progress against NCDs.

Setting up a strong surveillance system is thus important to underpin any programme on NCD control, but it will be equally important for the dissemination of quality health promotion messages to the population. In most LMICs where the burden of NCDs is increasing, there are strong belief systems that militate against good individual control, be it for cancer chemotherapy or lifelong anti-hypertensive treatment. A strong programme on communicating the exposure risks should be instituted and disseminated with the use of current media. This information may be stratified to different age brackets, e.g. social media may be used to reach the young who seem to obtain most of their information in this manner.

10.2.4 Access to essential medicines

For effective control of NCDs beyond primary prevention strategies such as changes in lifestyle and diet modification, the use of medicines will be critical in any programme. Thus, each control programme should have a strategy to include access to health technologies and essential medicines that will promote the widest access to use of cost-effective medications. Recently, the WHO set a target of 80% availability of essential drugs for those in need [42]. As drug treatment is likely to be lifelong, sustainable healthcare financing that will ensure adequate procurement of basic healthcare technologies and essential medicines will be critical. Countries should develop programmes that focus on improved access to basic health technologies and NCD medicines, e.g. with a focus on well-controlled generic procurement/production. The mechanisms for regulating the generic market should be strengthened to ensure the availability of quality medicines and to engender trust in the health system. National essential medicine lists should be strictly adhered to in order to limit costs, but allowance should be made for those who may need some other medications besides the most commonly used ones.

Countries should establish the local evidence to underlie promotion and implementation of evidence-based treatment policies useful for the population. For this to work, it will be essential to engender the confidence of prescribers and consumers alike in any such programme with a well-thought-out educational programme. Subregional or regional programmes may be promoted to ensure the availability of drugs. Partnerships with drug-development firms may be established, especially in the area of developing generics to ensure widespread availability. In the long term, local research capacity should be strengthened to explore the rich natural resources available in LMICs. Provision of adequate and affordable treatment will contribute to reductions in the prevalence of hypertension and other NCDs and ultimately in reducing premature mortality from NCDs.

10.2.5 Financing

The projected loss of income in developing countries over the next two decades is US$21.3 trillion, almost the same as the total aggregate income of US$24.5 trillion of these same countries in 2013 [43]. This is understandable considering that younger persons are more affected in LMICs and may suffer chronic disability or die prematurely. The resultant loss of livelihood, decreased earnings and premature retirement has been associated with the increased likelihood of poverty [44]. LMICs stand to lose the most economically, yet the loss will be a huge burden on all and inimical to the entire global community rather than to LMICs alone.

Prioritization of IDs in the past has been successful in quantifying the associated financial losses as well as the gains to be made following control. These have been determined for various IDs such as malaria [36], HIV/AIDS [45, 46] and tuberculosis [47], as well as neglected tropical diseases such as guinea worm infection [48]. Such economic evaluation of IDs has been carried out at various levels including community [49, 50], national [51], subregional [52] and even global [53] levels.

This is particularly relevant in NCDs to justify the substantial economic investments that NCD prevention and control might require and the length of time it would take to observe any impact thereof.

Focusing on NCDs as a developmental challenge rather than just a health issue makes it possible to use it as a tool for advocacy from the community level, explaining household income loss, up to the national on why to invest the limited available resources or convincing more developed countries to support the budgets of LMICs to tackle NCDs. By limiting the focus to health, NCDs will fail to garner the much-needed attention and resources for effective control.

10.3 Key Elements for NCD Control

In addition to addressing the strengthening of the above-mentioned elements of health system building blocks, critical consideration needs to be given to overarching elements such as research and development, partnerships, advocacy, and individual and community empowerment (Fig. 10.1) (see Mendis and Chestnov, Chapter 12, this volume). These elements working in synergy with a functioning health system will yield the anticipated results for sustainable NCD control.

10.3.1 Partnerships

ID control has enjoyed several partnerships at all levels. These partnerships include country donors, research institutions and practitioners, subregional governments and civil society organizations.

The HIV response to a large extent was reliant on partnerships between health services and individuals, groups and society. This was exhibited as patient support groups and advocates for instance, and was associated with significant positive change in the AIDS response [54]. In scaling up HIV treatment, the inputs of international organizations such as the WHO as well as governments, charity organizations such as the Global Fund to Fight AIDS, Tuberculosis and Malaria and civil society organizations were instrumental in ensuring that this was made possible.

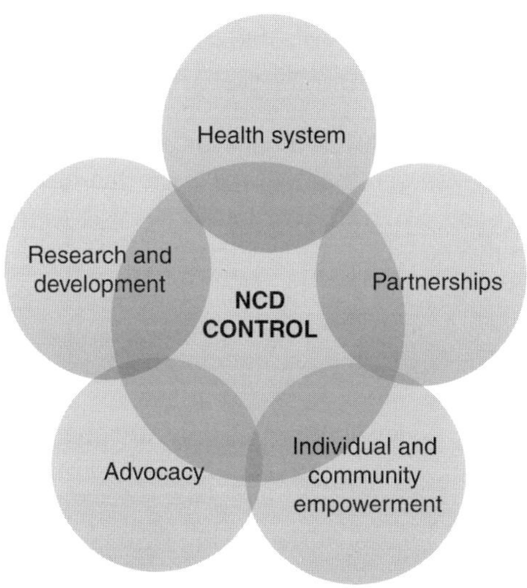

Fig.10.1. Key elements for NCD control.

10.3.2 Research and development

In most LMICs, there is very limited research on NCDs [55], and even when available, it is mostly epidemiological research. Although epidemiological or descriptive studies give some indication of the burden of the problem of NCDs, the lack of biomedical research and operational research on NCDs in LMICs needs to be addressed. One of the reasons underlying the low output of NCD research in LMICs is the lack of dedicated funding for NCD activity. Research on Malaria, HIV/AIDS and tuberculosis has been buoyed by the establishment of the Global Fund to Fight AIDS, Tuberculosis and Malaria in 2002. Significant improvements in the control of these diseases have followed increased spending on research and development of novel tools and improved delivery of known interventions. Besides the availability of global resources, the establishment of local or regional research and development programmes are bound to yield results. One of the most successful countries in managing vaccine-preventable diseases is Brazil, which has achieved more than 80% coverage of immunization. This success is linked to the domestic production of vaccines; as much as 70% of the vaccines used in Brazil as of 2002 were produced locally. Similarly, despite the rising cost of antiretroviral treatment globally, Brazil has experienced a decrease in this cost because of its ability to produce generic antiretrovirals [56]. In encouraging research practice, one of the skills that needs developing is the analytical skills of line managers to enable them to analyse routine data to inform on programme delivery. This has been shown to be inspirational to frontline workers when it has been done properly [57].

One of the challenges that primary healthcare encountered when it was initially mooted in 1978 (Alma-Ata Declaration) was that the goals appeared unattainable [58]. Proponents of selective primary healthcare were successful in part because of the evidence generated on the cost-effectiveness of their options [59]. While many interventions are available for controlling NCDs, it will be useful to assess the cost-effectiveness of the proposed interventions and also to identify high-impact options in order for them to enjoy much support. In ID control, an example of a high-impact intervention is oral rehydration therapy, and the significant reduction in diarrhoea-related deaths in the 1980s has been attributed to this intervention [60].

Advocating for the identification and use of high-impact and cost-effective interventions does not mean that other interventions should be ignored. For instance, in the above example on diarrhoea, in Brazil, piped drinking water and hygienic sewage disposal have remarkably decreased the incidence of diarrhoea, while the decrease in mortality was also made possible because of the increased access to health services. Today, the profile of diarrhoea has changed such that the leading cause of diarrhoea is viral, leading to the introduction of rotavirus vaccine in children who are more vulnerable. Finally, even in instances where there is active research, there appears to be a divide between science and practice. This is to the detriment of the NCD response.

10.3.3 Patient and community involvement/empowerment

HIV and NCDs are thought of as quite different challenges and tend to be addressed separately. However, both are linked in terms of the central role of individual behaviours and lifestyles. Preventative efforts for both HIV and NCDs primarily involve behaviour change directed at modifying risky behaviours. In HIV control, condom use, abstinence and avoidance of sharing needles were initiatives that were dependent on patient involvement. The need for patient involvement has been crucial in care and compliance with antiretrovirals.

By virtue of the crucial role played by lifestyle-related factors as risk factors for NCDs, intervention strategies need to recognize the importance of involving patients in their management and care. It is individuals and patients who will need to quit smoking, maintain a healthy diet, reduce salt and alcohol intake, and exercise regularly. Empowerment of the community is crucial in ensuring the success of the NCD response (see also de-Graft Aikins *et al.*, Chapter 9, this volume). Individuals need to be aware of the NCD threat and the options available to them to prevent and manage NCDs and their associated complications. What this stands to achieve is a core of NCD advocates at all levels. Individuals and communities are also more likely to demand and opt for changes to prevent NCDs. An empowered patient is an invaluable partner in care and is more likely to be adherent to treatment and care and to minimize their risk of disability and other negative health outcomes.

10.4 Conclusion

NCDs are already major causes of morbidity and mortality in LMICs, and the current health and economic costs need to be contained with robust control programmes. The priority areas for action include the establishment of strong surveillance systems to monitor exposure to risks, prevalence of the common conditions and programme performance. Health information, as well as the implementation of cost-effective and high-impact interventions that are sustainable in the specific conditions, will be important in the fight against NCDs. Programmes will need to be anchored in well-integrated healthcare systems that place the individual at the centre. In the long run, empowered individuals and communities that appreciate the risk and dangers imposed by NCDs will be the best agents for stemming the tide of the current NCD epidemic in LMICs.

References

1. Gaziano, T., Srinath, R.K., Paccaud, F., Horton, S. and Chaturvedi, V. (2005) Cardiovascular disease. In: Jamison, D.T., Breman, J.G., Measham, A.R., Alleyne, G., Claeson, M., Evans, D.B., Jha, P., Mills, A. and Musgrove, P. (eds) *Disease Control Priorities in Developing Countries*, 2nd edn. World Bank, Washington, DC, pp. 645–662.

2. de-Graft Aikins, A. (2007) Ghana's neglected chronic disease epidemic: a developmental challenge. *Ghana Medical Journal* 14, 154–159.
3. WHO (2013) *Global Action Plan for the Prevention and Control of Noncommunicable Diseases*. World Health Organization, Geneva, Switzerland <http://www.who.int/global-coordination-mechanism/publications/global-action-plan-ncds-eng.pdf?ua=1>.
4. WHO (2015) *Integrated Chronic Disease Prevention and Control*. World Health Organization, Geneva, Switzerland <http://www.who.int/chp/about/integrated_cd/en>.
5. Gaziano, T.A., Bitton, A., Anand, S., Abrahams-Gessel, S. and Murphy, A. (2010) Growing epidemic of coronary heart disease in low- and middle-income countries. *Current Problems in Cardiology* 35, 72–115.
6. Bloom, D.E., Cafiero, E.T., Jané-Llopis, E., Abrahams-Gessel, S., Bloom, L.R., Fathima, S., Feigl, A.B., Gaziano, T., Mowafi, M., Pandya, A., Prettner, K., Rosenberg, L., Seligman, B., Stein, A.Z. and Weinstein, C. (2011) *The Global Economic Burden of Noncommunicable Diseases*. World Economic Forum, Geneva, Switzerland <http://www3.weforum.org/docs/WEF_Harvard_HE_GlobalEconomicBurdenNonCommunicableDiseases_2011.pdf>.
7. WHO (2010) *Monitoring the Building Blocks of Health Systems: a Handbook of Indicators and Their Measurement Strategies*. World Health Organization, Geneva, Switzerland <http://www.who.int/healthinfo/systems/WHO_MBHSS_2010_full_web.pdf>.
8. Barreto, M.L., Teixeira, M.G. and Carmo, E.H. (2006) Infectious diseases epidemiology. *Journal of Epidemiology and Community Health* 60, 192–195.
9. Cohen, M.L. (1998) Resurgent and emergent disease in a changing world. *British Medical Bulletin* 54, 523–532.
10. Hardy, A. (1988) Urban famine or urban crisis? Typhus in the Victorian city. *Medical History* 32, 401–425.
11. Riedel, S. (2005) Edward Jenner and the history of smallpox and vaccination. *Baylor University Medical Center Proceedings* 18, 21–25.
12. United Nations (2009) *Achieving the Global Public Health Agenda*. Department of Economic and Social Affairs, United Nations, New York <http://www.un.org/en/ecosoc/docs/pdfs/achieving_global_public_health_agenda.pdf>.
13. United Nations (2008) *Achieving Sustainable Development and Promoting Development Cooperation*. Department of Economic and Social Affairs, United Nations, New York <http://www.un.org/en/ecosoc/docs/pdfs/fina_08-45773.pdf>.
14. WHO (2013) *Polio Eradication and Endgame Strategic Plan 2013–2018*. World Health Organization, Geneva, Switzerland <http://www.polioeradication.org/Portals/0/Document/Resources/StrategyWork/PEESP_EN_US.pdf>.
15. Uchoa, E., Barreto, S.M., Firmo, J.O., Guerra, H.L., Pimenta, F.G. Jr and Lima Costa, M.F. (2000) The control of schistosomiasis in Brazil: an ethnoepidemiological study of the effectiveness of a community mobilization program for health education. *Social Science & Medicine* 51, 1529–1541.
16. Gillespie, S. (ed.) (2006) *AIDS, Poverty, and Hunger: Challenges and Responses*. International Food Policy Research Institute, Washington, DC <http://www.ifpri.org/sites/default/files/publications/oc50.pdf>.
17. Hopkins, D.R., Richards, F.O., Ruiz-Tiben, E., Emerson, P. and Withers, C. (2008) Dracunculiasis, onchocerciasis, schistosomiasis, and trachoma. *Annals of the New York Academy of Sciences* 1136, 45–52.
18. Atun, R., Jaffar, S., Nishtar, S., Knaul, F.M., Barreto, M.L., Nyirenda, M., Banatvala, N. and Piot, P. (2013) Improving responsiveness of health systems to non-communicable diseases. *Lancet* 381, 690–697.
19. Connolly, M.A., Gayer, M., Ryan, M.J., Salama, P., Spiegel, P. and Heymann, D.L. (2004) Communicable diseases in complex emergencies: impact and challenges. *Lancet* 364, 1974–1983.

20. CDC (2013) *CDC Framework for Preventing Infectious Diseases: Sustaining the Essentials and Innovating for the Future*. Centres for Disease Control and Prevention, Atlanta, Georgia <http://www.cdc.gov/oid/framework.html>.
21. Srivastava, R.K. and Bachani, D. (2011) Burden of NCDs, policies and programme for prevention and control of NCDs in India. *Indian Journal of Community Medicine* 36, 7–12.
22. NCD Alliance (2012) *Post 2015 development goals: lessons learned from the adoption of the International Development Targets and the Millennium Development Goals, in particular how effective has the MDG process been to date?* <http://www.publications.parliament.uk/pa/cm201213/cmselect/cmintdev/writev/post2015/m67.htm>.
23. Stenberg, K. and Chisholm, D. (2012) Resource needs for addressing noncommunicable disease in low-and-middle income countries. *Global Heart* 7, 53–60.
24. WHO (2011) *WHO Global Coordination Mechanism on the Prevention and Control of Noncommunicable Diseases*. Policy brief by R. Nugent. World Health Organization, Geneva, Switzerland <http://www.who.int/nmh/ncd-coordination-mechanism/Policybrief5.2docx.pdf>.
25. Population Reference Bureau (2006) *Chronic Diseases Beleaguer Developing Countries* <http://www.prb.org/Publications/Articles/2006/ChronicDiseasesBeleaguerDevelopingCountries.aspx>.
26. Maher, D., Ford, N. and Unwin, N. (2012) Priorities for developing countries in the global response to non-communicable diseases. *Globalization and Health* 8, 14.
27. WHO (2010) *Global Status Report on Non-communicable Diseases*. World Health Organization, Geneva, Switzerland <http://www.who.int/nmh/publications/ncd_report_full_en.pdf>.
28. Reynolds, H.W. and Sutherland, E.G. (2013) A systematic approach to the planning, implementation, monitoring and evaluation of integrated health services. *BMC Health Services Research* 13, 168–178.
29. WHO (2012) *Service Delivery Approaches to HIV Testing and Counselling (HTC): a Strategic HTC Programme Framework*. World Health Organization, Geneva, Switzerland <http://apps.who.int/iris/bitstream/10665/75206/1/9789241593877_eng.pdf>.
30. UNAIDS (2012) *Delivering Antiretroviral Therapy in the Community: Experience from Four Countries in Southern Africa* <http://www.lekari-bez-hranic.cz/sites/czech/files/cz/downloads/Closer-to-Home-FINAL-July-2012.pdf>.
31. Miller, M.A. and Sentz, J.T. (2006) Vaccine-preventable diseases. In: Jamison, D.T., Feachem, R.G., Makgova, M.W., Bos, E.R., Baingana, F.K., Hofman, K.J. and Rogo, K.O. *Disease and Mortality in Sub-Saharan Africa*, 2nd edn. World Bank, Washington, DC.
32. Schlipköter, U. and Flahault, A. (2010) Communicable diseases: achievements and challenges for public health. *Public Health Reviews* 32, 90–119.
33. Global Fund (2001) *The Global Fund to fight AIDS, Tuberculosis and Malaria: the Framework Document* <http://www.theglobalfund.org/en/documents/governance>.
34. Pearce, N., Asher, I., Billo, N., Bissell, K., Ellwood, P., El Sony, A., García-Marcos, L., Chiang, C.Y., Mallol, J., Marks, G. and Strachan, D. (2013) Asthma in the global NCD agenda: a neglected epidemic. *Lancet Respiratory Medicine* 1, 96–98.
35. World Malaria Report (2009) Interventions to control malaria <http://www.who.int/malaria/world_malaria_report_2009/mal2009_rep_chap3_v2.pdf>
36. Roll Back Malaria (2008) *Global Malaria Action Plan* <http://www.rollbackmalaria.org/microsites/gmap>.
37. Al-Awadi, A.R., Karam, M.V., Molyneux, D.H. and Breman, J.G. (2007) The other 'neglected' eradication programme: achieving the final mile for Guinea worm disease eradication? *Transactions of the Royal Society of Tropical Medicine and Hygiene* 101, 741–742.
38. Expanded Programme on Immunization (1998) The Social Science and Immunization Research Project. *Weekly Epidemiological Record* 73, 285–288.
39. Nichter, M. (1990) Vaccination in South Asia: false expectations and commanding metaphors. In: Coreil, J. (ed.) *Anthropology and Primary Health Care*. Westview Press, Oxford, UK, pp. 196–221.

40. Streefland, P.H. (1995) Enhancing coverage and sustainability of vaccination programs: an explanatory framework with special reference to India. *Social Science and Medicine* 41, 647–656.
41. Jheeta, M. and Newell, J. (2008) Childhood vaccination in Africa and Asia: the effects of parents' knowledge and attitudes. *Bulletin of the World Health Organization* 86, 419.
42. WHO (2014) *Global Status Report on NCDs; Attaining the Nine Global Noncommunicable Diseases Targets; a Shared Responsibility*. World Health Organization, Geneva, Switzerland <http://reliefweb.int/report/world/global-status-report-noncommunicable-diseases-2014-attaining-nine-global>.
43. Uri, D. and Bennett, S. (2010) *The World Order in 2050* <http://carnegieendowment.org/files/World_Order_in_2050.pdf>.
44. International Labour Organization (2011) The great recession and the jobs crisis. In: *The Global Social Crisis: Report on the World Social Situation 2011*. United Nations, New York, pp. 27–48. <http://www.un.org/esa/socdev/rwss/docs/2011/chapter2.pdf>.
45. Population Council (2001) *Economic Evaluations of HIV/AIDS Interventions* <http://www.popcouncil.org/uploads/pdfs/horizons/rs/re_cost.pdf>.
46. Trapero-Bertran, M. and Oliva-Moreno, J. (2014) Economic impact of HIV/AIDS: a systematic review in five European countries. *Health Economics Review* 4, 15.
47. Menzies, N.A., Cohen, T., Lin, H., Murray, M. and Salomon, J.A. (2012) Population health impact and cost-effectiveness of tuberculosis diagnosis with Xpert MTB.RIF: a dynamic simulation and economic evaluation. *PLOS Medicine* 9, 1–17.
48. CDC (2013) *Parasites – Dracunculiasis (Also Known as Guinea Worm Disease)*. Centres for Disease Control and Prevention, Atlanta, Georgia <http://www.cdc.gov/parasites/guineaworm/disease.html>.
49. University of California, San Francisco (UCSF) Division of HIV/AIDS (2015) *Sustainable East Africa Research of Community Health – Uganda and* Kenya <http://hiv.ucsf.edu/research/international/search.html>.
50. Thirumurthy, H., Jain, V., Chamie, G., Geng, E., Kabami, J., Kwarisiima, D., Clark, T.D., Geng, E., Petersen, M.L., Charlebois, E.D., Kamya, M.R., Havlir, D.V. and the SEARCH Collaboration (2013) Improved employment, education, and economic outcomes in households of HIV-positive adults with high CD4 counts: evidence from a community-wide health campaign in Uganda. *AIDS* 27, 627–634.
51. WHO (2005) *Evaluating the Costs and Benefits of National Surveillance and Response Systems*. World Health Organization, Geneva, Switzerland <http://www.who.int/csr/resources/publications/surveillance/WHO_CDS_EPR_LYO_2005_25.pdf>.
52. Carpenter, G. and Wyman, O. (2008) The economic and social impact of emerging infectious disease: mitigation through detection, research, and response. Marsh, Mercer and Kroll. <http://www.healthcare.philips.com/main/shared/assets/documents/bioshield/ecoandsocialimpactofemerginginfectiousdisease_111208.pdf>.
53. Barret, S. (2004) Eradication versus control: the economics of global infectious disease policies. *Bulletin of the World Health Organization* 82, 639–718.
54. United Nations (2011) *UNAIDS Guidance for Partnerships with Civil Society, Including People Living with HIV and Key Populations* <http://www.unaids.org/sites/default/files/en/media/unaids/contentassets/documents/unaidspublication/2012/JC2236_guidance_partnership_civilsociety_en.pdf>.
55. Reidpath, D.D. and Allotey, P. (2012) The burden is great and the money little: changing chronic disease management in low- and middle-income countries. *Journal of Global Health* 2, 020301.
56. Nunn, A.S. Fonseca, E.M., Bastos, F.I., Gruskin, S. and Salomon, J.A. (2007) Evolution of antiretroviral drug costs in Brazil in the context of free and universal access to AIDS treatment. *PLoS Medicine* 4, e305.

57. Zachariah, R., Ford, N., Maher, D., Bissell, K., Van den Bergh, R., van den Boogaard, W., Reid, T., Castro, K.G., Draguez, B., von Schreeb, J., Chakaya, J., Atun, R., Lienhardt, C., Enarson, D.A.and Harries, A.D. (2012) Is operational research delivering the goods? The journey to success in low-income countries. *Lancet Infectious Diseases* 12, 415–421.
58. WHO (1978) *Primary Health Care.* Report of the International conference on primary health care in Alma-Ata, USSR, 6–12 September 1978. World Health Organization, Geneva, Switzerland <http://www.hauora.co.nz/assets/files/PHO%20Info/Alma_Ata_conference_1978_report%20and%20declaration.pdf>.
59. Cueto, M. (2004) The origins of primary health care and selective primary health care. *American Journal of Public Health* 94, 1864–1874.
60. Keusch, G.T., Fontaine, O., Bhargava, A., Boschi-Pinto, C., Bhutta, Z.A., Gotuzzo, E., Rivera, J., Chow, J., Shahid-Salles, S. and Laxminarayan, R. (2006) Diarrheal diseases. In: Jamison, D.T., Breman, J.G., Measham, A.R., Alleyne, G., Claeson, M., Evans, D.B., Jha, P., Mills, A. and Musgrove, P. (eds) *Disease Control Priorities in Developing Countries.* World Bank, Washington, DC.

11 Prevention and Control of Chronic Non-communicable Diseases: Lessons from High-income Countries

Charles Agyemang[1]*, Pietro Amedeo Modesti[2], Ricardo Queiroz Gurgel[3] and Gbenga Ogedegbe[4]

[1]*Department of Public Health, Academic Medical Centre, University of Amsterdam, Amsterdam, Holland;* [2]*Clinica Medica Generale e Cardiologia, University of Florence, Florence, Italy;* [3]*Universidade Federal de Sergipe, Aracaju, Sergipe, Brazil;* [4]*Center for Healthful Behavior Change, New York University School of Medicine, New York, USA*

11.1 Introduction

Non-communicable diseases (NCDs) are the leading causes of death worldwide. Of the 57 million total global deaths in 2008, 36 million (63%) deaths were attributed to NCDs, primarily cardiovascular diseases (CVDs), diabetes, cancer and chronic respiratory diseases [1]. About a quarter of worldwide NCD-related deaths were among people below 60 years of age, clearly indicating the importance of the economic cost associated with NCDs, particularly for low- and middle-income countries (LMICs) [2]. Global estimates indicate that LMICs are the most affected, with nearly 80% (29 million) of all NCD deaths occurring in LMICs [1]. NCDs are the most common causes of death in all world regions, and in the World Health Organization (WHO) Africa Region NCD mortality exceeds that of communicable, maternal, perinatal and nutritional conditions combined. The WHO forecasts further indicate that NCDs will account for a significant increase in the total number of deaths in the next decade. For example, NCD-related deaths are expected to increase by 17% globally between 2010 and 2020. The highest increases are expected to be in the WHO Africa Region (27%), followed by the eastern Mediterranean (25%) and South-east Asia (21%) [1]. The three leading causes of NCD deaths in 2008 were CVDs (17 million), cancer (7.6 million) and respiratory diseases (4.2 million). Diabetes caused an additional 1.3 million deaths [1].

*E-mail: c.o.agyemang@amc.uva.nl

11.2 History of the Epidemiology of Non-communicable Diseases in High-income Countries

Industrialization and technological advances in the last two centuries have led to improvements in sanitation, housing, nutrition and better treatment in most high-income countries. This, in turn, has resulted in a dramatic change in the cause of death from a predominance of infectious diseases, such as diarrhoea, pneumonia and tuberculosis, and malnutrition. At the beginning of the 20th century, NCDs were responsible for less than 10% of all deaths worldwide compared with 63% in 2008 [1]. This change has been named an epidemiological transition [3]. Omran categorized this epidemiological transition into three basic stages: pestilence and famine, receding pandemics, and degenerative and man-made diseases [3]. Olshansky and Ault [4] added delayed degenerative diseases as a fourth stage (Fig. 11.1). The first stage (i.e. age of pestilence and famine) is characterized by the predominance of malnutrition and infectious disease. At this stage, the average life expectancy at birth is mostly below 40 years. During the second stage (age of receding pandemics), the burden of infectious disease reduces and nutrition status improves due to increases in wealth leading to better availability of food, improved sanitation, and access to vaccines and antibiotics. These changes along with increased life expectancy at birth (30–50 years) eventually lead to a greater incidence of diseases related to hypertension such as haemorrhagic stroke and hypertensive heart disease. During the third stage (i.e. age of degenerative man-made diseases), life expectancy at birth continues to improve gradually until it exceeds 50 years and it is characterized by widespread high-fat diets, smoking and physical inactivity. NCDs dominate, with the highest deaths caused by atherosclerosis. In the course of the fourth stage (i.e. age of delayed degenerative diseases), NCD deaths tend to decline because of common primary and secondary prevention efforts. The congestive heart failure rate increases because of the improved survival of those with ischaemic heart diseases [5].

Comprehensive NCD prevention programmes in high-income countries have prevented or postponed NCDs to older ages. The increases in life expectancy at

Stage	Description	Life expectancy
Pestilence and famine	Predominance of malnutrition and infectious diseases	20–40 years
Receding pandemics	Improved nutrition and public health leads to increase in chronic diseases and hypertension	30–50 years
Degenerative and man-made diseases	Increased fat and caloric intake; widespread tobacco use; chronic disease deaths exceed mortality from infections and malnutrition	60 years
Delayed degenerative diseases	CVD and cancer are leading causes of morbidity and mortality; prevention and treatment avoids death and delays onset; age-adjusted CVD declines	>70 years

Fig. 11.1. Stages of the epidemiological transition. CVD, cardiovascular disease.

birth that have occurred during the last few decades have been largely due to improvements in medical care [6]. The notion of NCD preventability comes from data and analyses at individual and population levels. During the early stage of CVD epidemiology and prevention, the main strategy was geared towards the detection of high-risk individuals in the population and designing effective screening programmes. The term 'risk factor' first appeared in 1961 in a publication from the Framingham Study [7]. In the late 1960s, it became apparent that prevention and control programmes could not focus exclusively on the detection and protection of high-risk individuals in the community but must be rooted in the whole community. The community-based approach was supported by the fact that most of the NCDs such as CVD events in the population also occur among individuals with moderate risk, indicating that focusing on the high-risk strategy alone would miss large proportion of susceptible individuals. Therefore, the entire population must embrace preventative measures [8]. This concept was endorsed by Rose in his 1981 influential paper on the 'Strategy of prevention' [9]. He eloquently defined the 'high-risk strategy' and the 'population strategy' [9]. This thesis had an immediate impact and has remained valid ever since.

It worth emphasizing that the fact that high-income countries are at the later stage of the epidemiological transition does not necessary mean that NCDs are not a problem in these countries. NCDs are still the leading cause of death in these countries and there are important differences across social and ethnic groups, suggesting that the epidemiological transition might also operate through different levels both within and across countries [5]. In most high-income countries, the epidemiological transitions start in the rich and later move on to the poor – what others refer to as the 'diffusion theory' of coronary heart disease. The 'diffusion theory' postulates that the rise in coronary heart disease started in the high socio-economic groups in high-income countries, because they were the first who could afford the behaviours that increase the risk of coronary heart disease [10]. With time, the disease spread to lower socio-economic groups as living standards improved. When the coronary heart disease epidemic started to decline, the higher socio-economic groups were once again the first groups to reap the benefit as they were the first to adopt the healthy behavioural changes. The diffusion theory clearly holds in high-income countries, with the poor being more affected by NCDs than the rich. Important differences are also observed across ethnic groups in high-income countries.

11.3 Ethnic Inequalities of NCDs and Risk Factors in High-income Countries

In high-income countries, particularly in Europe and North America, the patterns of NCD morbidity and mortality differ substantially among ethnic groups. By ethnicity, we mean the group individuals belong to as a result of their roots, which includes language, religion, diet and ancestry [11]. Because people with similar ethnic backgrounds tend to live in diverse world regions and societies, differences in disease experience by ethnicity are also intertwined with geographical variations [5]. In addition, migration to different geographical locations can lead to different environmental exposures and subsequently may lead to considerable differences in lifestyle, even among people with similar ethnic backgrounds [12]. Some of these behaviours can persist for generations and shape their risk profiles and subsequently disease outcomes. The ethnic differences in disease outcomes may also reflect the different stages of the epidemiological transition among ethnic minority groups living in high-income countries. Indeed, ethnic minority populations (predominantly from LMIC origins) in high-income countries have different NCD outcomes from the local-born European populations [13–15]. For some NCDs such as CVD and diabetes, they generally have worse outcomes, whereas for other conditions such as cancer, their outcomes are better than the local-born populations [14, 15]. The relative differences in NCDs between the ethnic minority and locally born European populations are largely dependent on ethnic background, the type of NCD and risk factors, the country of residence and the length of stay in the host country. South-Asian born (India, Pakistani, Bangladeshi and Sri Lanka) people who have migrated to England and Wales, for example, have higher mortality from both stroke and ischaemic heart disease than the England and Wales national average [13]. People born in the West Indies/Caribbean or West Africa but residing in England and Wales have lower mortality from ischaemic heart disease but higher mortality from stroke than the England and Wales national average. Similar consistent findings have also been reported among South-Asian and African origin populations living in other European countries [16, 17]. In addition, Turkish-born and Polish-born populations have a higher risk of death from circulatory diseases than the local-born populations [18]. By contrast, low CVD mortality rates have been reported in some migrant populations such as Moroccans [16, 19, 20].

The prevalence of type 2 diabetes, for example, is about three to five times greater in some groups compared with the host European populations [21, 22]. They also develop type 2 diabetes at a younger age, and have higher morbidity and mortality from type 2 diabetes and related complications than European host populations. A recent report by Ujcic-Voortman *et al.* [22] showed that the typical age of onset of type 2 diabetes in Turkish and Moroccan ethnic groups was one and two decades younger than in European–Dutch populations, respectively. These differences correlate with the higher type 2 diabetes mortality among ethnic minority groups relative to the European local-born populations [23, 24]. By contrast, studies in many European countries have revealed a lower incidence and mortality rates of major cancer types including cancers of the lung, breast, ovary, prostate, colon, kidney and bladder among ethnic minority and migrant groups compared with host European populations. In most studies, ethnic minority groups have 20–50% lower incidence and mortality rates than the European host populations [25–29]. Although the risks of major cancer types are low in most ethnic minority and migrant groups, the magnitude of the differences varies substantially among groups. For example, compared with the local-born Dutch population, breast cancer mortality was 53% lower among Moroccan-born compared with 17% lower among Surinamese-born migrants living in the Netherlands [25]. These differences might reflect differences in the degree of exposure to specific risk factors [14]. Furthermore, cancers caused by communicable diseases, such as stomach cancer, nasopharyngeal cancer, hepatic cancer, Kaposi's sarcoma, cervical cancer and some lymphomas, are generally more common among ethnic minority and migrants groups than among local-born European populations [30]. A general explanation is that ethnic minority and migrant groups from LMICs had a high risk of exposure to these infections, such as *Helicobacter pylori* bacterium, an important risk factor for developing stomach cancer, in their homelands before migration [31].

Recent evidence seems to suggest that the diffusion theory of CVD is emerging in migrant populations in high-income countries in line with the general populations. In a recent study in the Netherlands, socio-economic inequalities in the incidence of stroke and acute myocardial infarction were found in both European–Dutch and all migrant groups [20, 32]. These findings contrast with the earlier studies where no relationships were observed between socio-economic status and CVDs in migrant groups [16, 33].

11.4 The Burden of NCDs in LMICs

NCDs are increasingly becoming a looming threat that is creating a double burden in LMICs [1, 34]. The high-level meeting on NCDs at the General Assembly of the United Nations in 2011 clearly underscored how NCDs now dominate health worldwide [35] (see Mendis and Chestnov, Chapter 12, this volume). This is rightly so because more than 60% of preventable deaths worldwide are now attributable to NCDs. In LMICs, 48% of such deaths occur in persons <70 years of age, compared with 26% in high-income countries [1, 36, 37]. In sub-Saharan Africa where infectious diseases are still the overall leading cause of death, the incidence of NCDs is increasing rapidly, a region in which urbanization and population growth are most extreme. In fact, in 2008, the age-standardized NCD mortality rates for all ages were highest in the WHO African Region compared with the overall NCD age-standardized death rates in LMICs [1]. CVD is the second leading killer overall and the leading cause of death among adults aged 30 years and older, who are in their most productive years of life in sub-Saharan Africa [37]. Over the next few years, sub-Saharan Africa is projected to experience one of the largest increases in death rates from NCDs [38]. NCDs are therefore no longer syndromes of wealthy societies; they are becoming just as dominant in LMICs [34].

The main drivers of the rising NCDs in LMICs are associated with urbanization and lifestyle changes, especially physical inactivity, unhealthy diet, smoking, excessive alcohol consumption and air pollution. Hypertension, type 2 diabetes, obesity and dyslipidaemia are important measurable indicators that predict adverse outcomes. The prevalence rates of type 2 diabetes and hypertension in many LMICs far exceed those reported in high-income countries [39–41]. The global estimates also indicate that the increases in the prevalence of hypertension and type 2 diabetes will be higher in LMICs than in high-income countries [39–41]. For instance, the estimates of Shaw *et al.* [41] indicate that, for LMICs, adult diabetes numbers are likely to increase by 69% from 2010 to 2030, compared with 20% for high-income countries. The estimates of Kearney *et al.* [39] also showed that the number of people with hypertension in LMICs will have increased by 80% in 2025, compared with 24% in high-income countries. Similarly, LMICs are projected to have a much larger proportional increase in the number of overweight and obese individuals than high-income countries between 2005 and 2030 [42]. Time trend analyses, for example, show that the prevalence of obesity in urban West Africa has more than doubled over the last 15 years [43]. More worryingly, large proportions of people with type 2 diabetes and hypertension are undiagnosed [39, 40]. This means that a large number of people with diabetes and hypertension are unaware that they are progressing towards complications.

The rising levels of CVDs in LMICs clearly reflects the changing lifestyles such as consumption of energy-dense foods and refined sugars complemented by less energy-demanding jobs particularly in urban centres, which are linked to structural factors such as urbanization and increasing globalization of the food market [44]. The burden is further compounded by weak health systems that are unable to cope with the double burden of CVD and infectious diseases [45]. The increasing burden of NCDs might exacerbate some of the progress made in combating communicable diseases due to interactions between some NCDs and communicable diseases. There is growing evidence, for example, that type 2 diabetes is an important risk factor for tuberculosis and might affect disease presentation and the response to treatment [46]. Additionally, tuberculosis might induce glucose intolerance and worsen glycaemic control in people with type 2 diabetes. With increasing rates of type 2 diabetes in LMICs, we can expect that the number of people who have both tuberculosis and type 2 diabetes will increase markedly in the coming years (see Oni and Unwin, Chapter 3, this volume).

11.5 Policy Initiatives for NCDs in High-income Countries

Declines in NCDs, particularly CVD mortality rates, occurred in most Western countries during the latter part of the 20th century. The decline has been attributed to population-wide primary prevention and treatment interventions [8]. Effective methods for NCD prevention comprise comprehensive tobacco and alcohol control through taxes and regulation of sales and advertising; reducing dietary salt, unhealthy fats and sugars through regulation and well-designed public education; increasing the consumption of fruit and vegetables, healthy fats and whole grains by lowering prices and improving availability; and the implementation of universal, effective and equitable primary care health systems that target NCD risk factors through clinical interventions [6]. Both prevention and treatment have contributed immensely to the decline in NCD mortality. In New Zealand, for example, a trends review of major risk factors and medical treatment found that primary prevention played a considerable role in the decline of coronary heart disease mortality from 1968 to 1978 [47]. It was estimated that medical treatment accounted for about 40% of the decline in coronary heart disease mortality from 1974 to 1981 in Auckland, New Zealand; and changes in lifestyle, particularly diet and smoking, accounted for 38–51% of the decline in coronary heart disease mortality in men aged 35–64 years from 1968 to 1980 [48]. In Australia, a reduction in the major risk factors, namely smoking, total cholesterol and blood pressure levels, explained much of the decline in major coronary events from 1985 to 1993 [49].

Several studies in Europe also indicate that much of the decline in CVD deaths was due to changes in major risk factors for CVDs [50–53]. In England and Wales, the coronary heart disease mortality rate in men peaked in the early 1970s, whereas in women the rate declined fairly steadily from the 1950s until the early 1970s and subsequently levelled off during much of the 1970s and part of the 1980s [54].

The decline of NCDs, especially CVDs, in high-income countries clearly suggests that it is feasible to prevent and reverse the rising prevalence of NCDs in LMICs through effective population-based prevention programmes. The successful population-based intervention programme in North Karelia, Finland, is a very good example [55]. In the 1960s, the coronary heart disease mortality rate in Finland was one of the highest in the world [56]. Given the high rate of coronary heart disease mortality in Finland, in 1972, the North Karelia Project was set up to lower these rates by improving the three fundamental risk factors for coronary heart disease, specifically smoking, total cholesterol and blood pressure [57]. Five key models – the behavioural change model, communication–behavioural change model, innovative-diffusion model, community organization model and unified model – were used for this study. Changes targeted both community and national levels. At the community level, stakeholders including health and other services, voluntary organizations, local media and businesses were engaged, and public policy was developed. At the national level, changes in public policy were put in place, industry's cooperation was increasingly sought and expert guidelines were established. These measures resulted in a huge decline in CVD risk factors and subsequent coronary heart disease incidence in Finland. The net reduction for smoking in North Karelia for the full 10-year period (1972–1982) was 27% for men and 14% for women; total cholesterol and systolic blood pressure was reduced by 3% each in men, and by 1 and 5%, respectively, in women [58]. The reduction in risk factors had a huge effect on coronary heart disease mortality rate in North Karelia with a reduction of 2.9% per year between 1969 and 1978 in men aged 35–64 years, compared with the national coronary heart disease mortality rate of 1.0% per year [55]. These findings encouraged more population-based efforts and resulted in further reductions in coronary heart disease mortality by 8.0% per year in North Karelia and by 6.5% per year at the national level in Finland from 1986 to 1995. A similar study in Stanford, USA, resulted in reductions in risk factors such as cholesterol (2%), blood pressure (4%) and smoking (13%) when compared with sites without the intervention, but there was no effect on disease endpoints [59, 60].

11.6 Policy Initiatives in LMICs

In 2008, the World Health Assembly endorsed an action plan for the implementation of a global NCD strategy [61]. One of the objectives of this action plan was to establish and strengthen national policies and strategies for the prevention and control of NCDs. Following the endorsement of the action plan, several LMICs have expanded their capacities to respond to the epidemic of NCDs. According to the WHO, about 92% of countries globally have developed at least one policy, plan or strategy to address NCDs and/or their risk factors [38]. Tobacco control policies and plans are available in more than 80% of countries, and policies and plans for addressing diet and physical inactivity are available in about 75% of countries. However, only a few countries have developed plans for tackling harmful alcohol consumption. Furthermore, a recent analysis by Rani *et al.* [62] showed that the priorities for establishing policies and plans are not always based on the disease burden and prevalence of the risk factor, as well as the availability of cost-effective interventions. Thus, the widespread presence of NCD policies or plans does not necessarily indicate that they are implemented or funded (see also Mendis and Chestnov, Chapter 12, this volume). The 2012 study of Rani *et al.* [62] also identified several areas of concern of governance response to NCDs in the western Pacific region. For instance, local evidence, even when acknowledged in situation analysis, was often ignored in favour of global priorities and goals. Furthermore, NCD-specific plans often have no information on financial and implementation feasibility and realistic quantifiable targets. Moreover, while the need for multi-sectorial coordination is acknowledged by most LMICs, the resources needed to organize and manage such coordination mechanisms were found to be inadequate.

Some LMICs such as Brazil have had some success in tackling NCDs [63]. Brazil, for example, has implemented major policies for the prevention of NCDs, and its NCD mortality is falling by 1.8% per year. The main policy comprises a series of actions in inter-sectorial articulation and policy development, health education, disease and risk factor monitoring, and healthcare provision centred on healthy diets, physical activity, smoking reduction and the reduction of harmful use of alcohol. The control of smoking has been the prominent success despite the fact that Brazil is the world's largest tobacco exporter and the second-largest tobacco producer, and has been suggested to be responsible for much of the decline in NCDs in Brazil. Smoking control is strongly supported by the government through legislations and ratification of the WHO Framework Convention on Tobacco Control [64]. However, the continued rapid increases in the prevalence and incidence of obesity, hypertension and diabetes seem to suggest the inadequacy of present strategies, and raise the challenge of implementing additional steps as recommended by the WHO's Global Strategy [65].

Several community intervention programmes have also proved to be successful in some LMICs such as the Mauritius project [66], the Tianjin project in China [67] and the Coronary Risk Factor Study in South Africa [68].

The Mauritius project was a government-led programme that changed the main cooking oil from a mostly saturated-fat palm oil to soybean oil high in unsaturated fatty acids. Overall, total cholesterol concentrations decreased by 14% during the 5-year study period from 1987 to 1992. These observations suggest that LMIC governments have an important role to play in tackling the burden of NCDs.

11.7 Lessons from High-income Countries

The reduction in NCD and particularly coronary heart disease mortality rates in high-income countries has been hailed as one of the greatest achievements in public health during the 20th century [69]. Improvements in risk factors, mainly smoking, total cholesterol and blood pressure, were the key milestones in the decline. Evidence from policy modelling efforts consistently indicates that further reductions in NCD mortality can be achieved if more aggressive targets for improving the distribution of risk factors in the population can be met and if compliance with evidence-based treatments can be improved [70, 71]. More importantly, most of these interventions have been shown to be cost-effective for wide application across the different levels of health systems in developed countries [72–74]. Furthermore, the four major NCDs – CVDs, cancer, diabetes and chronic respiratory disease – share common behavioural risk factors, including tobacco use, unhealthy diets and physical inactivity. Therefore, any effort to address these common risk factors would have a major impact in reducing NCDs in LMICs.

The key question is how NCD-related lifestyles and risk factors can be permanently achieved and maintained in the entire population in a cost-effective way, particularly in LMICs. The answer from the North Karelia Project in Finland, supported by the results from the Stanford Study in the USA, calls for a broad-ranging and determined intervention in the whole community. Practical activities integrated with the existing community organizations should be based on sound theoretical principles. This is particularly important in LMICs where the options are more limited owing to constraints in resources and weak health systems. Competing health priorities additionally complicate the prioritization of health interventions in LMIC contexts. Given these constraints, and the urgent need to address the rising epidemic of NCDs, LMICs need to prioritize investment of available resources in interventions that will provide a good return – cost-effective interventions that are feasible for implementation on a wide scale with a high impact [65]. Gazanio *et al.* [37] proposed four key factors that need to be taken into account: (i) the intervention must target behaviours or risk factors that have been causally associated with NCDs; (ii) there should be some knowledge that the intervention will probably lead to favourable changes in behaviours or risk factors, which should subsequently lead to reductions in NCD morbid or fatal events; (iii) evidence should show that the intervention is cost-effective in the settings in which it is implemented; and (iv) there should be evidence that the scaling up of the intervention is financially feasible in resource-constrained countries. Taking these factors into account, Gaziano *et al.* [37] reviewed data from LMICs, which suggested that tobacco control, salt reduction and a multi-drug strategy to treat individuals with high-risk NCDs are three interventions that have strong cost-effectiveness data for scaling up in LMICs.

There are, however, limited data for structural interventions directed at the social determinants of NCDs, including health systems in LMICs. This suggests that a detailed knowledge of the social determinants of NCDs is urgently needed in LMICs. Much of the work concerning prevention of NCDs has concentrated on the link between the agents (i.e. risk factors) and the host (i.e. people) [55]. To make a significant impact, we need to take account of the deep-rooted wisdom of public health by considering the totality of host, agent and environment. Most of the great achievements in public health have involved major emphasis on the environment. This link to the environment also applies to the control of NCDs and is a major rationale behind the community-based approach. The behaviours or risk factors for NCDs are largely determined by social forces and other environmental factors [75, 76]. Any major progress in influencing the NCD rates therefore has to deal with these environmental forces and structures.

References

1. World Health Organization (2011) *Global Status Report on Noncommunicable Diseases 2010*. World Health Organization, Geneva, Switzerland <http://www.who.int/nmh/publications/ncd_report2010/en>.
2. Suhrcke, M., Nugent, R.A., Stuckler, D. and Rocco, L. (2006) *Chronic Disease: an Economic Perspective*. Oxford Health Alliance, London, UK.
3. Omran, A.R. (1971) The epidemiologic transition: a theory of the epidemiology of population change. *Milbank Quarterly* 49, 509–538.
4. Olshansky, S.J. and Ault, A.B. (1986) The fourth stage of the epidemiologic transition: the age of delayed degenerative diseases. *Milbank Quarterly* 64, 355–391.
5. Yusuf, S., Reddy, S., Ounpuu, S. and Anand, S. (2001) Global burden of cardiovascular diseases: part I: general considerations, the epidemiologic transition, risk factors, and impact of urbanization. *Circulation* 104, 2746–2753.
6. Ezzati, M. and Riboli, E. (2012) Can noncommunicable diseases be prevented? Lessons from studies of populations and individuals. *Science* 337, 1482–1487.
7. Kannel, W.B., Dawber, T.R., Kagan, A., Revotskie, L. and Stokes, J. III (1961) Factors of risk in the development of coronary heart disease: six-year follow-up experience. *Annals of Internal Medicine* 55, 33–50.
8. Epstein, F.H. (1973) Coronary heart disease epidemiology revisited: clinical and community aspects. *Circulation* 48, 185–194.
9. Rose, G. (1981) Strategy of prevention: lessons from cardiovascular disease. *British Medical Journal* 282, 1847–1851.
10. Mackenbach, J.P., Cavelaars, E.J.M., Kunst, A.E. and Groenhof, F. (2000) Socioeconomic inequalities in cardiovascular disease mortality. An international study. *European Heart Journal* 21, 1141–1151.
11. Bhopal, R. (2004) Glossary of terms relating to ethnicity and race: for reflection and debate. *Journal of Epidemiology & Community Health* 58, 441–445.
12. Agyemang, C., de-Graft Aikins, A. and Bhopal, R. (2012) Ethnicity and cardiovascular health research: pushing the boundaries by including comparison populations in the countries of origin. *Ethnicity and Health* 17, 579–596.
13. Gill, P., Kai, J., Bhopal, R. and Sarah, W. (2007) The epidemiologically based NHS health needs assessment reviews. In: Raftery, J. (ed.) *Health Care Needs Assessment of Black & Minority Ethnic Communities*. Radcliffe Publishing, Abingdon, UK, pp. 227–399.
14. Agyemang, C., Addo, J., Bhopal, R., de-Graft Aikins, A. and Stronks, K. (2009) Cardiovascular disease, diabetes and established risk factors among populations of sub-Saharan African descent in Europe: a literature review. *Global Health* 5, 7.
15. Kunst, A.E., Stronks, K. and Agyemang, C. (2011) Non-communicable diseases. In: Rechel, B., Mladocsky, P., Devillé, W., Rijks, B., Petrova-Benedict, R. and McKee, M. (eds) *Migration and Health in the European Union*. Open University Press McGrawHill, Berkshire, UK, pp. 101–120.
16. Bos, V., Kunst, A.E., Garssen, J. and Mackenbach, J.P. (2005) Socioeconomic inequalities in mortality within ethnic groups in the Netherlands, 1995–2000. *Journal of Epidemiology and Community Health* 59, 329–335.
17. Regidor, E., Astasio, P., Calle, M.E., Martínez, D., Ortega, P. and Domínguez, V. (2009) The association between birthplace in different regions of the world and cardiovascular mortality among residents of Spain. *European Journal of Epidemiology* 24, 503–512.

18. Bhopal, R.S., Rafnsson, S.B., Agyemang, C., Fagot-Campagna, A., Giampaoli, S., Hammar, N., Harding, S., Hedlund, E., Juel, K., Mackenbach, J.P., Primatesta, P., Rey, G., Rosato, M., Wild, S. and Kunst, A.E. (2012) Mortality from circulatory diseases by specific country of birth across six European countries: test of concept. *European Journal of Public Health* 22, 353–359.
19. van Oeffelen, A.A., Agyemang, C., Stronks, K., Bots, M.L. and Vaartjes, I. (2014) Incidence of first acute myocardial infarction over time specific for age, sex, and country of birth. *Netherlands Journal of Medicine* 72, 20–27.
20. Agyemang, C., van Oeffelen, A.A., Bots, M.L., Stronks, K. and Vaartjes, I. (2014) Socioeconomic inequalities in acute myocardial infarction incidence in migrant groups: has the epidemic arrived? Analysis of nation-wide data. *Heart* 100, 239–246.
21. Oldroyd, J., Banerjee, M., Heald, A. and Cruickshank, K. (2005) Diabetes and ethnic minorities. *Postgraduate Medical Journal* 81, 486–490.
22. Ujcic-Voortman, J.K., Schram, M.T., Jacobs-van der Bruggen, M.A., Verhoeff, A.P. and Baan, C.A. (2009) Diabetes prevalence and risk factors among ethnic minorities. *European Journal of Public Health* 19, 511–515.
23. Vandenheede, H., Deboosere, P., Stirbu, I., Agyemang, C.O., Harding, S., Juel, K., Rafnsson, S.B., Regidor, E., Rey, G., Rosato, M., Mackenbach, J.P. and Kunst, A.E. (2012) Migrant mortality from diabetes mellitus across Europe: the importance of socio-economic change. *European Journal of Epidemiology* 27, 109–117.
24. Mather, H.M., Chaturvedi, N. and Fuller, J.H. (1998) Mortality and morbidity from diabetes in South Asians and Europeans: 11-year follow-up of the Southall Diabetes Survey, London, UK. *Diabetic Medicine* 15, 53–59.
25. Bos, V., Kunst, A.E., Keij-Deerenberg, I.M., Garssen, J. and Mackenbach, J.P. (2004) Ethnic inequalities in age- and cause-specific mortality in The Netherlands. *International Journal of Epidemiology* 33, 1112–1119.
26. Courbage, Y. and Khlat, M. (1996) Mortality and causes of death of Moroccans in France, 1979–91. *Population* 8, 59–94.
27. Hemminki, K., Li, X. and Czene, K. (2002) Cancer risks in first-generation immigrants to Sweden. *International Journal of Cancer* 99, 218–28.
28. Spallek, J., Arnold, M., Hentschel, S. and Razum, O. (2009) Cancer incidence rate ratios of Turkish immigrants in Hamburg, Germany: a registry based study. *Cancer Epidemiology* 33, 413–418.
29. Stirbu, I., Kunst, A.E., Vlems, F.A., Visser, O., Bos, V., Deville, W., Nijhuis, H.G. and Coebergh, J.W. (2006) Cancer mortality rates among first and second generation migrants in the Netherlands: convergence toward the rates of the native Dutch population. *International Journal of Cancer* 119, 2665–2672.
30. Arnold, M., Razum, O. and Coebergh, J.W. (2010) Cancer risk diversity in non-western migrants to Europe: an overview of the literature. *European Journal of Cancer* 46, 2647–2659.
31. Fischbacher, C.M., Blackwell, C.C., Bhopal, R., Ingram, R., Unwin, N.C. and White, M. (2004) Serological evidence of *Helicobacter pylori* infection in UK South Asian and European populations: implications for gastric cancer and coronary heart disease. *Journal of Infection* 48, 168–174.
32. Agyemang, C., van Oeffelen, A.A., Norredam, M., Kappelle, L.J., Klijn, C.J., Bots, M.L., Stronks, K. and Vaartjes, I. (2014) Socioeconomic inequalities in stroke incidence among migrant groups: analysis of nationwide data. *Stroke* 45, 2397–2403.
33. Marmot, M. and Mustard, J. (1994) Coronary heart disease from a population perspective. In: Evans, R., Barer, M. and Marmor, T (eds) *Why Are Some People Healthy and Others Not?* Aldin de Gruytere, New York, pp. 189–214.
34. de-Graft Aikins, A., Unwin, N., Agyemang, C., Allotey, P., Campbell, C. and Arhinful, D. (2010) Tackling Africa's chronic disease burden: from the local to the global. *Global Health* 6, 5.

35. Angell, S.Y., Danel, I. and De Cock, K.M. (2012) Global health. Global indicators and targets for noncommunicable diseases. *Science* 337, 1456–457.
36. Abegunde, D.O., Mathers, C.D., Adam, T., Ortegon, M. and Strong, K. (2007) The burden and costs of chronic diseases in low-income and middle-income countries. *Lancet* 370, 1929–1938.
37. Gaziano, T.A., Galea, G. and Reddy, K.S. (2007) Scaling up interventions for chronic disease prevention: the evidence. *Lancet* 370, 1939–1946.
38. WHO (2008) *The Global Burden of Disease: 2004 Update*. World Health Organization, Geneva, Switzerland <http://www.who.int/healthinfo/global_burden_disease/GBD_report_2004update_full.pdf>.
39. Kearney, P.M., Whelton, M., Reynolds, K., Muntner, P., Whelton, P.K. and He, J. (2005) Global burden of hypertension: analysis of worldwide data. *Lancet* 365, 217–223.
40. IDF (2013) *IDF Diabetes Atlas*, 6th edn. International Diabetes Federation, Brussels, Belgium.
41. Shaw, J.E., Sicree, R.A. and Zimmet, P.Z. (2010) Global estimates of the prevalence of diabetes for 2010 and 2030. *Diabetes Research and Clinical Practice* 87, 4–14.
42. Kelly, T., Yang, W., Chen, C.S., Reynolds, K. and He, J. (2008) Global burden of obesity in 2005 and projections to 2030. *International Journal of Obesity* 32, 1431–1437.
43. Abubakari, A.R., Lauder, W., Agyemang, C., Jones, M., Kirk, A. and Bhopal, R.S. (2008) Prevalence and time trends in obesity among adult West African populations: a meta-analysis. *Obesity Reviews* 9, 297–311.
44. van de Vijver, S., Oti, S., Addo, J., de Graft-Aikins, A. and Agyemang, C. (2012) Review of community-based interventions for prevention of cardiovascular diseases in low-and middle-income countries. *Ethnicity and Health* 17, 651–776.
45. Mendis, S. and Fuster, V. (2009) National policies and strategies for noncommunicable diseases. *Nature Reviews Cardiology* 6, 723–727.
46. Dooley, K.E.and Chaisson, R.E. (2009) Tuberculosis and diabetes mellitus: convergence of two epidemics. *Lancet Infectious Diseases* 9, 737–746
47. Beaglehole, R., Hay, D.R., Foster, F.H. and Sharpe, D.N. (1981) Trends in coronary heart disease mortality and associated risk factors in New Zealand. *New Zealand Medical Journal* 93, 371–375
48. Beaglehole, R. (1986) Medical management and the decline in mortality from coronary heart disease. *British Medical Journal (Clinical Research Edition)* 292, 33–35.
49. Dobson, A.J., McElduff, P., Heller, R., Alexander, H., Colley, P. and D'Este, K. (1999) Changing patterns of coronary heart disease in the hunter region of New South Wales, Australia. *Journal of Clinical Epidemiology* 52, 761–771.
50. Menotti, A. and Scanga, M. (1992) Trends in coronary risk factors in Italy. Responsible Investigators of the RF2, OB43 and MICOL Research Groups. *International Journal of Epidemiology* 21, 883–892.
51. Laatikainen, T., Critchley, J., Vartiainen, E., Salomaa, V., Ketonen, M. and Capewell, S. (2005) Explaining the decline in coronary heart disease mortality in Finland between 1982 and 1997. *American Journal of Epidemiology* 162, 764–773
52. Sigfusson, N., Sigvaldason, H., Steingrimsdottir, L., Gudmundsdottir, I.I., Stefansdottir, I., Thorsteinsson, T. and Sigurdsson, G. (1991) Decline in ischaemic heart disease in Iceland and change in risk factor levels. *British Medical Journal* 302, 1371–1375.
53. Vartiainen, E., Laatikainen, T., Peltonen, M., Juolevi, A., Männisto, S., Sundvall, J., Jousilahti, P., Salomaa, V., Valsta, L. and Puska, P. (2009) Thirty-five-year trends in cardiovascular risk factors in Finland. *International Journal of Epidemiology* 39, 504–518.
54. Dwyer, T. and Hetzel, B.S. (1980) A comparison of trends of coronary heart disease mortality in Australia, USA and England and Wales with reference to three major risk factors – hypertension, cigarette smoking and diet. *International Journal of Epidemiology* 9, 65–71.
55. Puska, P., Nissinen, A., Tuomilehto, J., Salonen, J.T., Koskela, K., McAlister, A., Kottke, T.E., Maccoby, N. and Farquhar, J.W. (1985) The community-based strategy to prevent coronary

heart disease: conclusions from the ten years of the North Karelia project. *Annual Review of Public Health* 6, 147–193.

56. Levi, F, Lucchini, F, Negri, E. and La Vecchia C. (2002) Trends in mortality from cardiovascular and cerebrovascular diseases in Europe and other areas of the world. *Heart* 88, 119–24.
57. Puska, P., Vartiainen, E., Tuomilehto, J., Salomaa, V. and Nissinen, A. (1998) Changes in premature deaths in Finland: successful long-term prevention of cardiovascular diseases. *Bulletin of the World Health Organization* 76, 419–425.
58. Vartiainen, E., Puska, P., Pekkanen, J., Tuomilehto, J. and Jousilahti, P. (1994) Changes in risk factors explain changes in mortality from ischaemic heart disease in Finland. *British Medical Journal* 309, 23–27
59. Farquhar, J.W., Fortmann, S.P., Flora, J.A., Taylor, C.B., Haskell, W.L., Williams, P.T., Maccoby, N. and Wood, P.D. (1990) Effects of communitywide education on cardiovascular disease risk factors. The Stanford Five-City Project. *Journal of the American Medical Association* 264, 359–365.
60. Farquhar, J.W., Maccoby, N., Wood, P.D., Alexander, J.K., Breitrose, H., Brown, B.W. Jr, Haskell, W.L., McAlister, A.L., Meyer, A.J., Nash, J.D. and Stern, M.P. (1977) Community education for cardiovascular health. *Lancet* 1, 1192–1195.
61. WHO (2008) *2008–2013 Action Plan for the Global Strategy for the Prevention and Control of Noncommunicable Diseases*. World Health Organization, Geneva, Switzerland <http://www.who.int/nmh/publications/ncd_action_plan_en.pdf>.
62. Rani, M., Nusrat, S. and Hawken, L.H. (2012) A qualitative study of governance of evolving response to non-communicable diseases in low-and middle- income countries: current status, risks and options. *BMC Public Health* 12, 877.
63. Schmidt, M.I., Duncan, B.B., Azevedo e Silva, G., Menezes, A.M., Monteiro, C.A., Barreto, S.M., Chor, D. and Menezes, P.R. (2011) Chronic non-communicable diseases in Brazil: burden and current challenges. *Lancet* 377, 1949–1961.
64. Iglesias, R., Jha, P., Pinto, M., Silva, V.L. and Godinho, J. (2008) Documento de discussão – saúde, nutrição e população (HNP) Controle do tabagismo no Brasil: resumo executive. *Epidemiologia e Serviços de Saúde* 17, 301–304 (in Portuguese).
65. WHO (2004) *Global Strategy for Diet, Physical Activity, and Health*. World Health Organization, Geneva, Switzerland <http://www.who.int/dietphysicalactivity/strategy/eb11344/strategy_english_web.pdf>.
66. Hodge, A.M., Dowse, G.K., Gareeboo, H., Tuomilehto, J., Alberti, K.G. and Zimmet, P.Z. (1996) Incidence, increasing prevalence, and predictors of change in obesity and fat distribution over 5 years in the rapidly developing population of Mauritius. *International Journal of Obesity and Related Metabolic Disorders* 20, 137–146.
67. Yu, Z., Song, G., Guo, Z., Zheng, G., Tian, H., Vartianinen, E., Puska, P. and Nissinen, A. (1999) Changes in blood pressure, body mass index, and salt consumption in a Chinese population. *Preventive Medicine* 29, 165–172.
68. Rossouw, J.E., Jooste, P.L., Chalton, D.O., Jordaan, E.R., Langenhoven, M.L., Jordaan, P.C., Steyn, M., Swanepoel, A.S. and Rossouw, L.J. (1993) Community-based intervention: the Coronary Risk Factor Study (CORIS). *International Journal of Epidemiology* 22, 428–438.
69. CDC (1999) Ten great public health achievements – United States, 1900–1999. *Morbidity and Mortality Weekly Report* 48, 241–243.
70. Capewell, S., Ford, E.S., Croft, J.B., Critchley, J.A., Greenlund, K.J. and Labarthe, D.R. (2010) Cardiovascular risk factor trends and potential for reducing coronary heart disease mortality in the United States of America. *Bulletin of the World Health Organization* 88, 120–130.
71. Capewell, S., Morrison, C.E. and McMurray, J.J. (1999) Contribution of modern cardiovascular treatment and risk factor changes to the decline in coronary heart disease mortality in Scotland between 1975 and 1994. *Heart* 81, 380–386.
72. Nissinen, A., Tuomilehto, J., Kottke, T.E. and Puska, P. (1986) Cost-effectiveness of the North Karelia hypertension program 1972–1977. *Medical Care* 24, 767–780.

73. Tosteson, A.N., Weinstein, M.C., Hunink, M.G., Mittleman, M.A., Williams, L.W., Goldman, P.A. and Goldman, L. (1997) Cost-effectiveness of populationwide educational approaches to reduce serum cholesterol levels. *Circulation* 95, 24–30.
74. Fortmann, S.P., Williams, P.T., Hulley, S.B., Haskell, W.L. and Farquhar, J.W. (1981) Effect of health education on dietary behavior: the Stanford Three Community Study. *American Journal of Clinical Nutrition* 34, 2030–2038.
75. Commission on Social Determinants of Health (2007) *A Conceptual Framework for Action on the Social Determinants of Health*. World Health Authority, Geneva, Switzerland <http://www.who.int/social_determinants/resources/csdh_framework_action_05_07.pdf>.
76. Samuels, T.A., Guell, C., Legetic, B. and Unwin, N. (2012) Policy initiatives, culture and the prevention and control of chronic non-communicable diseases (NCDs) in the Caribbean. *Ethnicity and Health* 17, 631–649.

12 The Global Response for Prevention and Control of Chronic Non-communicable Diseases: Key Milestones and Outcomes

SHANTHI MENDIS* AND OLEG CHESTNOV

World Health Organization, Geneva, Switzerland

12.1 Key Milestones in the Global Response for Prevention and Control of Non-communicable Diseases

Non-communicable diseases (NCDs) currently cause more deaths than all other causes combined. The human, social and economic consequences of NCDs are felt by all countries. As the leading cause of death globally, NCDs were responsible for 38 million (68%) of the world's 56 million deaths in 2012 [1]. Four major NCDs (cardiovascular disease, cancer, chronic respiratory disease and diabetes) were responsible for 82% of these NCD deaths. These four NCDs can largely be prevented or controlled by means of effective policies that address shared risk factors, namely tobacco use, an unhealthy diet, physical inactivity and harmful use of alcohol, and by cost-effective early detection and treatment interventions [2].

More than 40% of all NCD deaths globally in 2012 occurred before the age of 70 years [1]. This represented about 16 million deaths – an increase from 2000 when there were 14.6 million NCD deaths before the age of 70 years. In 2012, the majority of these premature deaths (82%) were in low- and middle-income countries (LMICs) [1]. Reducing the NCD burden is an overriding development priority for all countries and is particularly critical for LMICs.

A sustainable public health model for addressing the NCD burden needs to underpin surveillance, population-wide prevention and cost-effective healthcare delivery within a multi-sectoral national policy framework (see Coast *et al.*, Chapter 6, and Kengne *et al.*, Chapter 7, this volume). These are the pillars of the global strategy for the prevention and control of NCDs and were endorsed by the World Health Assembly in 2000 (resolution WHA53.17) [3]. Since then, several Health

*E-mail: mendiss@who.int

Assembly resolutions have been adopted or endorsed in support of NCD prevention and control including:

- the World Health Organization (WHO) Framework Convention on Tobacco Control (resolution WHA56.1) [4];
- the Global Strategy on Diet, Physical Activity and Health (resolution WHA57.17) [5];
- a global strategy to reduce harmful use of alcohol (resolution WHA63.13) [6]; and
- sustainable health financing structures and universal coverage (resolution WHA64.9) [7].

In 2008, the Health Assembly endorsed the action plan for the global strategy for the prevention and control of NCDs, covering the period 2008–2013 [2]. Despite these developments, the NCD epidemic has grown steadily and is spreading worldwide. Under a 'business as usual' scenario, for the period 2011–2025, cumulative economic losses due to NCDs in LMICs alone have been estimated at US$7 trillion [8].

On 19 September 2011, the Heads of State and Government adopted the Political Declaration of the High-level Meeting of the United Nations General Assembly on the Prevention and Control of NCDs [9]. For the first time, all Member States of the United Nations agreed that NCDs constitute a major challenge to socio-economic development, environmental sustainability and poverty alleviation. This recognition helped to galvanize the global struggle against NCDs and move it forward.

The UN Political Declaration on NCDs makes a clear call for including NCDs in health planning processes and the development agenda of each Member State. It committed governments to a series of multi-sectoral actions and to exploring the provision of predictable and sustained resources through domestic, bilateral and multilateral channels. Among the many commitments for prevention and control of NCDs, a time-bound commitment was made to establish and strengthen, by 2013, multi-sectoral national policies and plans for the prevention and control of NCDs.

In addition, a number of global assignments were given to the WHO to operationalize the vision of the 2011 Political Declaration to support Member States in their national efforts. These global assignments have now been completed and include the following:

- The comprehensive global monitoring framework, including the set of nine voluntary global targets for achievement by 2025 and a set of 25 indicators in order to monitor trends in NCDs and NCD risk factors [2].
- The Global Action Plan for the Prevention and Control of NCDs 2013–2020 underpinned by the global monitoring framework [2].
- The establishment of the United Nations Inter-Agency Task Force on the Prevention and Control of NCDs and the endorsement of its terms of reference by the Economic and Social Council on 13 June 2014 [10].
- The terms of reference for the comprehensive global coordination mechanism for the prevention and control of NCDs [11].

The Inter-Agency Task Force has been established to facilitate the response of the United Nations system to country demand for technical assistance. It will be convened by the WHO and will report to the Economic and Social Council through the Secretary-General [10].The purpose of the global coordination mechanism is to facilitate and enhance coordination of activities, multi-stakeholder engagement and action across sectors at global, regional and national levels. The aim will be to contribute to the implementation of the Global NCD Action Plan while avoiding duplication of efforts and using resources efficiently [11].

The impact of the Political Declaration includes an increase in the number of countries that have an operational national NCD policy with a budget for implementation, from 32% of countries in 2010 to 50% of countries in 2013. However, progress in implementing the commitments of the Political Declaration has been insufficient and highly uneven. In 2013, for example, only 69 countries had an operational policy to reduce the burden of tobacco use in line with the WHO Framework Convention on Tobacco Control. An operational policy to reduce harmful use of alcohol within the national context was in place in only 52 countries. Only 56 and 60 countries, respectively, had operational policies to reduce physical inactivity and an unhealthy diet. Evidence-based national guidelines for the management of major NCDs through a primary care approach were being implemented only in 64 countries [1].

12.2 Challenges in Implementing a Comprehensive Public Health Response to Address NCDs

NCDs and their risk factors adversely affect the quality of life of people. Long-term treatment, care costs and loss of productivity threaten household income and lead to productivity losses for individuals and their families and for the economies of Member States. In countries with weak health systems, NCDs and poverty work in tandem to contribute to a vicious cycle that often entrenches people in poverty.

There are many challenges that need to be overcome for NCD prevention and control. First, the effects of globalization of marketing and trade, rapid urbanization and population ageing are powerful forces that drive the burden of NCDs. Secondly, the prevalence of behavioural risk factors is increasing due to industry influence and a lack of physical and policy environments that facilitate healthy behaviours. Thirdly, only a comprehensive policy response can address the NCD epidemic in a sustainable manner. The policy response needs to address health inequities that arise from the societal conditions in which people live, work and age. These social determinants of health include early years' experiences, education, economic status, employment, housing and environment, and effective systems of preventing and treating ill health. Fourthly, prevention of NCDs require difficult work across different sectors and levels of government that influence public policies in sectors such as agriculture, communication, education, employment, energy, environment, finance, industry, labour, sports, trade, transport, urban planning, and social and economic development.

As outlined in the UN Political Declaration, a comprehensive policy response to address the NCD epidemic needs to operationalize [9]:

- a whole-of-government and a whole-of-society effort;
- action to reduce risk factors and create health-promoting environments;
- action to strengthen national multi-sectoral policies and health systems;
- research and development; and
- monitoring and evaluation.

12.3 The Global NCD Action Plan 2013–2020

The Global NCD Action Plan 2013–2020 provides a roadmap to operationalize the commitments of the Political Declaration [2]. The plan is organized around six objectives (Box 12.1). The overall aim of the action plan is to provide direction and support for the implementation of national policies, strategies and action plans.

It comprises a set of actions that, when performed collectively by Member States and other stakeholders, would tackle the growing public health burden imposed by NCDs. The set of actions focus on strengthening international cooperation, advocacy and national capacity, reducing exposure to NCD risk factors and their determinants, driving health systems towards universal health coverage, operational research, and monitoring progress in prevention and control of NCDs.

The plan recognizes that a life course approach is key to the prevention and control of NCDs. Such an approach starts with maternal health and nutrition, and continues through proper infant feeding practices, including the promotion of breastfeeding and health promotion for children, adolescents and youths, followed by the promotion of a healthy working life, healthy ageing and care for people with NCDs in later life.

Box 12.1. Objectives Global NCD Action Plan 2013–2020.

Objective 1: To strengthen international cooperation and advocacy to raise the priority accorded to prevention and control of NCDs in the development agenda and in internationally agreed development goals.

Objective 2: To strengthen national capacity, leadership, governance, multi-sectoral action and partnerships to accelerate the country response for prevention and control of NCDs.

Objective 3: To reduce exposure to modifiable risk factors for NCDs through the creation of health-promoting environments.

Objective 4: To strengthen and reorient health systems to address the prevention and control of NCDs through people-centred primary healthcare and universal health coverage.

Objective 5: To promote and support national capacity for high-quality research and development for prevention and control of NCDs.

Objective 6: To monitor the trends and determinants of NCDs and evaluate progress in their prevention and control.

There has been remarkable progress in implementing the first objective of the plan. International cooperation and advocacy have raised the priority accorded to prevention and control of NCDs. Addressing NCDs is now recognized as a priority not only for health but also for sustainable development [1]. An NCD target has been incorporated in the sustainable development goals and NCDs are poised to be an integral component of the post-2015 development agenda [10]. Progress in the implementation of the other objectives of the Global NCD Action Plan and attainment of the global targets are largely determined by target-oriented action, capacity and resources at country level [1, 2].

Objective 3 of the global action plan lists a range of policy measures to reduce exposure to risk factors [2]. For tobacco, they include raising taxes and inflation-adjusted prices on all tobacco products, legislation for tobacco smoke-free environments, warning people about the dangers of tobacco, implementing comprehensive bans on tobacco advertising, promotion and sponsorship, and offering help to people who want to stop using tobacco.

National policies to reduce harmful use of alcohol are directed to target drink-driving policies and countermeasures, pricing policies to reduce availability of alcohol, marketing of alcoholic beverages, policies to reduce the negative consequences of drinking and alcohol intoxication, and the public health impact of illicit alcohol and informally produced alcohol and the health systems response.

To address unhealthy diet and physical inactivity, countries are advised to implement national policies and action plans to advance the global strategy on diet, physical activity and health, the global strategy for infant and young child feeding, and a comprehensive implementation plan on maternal, infant and young child nutrition, and implementation of the WHO's set of recommendations on the marketing of foods and non-alcoholic beverages to children [2].

Objective 4 of the action plan highlights the importance of governments exercising responsibility and accountability for ensuring the availability of NCD services within the context of overall health system strengthening. Appropriate policies are required to orient health systems towards addressing social determinants of health and universal health coverage. All countries can make gradual progress towards universal health coverage through a combination of domestic revenues, innovative financing and external financial assistance, giving priority to financing a combination of cost-effective preventative and curative interventions at different levels of healthcare covering major NCDs and co-morbidities [1, 2]. Policy measures to ensure sufficient and competent human resources, particularly at the primary care level, and equitable access to essential medicines and basic technologies need to be accorded high priority.

12.4 Global NCD Targets and Monitoring Framework

The nine global voluntary targets of the Global NCD Action Plan give a clear indication of where we want to be globally by 2025 (Box 12. 2). At the country level, national targets need to be set, consistent with global targets and based on what is

Box 12.2. Voluntary global targets for prevention and control of NCDs to be attained by 2025.

1. A 25% relative reduction in overall mortality from cardiovascular diseases, cancer, diabetes or chronic respiratory diseases.
2. At least a 10% relative reduction in the harmful use of alcohol, as appropriate, within the national context.
3. A 10% relative reduction in prevalence of insufficient physical activity.
4. A 30% relative reduction in the mean population intake of salt/sodium.
5. A 30% relative reduction in the prevalence of current tobacco use in persons aged 15 years and over.
6. A 25% relative reduction in the prevalence of raised blood pressure or containing the prevalence of raised blood pressure, according to national circumstances.
7. Halt the rise in diabetes and obesity.
8. At least 50% of eligible people to receive drug therapy and counselling (including glycaemic control) to prevent heart attacks and strokes.
9. An 80% availability of the affordable basic technologies and essential medicines, including generics, required to treat major NCDs in both public and private facilities.

feasible in the national context. Policies and interventions to attain the nine targets need to be given high priority and budgeted in national multi-sectoral NCD action plans [1].

12.4.1 Global target 1: A 25% relative reduction in overall mortality from cardiovascular diseases, cancer, diabetes or chronic respiratory diseases by 2025

Progress in attaining all other targets contributes to the attainment of this overarching target on premature mortality. The ability of countries to meet this target will vary greatly across the world. Comprehensive, multi-sectoral policy actions and interventions and country capacity including civil/vital registration and surveillance systems are essential to attain this target. The shortage of resources in many countries means that, to attain this target, implementation of a set of very cost-effective policy options and interventions ('best buys') would have to be accorded the highest priority. The Global Status Report 2014 provides further guidance on how this could be accomplished [1].

12.4.2 Global target 2: At least a 10% reduction in the harmful use of alcohol by 2025

In 2012, an estimated 5.9% (3.3 million) of all deaths worldwide, and 5.1 of disability-adjusted life years (DALYs) were attributable to alcohol consumption [1]. More than half of these deaths resulted from NCDs.

The level of alcohol consumption worldwide in 2010 was estimated at 6.2 l of pure alcohol per person aged 15 years and over (equivalent to 13.5 g of pure alcohol per day). As alluded to above, there are cost-effective policy options that need to be implemented to attain this target on reducing harmful use of alcohol.

12.4.3 Global target 3: A 10% reduction in prevalence of insufficient physical activity by 2025

Insufficient physical activity contributes to 69.3 million DALYs (2.8% of the total) and 3.2 million deaths each year [1]. Adults who are insufficiently physically active have a higher risk of all-cause mortality compared with those who do at least 150 min of moderate-intensity physical activity per week, or equivalent, as recommended by the WHO. In 2010, 23% of adults aged 18 years and over were insufficiently physically active. Globally, 81% of adolescents aged 11–17 years were insufficiently physically active in 2010.

Several developed countries have reported increased physical activity over the last decade as a result of the implementation of national policies and programmes to improve physical activity. In recent years, more LMICs also have set up initiatives to address physical inactivity. Reaching the physical activity target requires collaboration between the Ministries of Health, Transport, Urban Planning, Sports and Education to create conducive and safe environments for physical activity for all age groups.

12.4.4 Global target 4: A 30% relative reduction in the mean population intake of salt by 2025

Excess consumption of dietary sodium is associated with increased risk of hypertension and cardiovascular disease. Globally, 1.7 million annual deaths from cardiovascular causes have been attributed to excess sodium intake [1]. Current estimates suggest that the global mean intake of salt is around 10 g of salt daily (4 g per day of sodium). The WHO recommends a reduction in salt intake to less than 5 g per day (sodium 2 g per day) to reduce blood pressure and the risk of coronary heart disease and stroke.

The main source of salt in many countries is processed foods and ready-made meals, while salt added during the preparation of food at home and at the table is significant in others. With the greater availability of processed foods in LMICs, sources of sodium are shifting rapidly towards these foods.

All Ministries of Health need to lead the development and implementation of policies aimed at reducing population-wide salt consumption. Food labelling, legislation, product reformulation and fiscal incentives that encourage the production and consumption of foods with reduced sodium content as well as consumer education are some of the measures that have been effective in reducing salt consumption in different settings [1].

12.4.5 Global target 5: A 30% relative reduction in prevalence of current tobacco use in persons aged 15 years and over by 2025

Approximately 6 million people are currently estimated to die from tobacco use per year [1]. Tobacco use accounts for 7% of all female and 12% of all male deaths globally.

As described above, there is a range of cost-effective policy measures that can be implemented to make progress on this target. Considerable progress has been made in global tobacco control in recent years in both the number of countries protecting their people and the number of people worldwide protected by effective tobacco control measures. However, more work is needed in many countries to pass and enforce effective tobacco-control measures.

12.4.6 Global target 6: A 25% relative reduction in the prevalence of raised blood pressure, or containing the prevalence of raised blood pressure, according to national circumstances by 2025

Raised blood pressure is estimated to have caused 9.4 million deaths and 7% of disease burden – as measured in DALYs – in 2010 [1]. If left uncontrolled, hypertension causes stroke, myocardial infarction, cardiac failure, dementia, renal failure and blindness. There is strong scientific evidence of the health benefits of lowering blood pressure through population-wide and individual (behavioural and pharmacological) interventions. The global prevalence of raised blood pressure (defined as systolic and/or diastolic blood pressure equal to or above 140/90 mmHg) in adults aged 18 years and over was around 22% in 2014.

Many modifiable factors contribute to the high prevalence rates of hypertension. They include eating food containing too much salt and fat, inadequate intake of fruits and vegetables, overweight and obesity, harmful use of alcohol, physical inactivity, psychological stress, socio-economic determinants and inadequate access to healthcare. In order to achieve this target, a comprehensive set of population-wide and individual interventions and policies are required to address these modifiable risk factors. In addition, integrated programmes need to be established at the primary care level to improve the efficiency and effectiveness of detection and management of hypertension and other cardiovascular risk factors through a total risk approach, as recommended by the WHO [11].

12.4.7 Global target 7: Halt the rise in diabetes and obesity by 2025

Obesity increases the likelihood of diabetes, hypertension, coronary heart disease, stroke and certain types of cancer. Worldwide, obesity has nearly doubled since 1980. In 2014, 11% men and 15% women aged 18 years and over were obese [1]. More than 42 million children under the age of 5 years were overweight in 2013. Obesity can be prevented through multi-sectoral population-based interventions throughout the life course [1].

The global prevalence of diabetes in 2014 was estimated to be 9%. Weight loss and physical activity reduce the risk of diabetes. Diabetes risk can be reduced by moderate weight loss and moderate daily physical activity in persons at high risk [1].

12.4.8 Global target 8: At least 50% of eligible people receive drug therapy and counselling (including glycaemic control) to prevent heart attacks and strokes by 2025

Cardiovascular disease was the leading cause of NCD deaths in 2012 and was responsible for 17.5 million deaths, or 46% of NCD deaths [1]. Of these deaths, an estimated 7.4 million were due to heart attacks (ischaemic heart disease) and 6.7 million were due to strokes.

This target to reduce heart attacks and strokes is aimed at improving the coverage of drug treatment and counselling to prevent heart attacks and strokes in people with raised cardiovascular risk and established disease. It is an affordable intervention that can be delivered through a primary healthcare approach, even in resource-constrained settings [12, 13]. This intervention to prevent heart attacks and strokes needs to be part of the basic benefits package for moving towards universal health coverage. In addition, context-specific strategies will be required to address multiple gaps in health systems related to access to basic technologies and medicines, the health workforce, service delivery, health information and referral with a special focus on primary care.

12.4.9 Global target 9: An 80% availability of the affordable basic technologies and essential medicines, including generics, required to treat major NCDs in both public and private facilities by 2025

The basic requirement of technologies and medicines for implementing cost-effective primary care interventions to address cardiovascular disease, diabetes and asthma are included in this target [1]. The essential medicines include aspirin, a statin, an angiotensin-converting enzyme inhibitor, a thiazide diuretic, a long-acting calcium-channel blocker, a long-acting blocker, metformin, insulin, a bronchodilator and a steroid inhalant. The basic technologies include at least a blood pressure measurement device, a weighing scale, blood sugar and blood cholesterol measurement devices with strips, and urine strips for an albumin assay.

These are minimum requirements without which even basic NCD interventions cannot be implemented in primary care. Currently, there are major gaps in the affordability and availability of basic health technologies and essential medicines, particularly in LMICs. Thus, national policies that encourage the availability of basic health technologies and essential medicines should be central to efforts focused on achieving universal health coverage.

12.5 High-level Meeting of the United Nations General Assembly 2014

On 10–11 July 2014, the United Nations General Assembly conducted a comprehensive review, taking stock of progress in implementing the commitments of the Political Declaration, identifying ways to address gaps, and reaffirming political commitment to respond to the challenge of NCDs [14]. The commitments made by countries in the outcome document aimed to build on the guidance provided by the WHO Global NCD Action Plan 2013–2020, and included the following:

- Integrate NCDs into health planning and national development plans.
- By 2015, set national NCD targets for 2025, consistent with voluntary global targets.
- By 2015, develop national NCD multi-sectoral plans to achieve the national targets.
- By 2016, implement policies and interventions to reduce NCD risk factors and underlying social determinants.
- By 2016, strengthen and orient health systems to address NCDs through people-centred primary healthcare and universal health coverage.
- Report on the progress in attaining the global targets using the established indicators in the global monitoring framework.

12.6 Moving the NCD Agenda Forward in LMICs

To contain the NCD epidemic through attainment of the global NCD targets by 2025, the above time-bound commitments made by countries have to be realized. There are many barriers to progress in prevention and control of NCDs, particularly in LMICs. Concrete actions are required to overcome these strategically by maximizing opportunities and synergies, as discussed below.

12.6.1 Build capacity for multi-sectoral collaboration

Action across sectors outside health is key to reducing exposure to behavioural risk factors and inequities. This work across different sectors and levels of government has to take into account their contribution to health and health equity, and pursue all necessary efforts to support nationally driven multi-sectoral action plans with the full and active participation of civil society and the private sector. Government leadership, responsible stewardship and management of conflict of interest and workforce capacity for forging a collaborative response are essential for the success of multi-sectoral action. Governments need to provide leadership in the development of a national policy framework for reducing risk factors through multi-sectoral action. Governments should be the key stakeholders of the multi-sectoral national action plan and allocate defined roles to other stakeholders, while protecting the public interest and avoiding conflicts of interest. Supportive environments that promote healthy behaviour need to be created using incentives and disincentives, regulatory and fiscal measures, laws and other policy options, and health education.

Mechanisms for multi-sectoral collaboration need to be embedded in the planning stage of prevention programmes and should continue into implementation, enactment of public policies and monitoring and evaluation. High-level, multi-sectoral structures are essential to curb childhood obesity, encourage healthy urban planning, promote physical activity or improve access to fruit and vegetables.

12.6.2 Intensify research for context-specific innovation

The capacity of LMICs needs to be strengthened for translational research for global application of proven cost-effective interventions. Priority should be given to health system research, and research to understand and influence multi-sectoral action and the macro-economic and social determinants of NCDs. Research is also required to enable expensive but effective interventions to become accessible and used appropriately in resource-constrained settings [13].

12.6.3 Invest in health systems

Investment in health systems is critical. NCDs require continuity of care and long-term care pathways rather than the episodic treatment of acute incidences that characterizes healthcare in most LMICs. Scaling up interventions against infectious diseases has already revealed the pressure points of health systems and the major constraints in capacity in LMICs (see Koram and Nimako, Chapter 10, this volume). Analysis of health systems shows that there are key components that present a challenge to scale-up and that these apply to NCDs as well. These areas are health financing, governance, the health workforce, health information, medical products and technologies, and health service delivery.

Where the global health community once advocated for better and more equitable access to healthcare, it has now coalesced around an even more ambitious goal: universal health coverage for all. The challenges of achieving such coverage are numerous, especially in LMICs, but working towards universal healthcare requires creating integrated and comprehensive health services that are rooted in people-oriented good-quality primary care, all of which are also necessary for scaling up NCD interventions. With this global momentum already in place, this is the ideal opportunity to understand how best to incorporate NCD interventions into existing health systems, to analyse what is financially feasible and to predict what the health impacts of investments in NCDs are likely to be.

12.6.4 Use existing resources more intelligently

Countries at all levels of development can begin to address NCDs if existing resources are used rationally and are invested in highly cost-effective interventions [1]. While secondary- and tertiary-level interventions are necessary for the care of advanced stages of NCDs, population-wide interventions and primary care interventions are more cost-effective and feasible and allow the prevention and treatment of early stages of NCDs. In many countries with a growing dual burden of infectious diseases and NCDs, large sections of rural populations have poor access to healthcare, and primary care systems are too overwhelmed to deliver effective treatment interventions. Crucially, the roll-out of highly cost-effective individual interventions relies on primary healthcare [1]. Currently, the poor quality of services at the primary level not only dissuades people from utilizing primary care but also delays diagnosis and treatment. If the quality of primary care services is improved, people will not bypass primary care and use secondary or tertiary services, which incur higher personal and health system costs. Furthermore, NCD programmes that are implemented in primary care need to be integrated programmes, as they are more cost-effective than vertical disease-specific programmes. For example, hypertension and diabetes could be entry points for a common total risk approach programme in primary care, the objective of which should be prevention of heart attacks, strokes and diabetes complications [13].

International aid has not kept pace with the growing need for NCD prevention and control. Prioritizing highly cost-effective interventions and integrated approaches is critical in order to get the best return on investment of domestic resources, particularly in LMICs. International financing for NCDs remains low, although in the recent past there have been encouraging developments. For instance, an estimated nine members of the Development Assistance Committee of the Organisation for Economic Co-operation and Development (OECD) have integrated NCDs into their bilateral and multilateral development policies (compared with one member in 2010). Some philanthropic foundations such as Bloomberg Philanthropies and the Bill & Melinda Gates Foundation have committed sizeable funds to support national efforts to implement proven tobacco-control policies.

12.6.5 Draw on lessons from the scale-up of other disease programmes

Global and national efforts to tackle disease are often vertical in terms of both governance and funding. Yet scaling up of action against NCDs does not present an entirely new challenge. Other major disease intervention scale-ups, such as those for maternal and child health and human immunodeficiency virus (HIV)/AIDS, have already struggled with many of the barriers facing NCD scale-up (see Koram and Nimako, Chapter 10, this volume). The scale-up of HIV/AIDS strategies has achieved remarkable results. The last 10 years showed a complete change in HIV care: prices of medicines have come down, treatment regimens have been simplified, thresholds of eligibility for care have been lowered and health systems have been strengthened.

Prevention is critical for both HIV and NCDs, and both disease areas rely on long-term continuity of care, strict adherence to treatment regimens and long-term behaviour change. An analysis of programmatic responses to HIV/AIDS shows that several approaches are also applicable to NCDs. These include: task sharing between doctors, nurses and allied health workers in the delivery of patient care, treatment adherence and community reach (which can extend to community-based and home-based care) (see Coast *et al.*, Chapter 6, and Addo and van de Vijver, Chapter 8, this volume); engagement of people living with the disease and of civil society in order to improve awareness and education, which is critical in bringing about behaviour change (see de-Graft Aikins *et al.*, Chapter 9, this volume); and better monitoring and evaluation systems with innovations that allow data entry at the facility level rather than only at the national level (see Kengne *et al.*, Chapter 7, this volume). Analysing lessons from other initiatives will allow policy makers to avoid potential stumbling blocks, and by understanding cross-cutting synergies they can harmonize NCD efforts with existing funding streams or scale-up.

12.6.6 Forge inter-sectoral partnerships

Partnerships with civil society organizations and the private sector are crucial in raising financial resources, capacity strengthening, supporting research, advocating for NCD prevention and control, and realization of multi-sectoral national policies (see de-Graft Aikins *et al.*, Chapter 9, this volume).

One of the reasons for the paucity of resources to address NCDs has been the lack of civil society pressure for urgent action. For instance, the political momentum around HIV/AIDs was driven by a group of activists, people with HIV/AIDs and volunteers. People living with NCDs need champions to advocate for the cause or to be activists themselves. Lack of social mobilization has allowed misconceptions – such as that NCDs chiefly affect people in developed countries and only the wealthy in developing countries – to remain uncontested. There is now an immense opportunity for non-governmental organizations (NGOs) to play a leadership role in lobbying and campaigning for a major shift in resources for NCDs. The Global NCD Action Plan outlines the role of NGOs in supporting national NCD efforts, including in capacity strengthening and research.

Synergies of the private sector (with the exception of the tobacco industry) need to be harnessed in support of national efforts for prevention and control of NCDs. The private sector has a social responsibility not to harm the health of populations, and particularly of children. A small number of private-sector entities have started to take measures to implement the WHO recommendations to reduce the impact of marketing of unhealthy foods and non-alcoholic beverages to children, while taking into account existing national legislation and policies. Similarly, a small number of private-sector entities have started working towards reducing the use of salt in the food industry in order to lower sodium consumption. Several entities have begun producing and promoting more food products consistent with a healthy diet, for example by reformulating products to provide healthier options and adherence to labelling standards, including information on sugars, salts, fats and *trans*-fat content. Unfortunately, these food products are not affordable, accessible or available in most LMICs.

All businesses depend on the health of their employees, their consumers and the communities in which they operate. Thus, it is also in the interests of the private sector to implement workplace and outreach programmes to promote the health of employees, families and communities.

12.6.7 Strengthen accountability

Accountability implies the existence of transparent processes of monitoring, review and action. At national level, a functioning health information system that collects, analyses and reports health and expenditure data is essential for monitoring progress. Reviews need to be based on evidence gathered through monitoring, including through vital registration and health information systems. Such reviews should also provide feedback on progress. To move the NCD agenda forward at the country level, the highest level of political engagement will be required to develop a country framework for accountability.

Acknowledgement

The authors contributed this chapter in their personal capacity. The contents of the paper do not necessarily represent the decisions and policies of the WHO.

References

1. WHO (2015) *Global Status Report on Noncommunicable Diseases 2014*. World Health Organization, Geneva, Switzerland <http://apps.who.int/iris/bitstream/10665/148114/1/9789241564854_eng.pdf>.
2. WHO (2013) *Global Action Plan for the Prevention and Control of Noncommunicable Diseases 2013–2020*. World Health Organization, Geneva, Switzerland <http://apps.who.int/iris/bitstream/10665/94384/1/9789241506236_eng.pdf?ua=1>.
3. WHO (2000) *Global Strategy for Prevention and Control of Noncommunicable Diseases*. World Health Organization, Geneva, Switzerland <http://apps.who.int/gb/archive/pdf_files/WHA53/ResWHA53/17.pdf>.
4. WHO (2003) *WHO Framework Convention on Tobacco Control*. World Health Organization, Geneva, Switzerland <http://whqlibdoc.who.int/publications/2003/9241591013.pdf>.
5. WHO (2004) Resolution WHA57.17. Global strategy on diet, physical activity and health. In: *57th World Health Assembly*, Geneva, 17–22 May 2004. World Health Organization, Geneva, Switzerland <http://apps.who.int/gb/ebwha/pdf_files/WHA57/A57_R17-en.pdf>.
6. WHO (2010) Resolution WHA63.13. Global strategy to reduce the harmful use of alcohol. In: *63rd World Health Assembly*, Geneva, 17–21 May 2010. World Health Organization, Geneva, Switzerland <http:// apps.who.int/gb/ebwha/pdf_files/WHA63/A63_R13-en.pdf>.
7. WHO (2011) Resolution WHA64.9. Sustainable health financing structures and universal health coverage. In: *64th World Health Assembly*, Geneva, 16–24 May 2011. World Health Organization, Geneva, Switzerland <http://apps.who.int/gb/ebwha/pdf_files/WHA64/A64_R9-en.pdf>.
8. WHO and World Economic Forum (2011) From burden to "best buys": reducing the economic impact of non-communicable diseases in low- and middle-income countries. World Health Organization and World Economic Forum, Geneva, Switzerland <http://www.who.int/nmh/publications/best_buys_summary>.

9. United Nations (2011) Resolution 66/2. Political Declaration of the High-level Meeting of the General Assembly on the Prevention and Control of Non-communicable Diseases. In: *66th Session of the United Nations General Assembly*. United Nations, New York <http://www.who.int/nmh/events/un_ncd_summit2011/political_declaration_en.pdf>.
10. United Nations Economic and Social Council (2013) *United Nations Inter-Agency Task Force on the Prevention and Control of Non-communicable Diseases*. United Nations, Geneva, Switzerland <http://www.who.int/nmh/events/2013/E.2013.L.23_tobacco.pdf>.
11. WHO (2014) Provisional agenda item 13.1. Prevention and control of noncommunicable diseases. Terms of reference for the global coordination mechanism on the prevention and control of noncommunicable diseases. In: *67th World Health Assembly*, 19–24 May 2014. World Health Organization, Geneva, Switzerland <http://apps.who.int/gb/ebwha/pdf_files/WHA67/A67_14Add1-en.pdf>.
12. WHO (2010) *Package of Essential Noncommunicable (PEN) Disease Interventions for Primary Health Care in Low-resource Settings*. World Health Organization, Geneva, Switzerland <http://whqlibdoc.who.int/publications/2010/9789241598996_eng.pdf>.
13. WHO (2013) *Implementation Tools: Package of Essential Noncommunicable (WHO-PEN) Disease Interventions for Primary Health Care in Low-resource Settings*. World Health Organization, Geneva, Switzerland <http://www.who.int/cardiovascular_diseases/publications/implementation_tools_WHO_PEN/en/>.
14. United Nations (2014) Outcome document of the high-level meeting of the General Assembly on the comprehensive review and assessment of the progress achieved in the prevention and control of non-communicable diseases. In: *68th Session of the United Nations General Assembly*, 7 July 2014. United Nations, New York <http://www.un.org/ga/search/view_doc.asp?symbol=A/68/L.53&L>.

Index

Note: **bold** page numbers indicate figures and tables.